Human Motivation and Interpersonal Relationships

Netta Weinstein
Editor

Human Motivation and Interpersonal Relationships

Theory, Research, and Applications

Springer

Editor
Netta Weinstein
Department of Psychology
University of Essex
Colchester, United Kingdom

ISBN 978-94-017-7833-6 ISBN 978-94-017-8542-6 (eBook)
DOI 10.1007/978-94-017-8542-6
Springer Dordrecht Heidelberg New York London

Printed on acid-free paper

Springer is part of Springer Science+Business Media (www.springer.com)

Contents

Part I
Introduction to the Study of Motivation in Relationships

Chapter 1
On the Mutuality of Human Motivation and Relationships

Netta Weinstein and Cody R. DeHaan

Motivation

Motivational processes are responsible for initiating and directing human activity; they energize behavior, generate and increase task engagement, and direct actions toward certain ends or goals. They are also inextricably linked with relational experiences. People bring their goals, values, hopes, and past regulatory experiences to bear on various types of relationships and interactions. The nature of these motivational forces that bring people into contact with each other, and that keep them interacting, plays a critical role in relationships. The chapters collected in this book describe the links between human motivation and the influential interactions and relationships that shape individuals' daily lives and long-term experiences.

The links between human motivation and relational experiences are not simple. As these chapters describe, social interactions and influential relationships shape the qualities and extent of motivation. Support for healthy motivation (or lack thereof) by important relationship figures (e.g., parents) as well as by individuals who have a specific social role (e.g., physicians) influences stable motivational orientations or dispositions over time, and shape one's sense of well-being, psychological growth, and resilience over the long term. Moreover, research conducted in this field shows that relational figures impact motivation through a number of identifiable interpersonal behaviors that communicate and provide support to a greater or lesser extent. For example, interactions may be characterized by the ways that feedback is given, the style by which opinions are expressed, or reactions to desirable and undesirable behaviors and values.

N. Weinstein (✉)
Department of Psychology, University of Essex, Colchester, UK
e-mail: netta@essex.ac.uk

C.R. DeHaan
Department of Clinical and Social Sciences in Psychology, University of Rochester, Rochester, NY, USA

N. Weinstein (ed.), *Human Motivation and Interpersonal Relationships: Theory, Research, and Applications*, DOI 10.1007/978-94-017-8542-6_1,

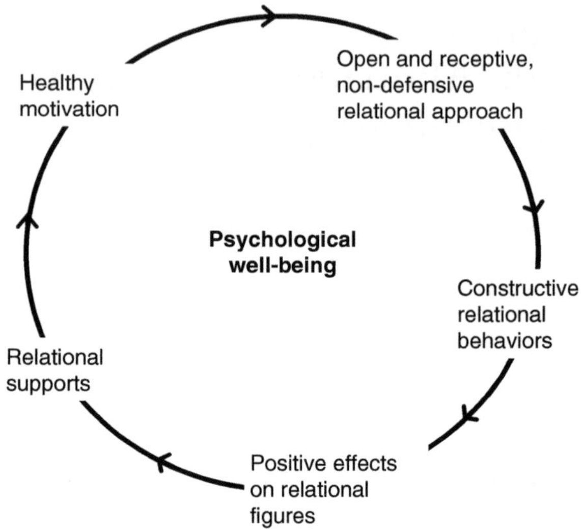

Fig. 1.1 Cyclical model depicting relations between human motivation and relationships

The ways in which relational figures communicate motivationally laden messages affect emotions, energy levels, and the quality of goal-directed behaviors in a given context (e.g., school, workplace, health care). However, these messages also provide input toward learning about interpersonal contexts as a whole, and as a result have impacts outside of any particular context; instead, affecting individuals across all life domains and throughout the lifespan. The psychological processes and interpersonal behaviors that result from past experiences shape adaptive or non-adaptive responding in interpersonal contexts. For example, an unhealthy relationship or series of experiences in an influential domain can give rise to a negative motivational style, leading to unhealthy behaviors in future relationships. It would seem then that these motivationally relevant communications (relational inputs) impact the qualities of interactions (relational outputs) by shaping motivation. The links between motivation and relationships may therefore be modeled by a cyclical series of effects wherein motivational styles are influenced by both early and adult relationships and interactions, and in turn impact individuals' behaviors in their relationships {Fig. 1.1 presents a broad representation of this cyclical model, summarizing the relations described in this book}. For example, behaviors of parents and early caregivers may influence tendencies or dispositions toward certain motivations as children develop into adulthood, carrying the lessons they have learned with early caregivers into new relationships and relational situations. Because of their continuing influence, these dispositions in turn shape childhood, adolescent, and adult interactions with parents, affecting negative tendencies toward conformity and self-suppression, rebelliousness and interpersonal distance, as well as positive trajectories toward closeness and trust in other cases.

In addition to the lifelong impacts that important relational figures have, experiences in particular life contexts often have an impact on future motivational tendencies specific to those contexts, and these tendencies in turn affect context-dependent relational behaviors in positive or negative ways. In the workplace, for example, the types of supports, feedback, or collaborations individuals have with colleagues shape motivation in the workplace environment; motivation in turn affects the ways in which individuals work alongside their colleagues. Motivationally supportive environments may inspire open and collaborative professional relationships that foster satisfaction and productivity in the workplace. Motivationally thwarting environments, on the other hand, may increase feelings of competitiveness and distrust, or may discourage sharing of ideas and reduce creativity; as a result they may undermine well-being in the workplace.

The chapters in this book employ a number of approaches and perspectives informed by the theoretical framework of self-determination theory (SDT, Deci & Ryan, 1985; Ryan & Deci, 2000a), an empirically grounded theory of human motivation, personality, and development in social contexts. SDT is built upon two basic assumptions: first, human beings are naturally active and growth-oriented. In other words, humans have an innate tendency toward growth and improvement unless derailed by thwarting interpersonal experiences. Second, SDT approaches assume that humans have a deep-rooted organismic tendency towards psychological integration, organization, and cohesiveness. Furthermore, through an empirical process, SDT has identified three distinct and universal basic psychological needs: the needs for competence, autonomy, and relatedness. The satisfaction of these needs is assumed to support healthy motivations and psychological well-being, and foster people's inherent activity, growth, and integrative tendency. In this chapter we discuss these concepts, each in turn, and explore their implications for relationships.

Organismic Integration

Central to growth and development is the human tendency toward integration and self-organization (e.g., Deci & Ryan, 2002; Ryan, 1993; Weinstein, Przybylski, & Ryan, 2012). As people engage new and diverse experiences, they are challenged to integrate them with existing aspects of themselves. This tendency to integrate experiences is thought to be innate and universal; people naturally organize and make sense of their experiences (Ryan & Deci, 2000b). Through engaging their integrative tendencies, individuals can make more sophisticated and sensitive connections between their experiences and existing ideas, values, and desires. This propensity allows individuals to develop self-structures that are increasingly complex and elaborate (Deci & Ryan, 1985; Hodgins & Knee, 2002; Ryan, Deci, Grolnick, & La Guardia, 2006). The inborn tendency to develop ever more elaborated, refined, and coherent internal processes and structures is the means through which values, regulatory processes, and other experiences introduced by the environment are internalized by the individual and effectively synthesized into an integrated sense of self. To the extent that individuals effectively assimilate, synthesize, and organize meaningful experiences, they become increasingly flexible and integrated, and their behaviors reflect their internal values, beliefs, and needs.

The integrative tendency allows people to understand more about themselves and their world and to develop greater clarity of purpose. It increases coherence among people's deeply held values, the goals and purposes that guide their behaviors, the relationships they develop and nurture, the responsibilities they take on, and the activities in which they engage autonomously. This sense of interested engagement and volitional persistence in interacting with individuals and engaging activities that are in accord with people's values and purposes contributes to their psychological health and well-being.

The integrative tendency is a process that occurs within individuals across time; it also takes place between an individual and others in his or her social sphere. Both internal and social integration processes are responsible for individuals continuing to pursue novel experiences and information that facilitates adaptive functioning within themselves and with larger social systems. Organismic integration thus refers to an increasingly elaborated and coherent set of processes and information that exists within people and between individuals and others in their social sphere.

People may be more or less successful in internalizing and integrating personal and social experiences. When the reasons for behaving and relating self-relevant information are well internalized or integrated, they drive *autonomous* self-regulation, which reflects individuals' personally held values, beliefs, and interests (Deci & Ryan, 2012). When motivation or regulations have been more fully internalized or integrated, actions emerge from people's sense of self and are self-consistent and volitional. Autonomous regulation promotes more adaptive and rewarding functioning; in the context of relationships it often drives pro-relatedness behaviors that foster intimacy and closeness. The result of autonomous regulation is a sense of psychological wellness, including deeper engagement with tasks and with the social world (Deci & Ryan, 1985), higher vitality (Ryan & Frederick, 1997), a tendency toward self-actualization (Shostrom, 1964), and positive and consistent self-esteem (Brown & Ryan, 2003; Ryan & Brown, 2003).

As previously mentioned, SDT maintains that individuals are by nature actively engaged in learning about and mastering their emotions and other self-relevant experiences, as well as their environments. White (1959) referred to this in terms of interacting effectively with the environment, and he said that this property might be thought of as effectance motivation; in the SDT literature this style of motivation is referred to as *intrinsic motivation* (Deci, 1975; Harlow, 1950) and is the motivational basis for mastery-oriented activities. Intrinsic motivation is experienced when engaging in activities because the activities—their intrinsic properties—are spontaneously rewarding and provide opportunities for exploration, interest-taking, enjoyment, and basic need satisfaction. Intrinsic motivation is a common and innate reason for children and people to play, explore, and be creative. It exposes individuals to new environments, engages new pursuit of challenges, and underlies the development of skills and knowledge. As such, intrinsic motivation is a basic and innate tool that individuals have that helps them to develop and grow, and to build new skills for responding to later challenges with mastery and the capacity for adaptation. Intrinsic motivation is present from birth and extends across the lifespan, encouraging people to explore, experiment, and master new skills. Studies have found, for example, that intrinsically motivated activities promote deep learning, creativity, exploration, independent mastery attempts, and psychological well-being (e.g., Amabile, 1983; Benware & Deci, 1984; Deci, Schwartz, Sheinman, & Ryan, 1981; Grolnick & Ryan, 1987). Stated differently, intrinsic motivation encourages meaningful engagement with the world that underlies much well-being and growth. As they engage the world in an interested, creative, and deeply thoughtful way, people find activities and goals that help them establish a sense of purpose and direction in their lives. Intrinsic motivation reflects the very definition of well-internalized motivation, in which behavior is experienced to be emanating from the self.

Intrinsic motivation is one type of highly internalized self-regulation that promotes psychological well-being. To the degree that experiences are not fully internalized, self-regulation may be driven by external or introjected reasons, in that individuals perceive external or poorly internalized contingencies such as rewards or punishments as driving their behavior. Social environments that attempt to shape desired behaviors by obligating, pressuring, or imposing implicitly or explicitly stated contingencies foster these more *controlled* forms of self-regulation. Such external and incompletely internalized contingencies represent unintegrated reasons for behavior engagement even when tasks are not personally compelling.

When people are pressured and controlled they may gradually take in the behavioral regulations but in a superficial way, and they lack a sense of ownership of the values and behaviors (Deci, Eghrari, Patrick, & Leone, 1994). In such cases, individuals undertake behaviors in order to feel a sense of self-approval or self-esteem, feel lovable or socially accepted, or in order to avoid feeling guilty or ashamed. This motivational phenomenon, known as *introjection*, reflects an incomplete internalization of values and regulations that are absent of personal value and not truly self-endorsed. Introjection reflects the presence of contingencies that have been partially internalized and pressure people to select options and behave in particular ways to attain feelings of worth within a system of unstable self-esteem (Deci & Ryan, 1985; Ryan & Brown, 2003; Ryan & Connell, 1989). When individuals act for reasons that have not been integrated, behavior is executed to *achieve* rather than to *experience*, and well-being is lower following engagement. For example, research in motivation around religious practices shows that churchgoers with less internalized and more introjected motivation for their religious behaviors reported lower well-being, including higher levels of depression, anxiety, and somatization, and less self-esteem and self-actualization (Ryan, Rigby, & King, 1993). Research in psychotherapy shows that depressed clients seeking treatment, who had poorly internalized motivation for doing so, showed poorer therapy outcomes than did clients with more fully internalized motivation (Zuroff et al., 2007). Finally, studies in the school context have shown that students whose reasons for learning were external or introjected displayed poorer understanding of learning materials, performed more poorly on exams, and had lower well-being as a result of school engagement: lower positive affect, less use of proactive coping approaches, and more anxiety about failing than did students with more internalized motivation for school (Black & Deci, 2000; Ryan & Connell, 1989). Thus, in both childhood and adulthood, the extent to which motivation is internalized or integrated is a critical feature in understanding the performance, functional, and well-being outcomes of engagement in any number of domains.

Social environments can shape the quality of self-regulation and influence the extent that it is characterized by high internalization or autonomy, or conversely by controlled regulation styles such as introjection. Hundreds of empirical studies emerging from the self-determination theory literature have pointed to the importance of perceiving one's social sphere to be supportive and accepting to internalization.

Environmental Supports

Many chapters in this book point to the importance of having *need satisfying* relationships with others. Need satisfactions are the nutriments necessary for psychological growth and integration, which are comprised of the three basic and universal psychological needs for competence, autonomy, and relatedness. These three needs have been identified from a body of empirical work, across which they emerged as being necessary to understanding human motivation and well-being (see Deci & Ryan, 2000, 2012, for a review). Moreover, these needs have emerged as being important universally, in both Western, individualistic cultures as well as Eastern, traditionalist and collectivist cultures (e.g., Chirkov, Ryan, Kim, & Kaplan, 2003; Ryan, La Guardia, Solky-Butzel, Chirkov, & Kim, 2005).

The need for *competence* refers to the necessity of people feeling effective in acting on the world (White, 1959). This involves the perceptions that actions will bring about desired outcomes, the expectation that one can master important challenges, and the belief that one has necessary or sufficient abilities. The social environment supports individuals' competence by providing positive and constructive feedback and by presenting with optimally challenging tasks that are difficult but not overly so. The need for *autonomy* refers to the experience that one is acting in choiceful ways and is able to endorse his or her behaviors, and the perception that regulation of these behaviors comes from within the self. When experiencing their behaviors as autonomous, individuals feel a sense of personal congruence—they experience their different thoughts, emotions, and behaviors as being in harmony with one another. The social environment supports people's autonomy by encouraging actions that are in accord with their true selves, or 'who they really are,' as opposed to those that merely serve others' desires or expectations. Finally, the need for *relatedness* refers to feeling close and connected to others in one's social sphere, and of caring for and being cared for by others. Relatedness is reflected in having trusting and satisfying relationships with significant others and having a sense of belonging to valued groups or organizations. Social environments provide relatedness need support when one relates to others in an open and authentic fashion.

According to self-determination theory, the integrative process is fostered and sustained by these three universal and basic need satisfactions. When individuals' needs are satisfied, they experience interest, enjoyment, and engagement, and they can become more psychologically organized, integrated, and cohesive. Empirically, numerous studies have shown that basic need satisfaction promotes both intrinsic motivation and integration (e.g., Deci, Koestner, & Ryan, 1999; Ryan & Deci, 2000b). Furthermore, studies have shown that need satisfaction leads individuals to experience a general sense of well-being (e.g., Baard, Deci, & Ryan, 2004; Brown & Ryan, 2003). When social environments encourage satisfaction of basic psychological needs, individuals experience feelings of energy and aliveness (e.g., Ryan & Frederick, 1997) over the long term, as well as from day to day. For example, studies employing diary designs demonstrate that on days when individuals experience more need satisfaction they also experienced higher well-being, including more positive affect and vitality (Reis, Sheldon, Gable, Roscoe, & Ryan, 2000; Sheldon, Ryan, & Reis, 1996). Accounting for daily effects of need satisfaction, greater overall need satisfaction also relates to higher well-being at the individual difference level. Over extended periods of time, the satisfaction of basic psychological needs has related to indicators of psychological health indicators including lower anxiety and higher self-esteem in a diversity of life domains, including work and home (Baard et al., 2004; Lynch, Plant, & Ryan, 2005; Niemiec, Lynch, Vansteenkiste, Bernstein, Deci, & Ryan, 2006). In the context of parent-child relationships, autonomy-supportive parenting is associated with a variety of positive outcomes for children, including higher well-being (Chirkov & Ryan, 2001), increased prosocial behavior (Gagné, 2003), and engagement with schoolwork (Assor, Kaplan, & Roth, 2002). As these studies demonstrate, basic psychological needs are essential for psychological health and well-being. When individuals' needs are satisfied over time, they also develop in ways that shape motivational orientations or individuals' tendencies toward certain, more or less adaptive styles of self-regulation and engagement.

Need Satisfaction Versus Need Thwarting

Social environments do not consistently succeed in satisfying basic psychological needs, and in the past, motivational literatures have compared occurrences when these needs are satisfied to relational experiences that are relatively low in need satisfaction. Recently, a different model of psychological need satisfaction has emerged, which argues that social environments can support or derail psychological growth and well-being by either actively satisfying the basic psychological needs, or actively thwarting them. This approach is supported by recent empirical work, and suggests that many social contexts can actively fulfill psychological needs to a lesser or greater extent, and independently, actively undermine psychological needs to a lesser or greater extent. For example, a parent may either actively support the psychological need for relatedness by offering warmth and affection, or he or she may actively undermine relatedness need satisfaction with hurtful language or overt expressions of rejection.

The extent to which social contexts either support or thwart basic psychological needs incurs distinct psychological outcomes. Recent work has shown when basic psychological needs are thwarted, individuals have worsening of health and increased ill-being (Pelletier, Dion, & Lévesque, 2004; Reinboth, Duda, & Ntoumanis, 2004), and to the extent psychological needs are supported individuals report higher well-being, vitality, and growth (e.g., Brown & Ryan, 2003). This literature indicates that the relations between actively thwarting psychological needs and indicators of ill-health are more robust than are the relations between need supports and ill-health; the same is true for relations between need supports and well-being. In other words, it appears that need supports actively facilitate growth and wellness, whereas need thwarting actively increases ill-being. For example, findings in sports contexts (e.g., examining relationships between coaches and athletes) show that need thwarting is linked to more exhaustion, depression, disordered eating, and burnout, whereas need satisfaction is linked to more vitality and positive affect (Bartholomew, Ntoumanis, Ryan, & Thøgersen-Ntoumani, 2011). In Chap. 12 of this book, the authors present an empirical model that supports need satisfaction and thwarting as having differential outcomes in the workplace. In their research (presented in Chap. 12), Dagenais-Desmarais and colleagues show that to the extent that workplace environments actively supported needs, employees reported higher self-esteem, social involvement, mental balance, control of self and events, sociability, and happiness. To the extent to which workplace environments actively thwarted psychological needs, increases in negative well-being indicators such as anxiety/depression, irritability, self-depreciation, and social disengagement were reported. The extent to which psychological supports and thwarts represent two ends of one continuum representing environmental support or two independent qualities of interacting is yet to be determined; for now, it appears that added variance may be explained by considering need thwarting and need supports separately.

Need Satisfaction Across Social Contexts

The work reviewed in this book suggests that satisfaction of basic psychological needs is critical for well-being and psychological growth, and that need supportive environments over time lead to more internalized motivational dispositions, that in turn improve relationships by encouraging responsive and close relational behaviors. This work also highlights the importance of need supports in predicting context-specific behavior and well-being. The dynamic process in which social relationships support basic psychological needs, furthering more internalized forms of motivation, and in turn fostering better social relationships, takes place across a wide number of relationships and contexts. As people develop they are exposed to greater numbers of increasingly varied social contexts; each of these has a role, small or large, in shaping general satisfaction or thwarting of basic psychological needs. In the subsequent chapters of this book, we learn that early relationships, primarily those with parents and caregivers, but also relationships with teachers and other important childhood figures, play a critical role in personal growth and well-being over time.

In early childhood, support for autonomy need satisfaction is first provided by caregiver-child interactions. Research on mother-child relationships shows that the ways in which mothers talk with their young children reflect their motivational approach and impacts children's behaviors in joint tasks (Grolnick & Ryan, 1987; Soenens, Vansteenkiste, & Niemiec, 2009; reviewed in Chap. 4). In this research, controlling parenting (styles of responding to children that undermines autonomy and self-expression) seems to have detrimental developmental and well-being consequences throughout childhood. In addition, parent-provided need supports predict healthy, adaptive behaviors higher and well-being in adolescence, whereas controlling, need thwarting parenting styles predict maladaptive and rebellious behaviors.

Several of the chapters explore caregiver relationship events in which parents may find it difficult to provide need support. These events are often characterized by a mismatch between parents' expectations and their children's, or between parents' personal values or beliefs and those of their children. In such cases, parents are challenged to provide need satisfaction under more demanding conditions that require openness, perspective taking, and trust in children. For example, children may fail to accept parents' religious views (Chap. 10) or they may hold LGBT identities that represent an unknown or threatening quality to parents living in a stigmatizing society (Chap. 9). In these cases, parents are challenged with communicating understanding and love, while accepting or internalizing their children's diverging paths. In sum, findings reviewed in these chapters indicate that in these difficult situations, it is *especially* important that parents are able to provide autonomy support for their children.

Caregiver relationships are among the most influential in shaping lifelong experiences of need satisfaction and in determining resulting relational behaviors and outcomes across throughout the lifespan. In adulthood, close peer relationships (including friendships and romantic relationships) are important sources of either need thwarting or need satisfying interactions, and in adolescence and early adulthood these relationships appear most influential in determining the quality of day-to-day experience. In adulthood, romantic relationships may be supportive or conflictual and defensive, and these qualities impact on relationship satisfaction and well-being in major ways (Patrick, Knee, Canevello, & Lonsbary, 2007; work reviewed in Chaps. 3, 4, and 7). Close and romantic relationships may be the most important contexts for receiving need supports in adulthood, but research has shown that daily interactions with strangers or acquaintances also influence people's well-being on a daily or context-specific level (Chaps. 2, 3, and 4). So far, research demonstrating the links between motivation, needs, and relationship quality has been conducted largely with laboratory experimental designs, and has demonstrated short-term though robust effects. Presumably, these interactions translate to short-term but frequent daily experiences that together affect our daily well-being.

Relationships with therapists may offer need satisfaction when it is not otherwise available in one's daily life, or may augment existing need supports from important peer and parent relationships. Optimally, therapist-client relationships provide a safe and encouraging environment for self-exploration and for experiencing relatedness, autonomy, and competence. Therapist relationships may even be reparative when they provide need support to individuals who may have been need thwarted in their other relationships. Chapter 14 reviews evidence in psychotherapy research that indicates healthy and productive therapist interactions take place when the therapeutic relationship satisfies basic psychological needs and when clients are autonomously motivated to engage with their therapists (in contrast to participating in therapy because of a controlling mandate, or as a result of pressure from friends or family).

Other specific social contexts provide opportunities for need support that shape the quality of experiences in those contexts. In important relational environments such as the workplace, employees are benefited from experiencing autonomy, competence, and relatedness support from colleagues and managers. Others in the workplace might satisfy needs, for example, by providing achievable and structured tasks, fostering generally trusting and communicative peer and managerial relationships, and offering opportunities for choice at work. These strategies and others reviewed in Chap. 12 enhance productivity at work, employees' commitment to the organization, and satisfaction at work. Work in health care contexts highlights the importance of physicians and family members supporting basic psychological needs. These figures may be challenged to support patients' autonomy need satisfaction around health care behavior engagement, especially when the patient has diverging intentions for how to respond to his or her health needs (Chaps. 13 and 15). According to this work, need supportive doctor-patient interactions are those in which doctors encourage individuals to engage their own health care choicefully, in a way that allows patients to feel a sense of ownership and volition in their health-care experiences.

In summary, both lifelong close relationships with parents and romantic partners, and context-specific but important relationships with colleagues and physicians, shape experiences of need satisfaction. Together, these types of relationships, as well as daily interactions with acquaintances and strangers that may influence short-term repeated responses, impact on the overall experiences the individual has of being need satisfied or thwarted. Both in-context and across-context (dispositional) levels of autonomous or controlled styles of motivation in turn drive individuals' responding to their social environments.

Dispositional Autonomy

The work we reviewed so far suggests individuals may be control or autonomously motivated for a certain task or class of tasks; over time, they also develop more stable tendencies to adopt one quality of motivation over the other. These individual differences in the propensity to act autonomously or with control over time are relationally driven and in turn they shape relational responding (e.g., Deci & Ryan, 1985; Koestner & Losier, 2002). When autonomous, people experience their behavior as self-endorsed and congruent with their values and interests; when controlled, individuals' behaviors are regulated or controlled by influences perceived as alien to the self, for example external contingencies, social pressure, or contingent regard (see Deci & Ryan, 2000; Ryan & Deci, 2000a).

Although the relative autonomy of an individual's motivation is often driven by situational and domain specific factors (Deci & Ryan, 2012; La Guardia & Ryan, 2007), over time the many relational experiences, which are described above, shape developmental trajectories that are stabilized into individual tendencies (e.g., Deci & Ryan's, 1985). These individual differences, in turn, can pervasively influence relational and task behaviors, and well-being in a multitude of ways (Deci & Ryan, 1985, 2000; Ryan & Deci, 2001; Ryan et al., 2006; Weinstein & Hodgins, 2009; Weinstein et al., 2012).

Autonomously oriented individuals generally experience their actions as self-endorsed and originating from the self. Individuals who are high in this individual difference can therefore generally stand behind their actions, and they select activities and styles of responding that are consistent with their values, beliefs, and needs (Deci & Ryan, 2000; Ryan, 1995; Weinstein et al., 2012). These individuals are relatively integrated and self-congruent, presumably because they pursue a trajectory of growth and self-coherence as a result of robust and consistent satisfaction of basic psychological needs. The autonomously oriented individual is, as a result, open to self-exploration and is willing to employ his or her own values, feelings, and needs in choosing how to engage and respond to social contexts. Alternatively, controlling influences such as internalized parental messages and other social pressures may regulate an individual through influences perceived as external to the self (Deci & Ryan, 1985). Because this is often a matter of degree, this construct spans from autonomous regulation by the self to increasingly controlled regulation by external influences (Deci & Ryan). In recent research (Weinstein et al.), three elements have emerged as being central for autonomous functioning. The first of these central characteristics of autonomous orientation is that when autonomous one experiences oneself as authoring or endorsing behavior volitionally, and undertakes behavior that is self-congruent and may be integrated with existing values and beliefs. Individuals who function autonomously engage in behaviors that are based on, in line with, and satisfying of their needs, feelings, and values (Ricoeur, 1966). A second facet of an autonomy disposition that was recognized in this work is interest-taking. Interest is the spontaneous and innate reflective capacity for open self-reflection exercised in the service of personality growth, and characterized by intrinsic motivation for self-understanding (Deci & Ryan, 1985; Flavell, 1977; Loevinger, 1976; Ryan & Deci, 2006; White, 1963). Individuals who are high in autonomy orientation tend to take an interest in their own emotions, reactions, and experiences, which informs their behaviors and facilitates down-regulation of negative relational responses particularly in the face of frustration or conflict. A final aspect of autonomy involves resilience in the face of pressuring influences, or capacity to avoid pressuring motives. This research and other work has noted that autonomous individuals tend to experience events as less pressuring; in addition, pressuring experiences were less powerful in influencing the behaviors of autonomously oriented individuals. In other words, autonomous individuals experience less pressure in situations, and are also more resilient to the pressure they do experience. Perceptions of pressure are notably different from the reality of being pressured by others (Ryan et al., 1997), and presumably autonomous individuals interpret similar situations differently, perceive a greater degree of personal choice and initiative, and avoid responding to coercive or controlling influences (Perls, 1973; Ryan & Connell, 1989).

Elements of Motivational Supports

The work reviewed in this chapter suggests relational figures can shape autonomous motivation for tasks and, over time, affect individuals' motivational dispositions. Such relational partners interact on a daily basis, and the qualities of those interactions influence the level of support for autonomy and facilitate or undermine the integrative process. The qualities of interactions that appear most influential in supporting autonomy include communicating a high level of support for self-expression and a fundamental acceptance and caring for the individual. Such interactions communicate that individuals are free to self-express and explore; whereas interactions that undermine autonomy and foster control communicate that individuals *must* behave, look, feel, or think in particular ways to be acceptable and lovable. In relationships, individuals who are autonomy supportive encourage their partners to actualize their capacity for being choiceful and congruent, and for understanding and endorsing their behaviors, decisions, and values. Recent work has examined the ways that relationship partners convey support for autonomy in particular ways.

Relationships may be most dangerous to one's autonomy when they parry satisfaction of the need for autonomy against that of relatedness—when the individual feels that to act autonomously would threaten his or her relationships. **Non-conditional regard** is one important way that relationships partners convey that one is *lovable and accepted* regardless of one's behavior, beliefs, and emotions. When partners are non-conditionally regarding they express warmth, convey their love, or offer their support independent of one's behaviors, thoughts, and feelings. Doing so does not necessitate partners to accept or approve of every behavior; rather, when partners are non-conditionally regarding they discriminate between the person as a growth-oriented and inherently valued individual, and his or her desirable or undesirable behavior. Non-conditional regard thus means that one's behavior does not determine one's lovability, and it promotes feelings that one's social environment is a safe space to which one can bring his or her authentic self, and which allows for honest self-expression and exploration of desirable and undesirable aspects of self and identity.

Perspective-Taking

Individuals can also support autonomy by taking their partners' perspectives. By taking an interest in partners' point of view rather than imposing their own view, partners express a willingness to see one as he or she *really is,* and they give credibility to one's subjective experiences. When individuals feel their perspectives are taken into account, they feel supported in the validity and relevance of their personally held thoughts and feelings, and they are encouraged to view their internal processes as a worthwhile space for exploration and inquiry. Perspective-taking thus encourages individuals' capacity and willingness to engage in their own exploration and grants legitimacy to personal experiences when undertaking such a journey. Research shows, for example, that teachers who take their students' perspectives encourage an autonomous form of education that increases well-being and an internalized form of sustained learning (Reeve, 2009). Taking the perspective of a relationship partner does not only encourage feelings of being more understood, but also provides the opportunity to truly understand a partner's perspective, fostering knowledge and understanding of the others' experience, perspectives and intentions.

Trust and Acceptance

The relation between trust and autonomy support is best characterized by a snowballing, cyclical effect wherein autonomous interactions foster trust, and additionally in long lasting, close relationships, where expressions of trust support further autonomy. When important partners express trust in one another, they encourage non-defensive open interactions in which individuals can express openly, share mistakes and fears, and explore failures. Like non-conditional regard, expressions of trust do not involve suppressing disagreements or naïve partner views that one can do no wrong. Instead, relationships that are trusting communicate the belief that the individual is inherently in a process of growth, and is attempting (and will continue) to do the best that he or he can, given the circumstances. Work with adolescents indicates that parents who do not trust their children are met with less self-disclosure from their adolescents (Kerr & Stattin, 2000; Kerr, Stattin, & Trost, 1999), undermining further relationship growth.

Relationship partners also support each other by offering **structure.** Structure is created when partners set clear expectations for behavior. Structure does not place judgment on the person who fails to meet expectations, but rather offers informational feedback about the natural outcomes of behaving or not behaving. Although it seems intuitive that communicating such expectations undermines people's autonomy, perhaps by seeming to restrict options in how to behave, research shows that structure can foster autonomy support (e.g., Jang, Reeve, & Deci, 2010). The key is not in whether structure is present or absent, but rather in the way that structure is framed. At its best, communicating structure is paired with trust and an expression of confidence in the individual, it employs meaningful rationales for limits on behaving, and it involves no pressure or contingent regard (Sierens, Vansteenkiste, Goossens, Soenens, & Dochy, 2007). Structure-promoting contingencies and expectations, so long as they are not pressuring or conditionally regarding, may be beneficial to certain relationships and can be differentiated from psychological control, which generally undermines autonomous motivation (Barber, Stolz, & Olsen, 2005). If communicated in the right way, structure-promoting relationships may also assist in learning and increase well-being (Grolnick & Ryan, 1989; Reeve, Jang, Carrell, Jeon, & Barch, 2004).

Transparency

The importance of transparency, the willingness to honestly and thoughtfully self-disclose to one's partner, has been discussed largely in the context of therapeutic relationships, but may also be important for promoting autonomy in other relationships. When partners are transparent, they model a way of expressing that is trusting and open and they demonstrate willingness to collaborative self-reflection. Transparency further supports the previously mentioned components of autonomy support, making it easier for the other to take a perspective when they understand your experience, and while doing that can also serve to enhance trust and acceptance. Carl Rogers proposed that this quality creates a space where one can openly share thoughts and feelings, and thus engage in a collaborative process of self-exploration resulting in greater awareness (Rogers, 1957).

Use of Reinforcements and Pressure

To the extent that relationships rely on performance-contingent and salient reinforcements of punishments, such as monetary rewards, to shape behavior, they may also undermine autonomy for certain tasks. Partners, teachers, parents, and employers may use reinforcements to motivate individuals toward desired behaviors. While they may be effective in changing behaviors for a short time (Alberto & Troutman, 1999; Bandura & McClelland, 1977), these techniques inhibit internalization of motivation for activities: whereas in the absence of reinforcements individuals may be motivated by their curiosity, interest, or personally held values, the use of reinforcements reorients motivational energy outside of the task to the external reward. The resulting behaviors—those motivated by reinforcement or pressures—are likely short-lived, and require continued or repeated reinforcements and pressure for behavior to be sustained. Indeed, a multitude of research has shown that when these external motivators are no longer present people cease to engage behavior. Monetary rewards are often used to encourage behavior; as well, partners often use pressuring language and tone of voice to induce behaviors. In the long-term, these strategies may reduce task motivation and engagement; studies testing parent-child interactions in the lab note that when mothers use controlling or pressuring language their children's intrinsic motivation for tasks is undermined (Deci, Driver, Hotchkiss, Robbins, & Wilson, 1993; Kochanska & Aksan, 1995; see Joussemet, Landry, & Koestner, 2008 for a review of other such studies).

Relational Outcomes of Autonomous Motivation

We have discussed a body of work that suggests that when relationships provide need supports, individuals develop more internalized and autonomous motivation over time, and we have argued that autonomous motivation in turn increases well-being. A recent literature has also focused on the *relational* outcomes of being autonomous, and this research has identified a number of interpersonal important outcomes of both state motivation and motivation orientation.

Some of the earliest work in this area explored the impact of autonomy and control on perceptions of personal threat and consequent defensiveness in relational responding. Experimental research using motivational primes and correlational work testing links with dispositional motivation has shown that people acting from a control orientation have higher readiness and propensity to perceive threat in the environment and are therefore more likely to respond defensively to potentially challenging elements in their social spheres. For example, these individuals may respond in more defensive and less honest ways when others disagree about a certain belief, when taking responsibility for errors or mistakes, or when disclosing secrets (Hodgins, 2008; Hodgins & Liebeskind, 2003; Hodgins et al., 2010). Presumably, because control oriented individuals are more defensive, they are also less able to process emotionally challenging materials. In two studies, Weinstein and Hodgins (2009) explored the links between motivation orientation and emotional integration of challenging material—in these studies video clips of the Hiroshima-Nagasaki bombings were used. Individuals who were high in trait autonomy or primed with autonomy, and were given the opportunity to integrate by expressing their feelings, were less defensive in response to materials and better able to integrate them. Further research by Weinstein, Deci, and Ryan (2011) extended this research to defensiveness in light of negative aspects of one's identity. The authors found that trait autonomy and autonomy priming (vs. control) facilitates integrating regretful negative past events and shameful personal characteristics. Other work in this area has shown that parent-provided non-conditional regard supported higher integration, less defense, and more awareness and ownership of negative emotions in kindergarteners showed higher integration, in terms of awareness and ownership of negative emotions (Roth & Assor, 2010).

Arguably, an autonomous orientation facilitates the integrative process by promoting a sense of openness, ownership to experience, and self-acceptance even in the face of threatening experiences. When material cannot be integrated, perhaps because the individual does not have the personal resources for the challenge of doing so, defensive processes occur as poorly guided attempts to cope. In operationalizing integrated regulation, researchers contrast awareness of emotions with suppressing, or actively defending against and avoiding them (e.g., Roth & Assor, 2010). Similarly, the mainstream coping literature has broadly classified two types of coping in response to stressful events: avoidant and approach (Roth & Cohen, 1986). Avoidant coping reflects a defensive form of regulation that involves ignoring, distorting, or escaping threatening stimuli (e.g., Stowell, Kiecolt-Glaser, & Glaser, 2001). In this literature, avoiding responding is contrasted with approach coping involving a cognitive, emotional, or behavioral 'turning toward' challenging situations (e.g., Fortune, Richards, Main, & Griffiths, 2002). Approach coping is generally considered adaptive in that effort is directed toward resolving challenging situations or overcoming the stress associated with them. As a result, these strategies are believed to facilitate the assimilation and transcendence of stress in a way that ultimately enhances well-being (Shontz, 1975).

Chapter 4 in this book reviews this literature in light of interpersonal interactions, and discusses a number of relational outcomes of defensive responses that result from autonomous motivation. Chapter 5 further explores defensive processes; in doing so, the author examines the links between defense and need supports (primarily autonomous need support), and focuses on outcomes for integration and coherent self-concepts. One of the mechanisms which has been more recently identified is the us-them divide, the division that is sometimes perceived to exist between 'me' and 'others'. In their Chap. 5, the authors describe the ways defensive processes elicit an artificial perceived divide between 'us' (ingroup/similar, close others) and 'them'. The authors argue that individuals high in control versus autonomous orientation are more likely to perceive an artificial 'us'–'them' divide, which increases defensive responding to others in one's social sphere. Whereas Chap. 5 explores this differentiation between individuals, in Chap. 8 the authors examine early work on ingroup/outgroup tensions at a group level. This chapter specifically reviews evidence that social environments that are need thwarting, namely autonomy thwarting, elicit more defensive and fragmented identification between members of different groups. Presumably, along with increasing aggressive responses, defensiveness also increases prejudiced behaviors by creating a sense of threat around and feelings of competition with others.

In close relationships, defensive processes lead to higher interpersonal conflict, and less responsive and empathic responding that reduces conflict once it starts. A body of work (e.g., Hodgins & Liebeskind, 2003; Knee, Lonsbary, & Canevello, 2005; Patrick et al., 2007; Weinstein, Hodgins, & Ryan, 2010) has demonstrated that in relationships driven by pressure and control, rather than by autonomous interest and valuing, interpersonal conflict between two partners is met with defensive and non-conciliatory behaviors that lengthen and exacerbate fights. This style of responding to conflict, in turn, results in negative affect and lower relationship satisfaction for both partners. Chapter 7 reviews this work in length, and examines the role of control or self-determination in conflict between romantic relationship partners. The authors argue that conflict is exacerbated when self-esteem is contingent on the relationship, a form of controlling regulation. In this chapter, the authors focus on romantic relationships; in Chap. 10, Assor et al. review processes of interpersonal conflict and consequences for well-being and behavior in parent-child relationships; they review research showing that parental autonomy support and non-conditional regard encourage children to express themselves honestly. Experimental research described across chapters also suggests that motivation carried into new interactions and relationships facilitates interpersonal openness and higher self-disclosure (e.g., Niemiec & Deci, 2012; Weinstein et al., 2010). Across parent, relationship, and acquaintance interactions, these processes of non-defense and openness are responsible for a sense closeness and intimacy. In contrast to higher defense that arises from control, the autonomous self is characterized by better ability for perspective taking and empathy. Chapter 3 makes the argument that this capacity for self-regulation that characterizes autonomy is extended to social integration, or more harmonious relationships with others in the social sphere.

Across this book, there are repeated examples of integrated motivational processes leading to warmth and closeness in relationships. For example, Chaps. 3 and 4 reviews evidence that motivation has an impact on behavioral and subjective/felt closeness across an array of relationships. This link is evident in romantic relationships, parent-child relationships, and initial interactions with strangers. Other chapters point to the relevance of human motivation for interpersonal closeness in professional relationships such as those between therapists and clients and health-care practitioners. Finally, Chap. 9 reviews implications for interpersonal closeness in the context of lesbian-gay-bisexual-transgendered (LGBT) identities.

Whereas motivational styles have an impact on the quality of relationships in the variety of ways discussed, relationships can in turn shape self-processes that are relevant for motivation, supporting a cyclical model of motivation and relationships. Self-concept, or the set of perceptions and definitions of oneself, is a particularly useful mark of integration and a robust predictor of psychological well-being. Chapter 6 argues that need thwarting social contexts and personal dispositions for control over autonomy both lead to problems relating to self-concept. Exploring these relations from multiple perspectives, the author reviews differences in self-concept consistency across time and contexts, and discrepancies between actual and ideal selves—how one perceives oneself and how one would ideally like to be. Complementary findings in LGBT groups (Chap. 9) indicate that supportive social contexts may have similar effects on specific self-concepts or identities. Recent work reviewed in these chapters has shown that motivationally supportive contexts shape self-concepts in ways that increase well-being and reduce ill-being. This work has implications for future research studying self-concept within the context of relationships. They also have implications for understanding the integrative process. For example, future studies may examine how being closer to one's ideal self in turn feeds into responsive and supportive relationships by promoting integration and non-defensive in relational contexts.

In Chap. 8, Legault et al. explored the relational outcomes of motivation by studying *group-level* motivation and intergroup relationships. In this new and exciting research, the authors aim to understand how people respond to both ingroup and outgroup members as a function of their motivation for social identity. The research reviewed in this chapter indicates that motivation can shape, either positively or negatively, the quality of relationships with outgroup members in particular. Previous research had tested the extent that the absence (amotivation) or presence of motivation to regulate one's prejudice impacts on discriminatory behaviors. This new work extends the previous model and distinguishes between autonomy and control motivation for prejudice regulation, and it shows external and introjected motivation to regulate prejudice leads to more implicit and behavioral forms of prejudice and poor prejudice regulation (inability to reduce bias, particularly when it is difficult to do so). Follow-up studies conducted by the authors explore potential underlying processes for these effects, and they identify autonomous regulation to be more automated and chronically accessible, whereas controlled motivation requires more energy and cognitive effort.

In Chap. 8, the authors also showed that autonomous motivation leads to more investment and stable self-inclusion in one's ingroup. In other words, when individuals identified autonomously with their ingroup, they were more committed to the group. Similar commitment-related outcomes were in evidence across different types of relationships at the individual level. In Chap. 3, the authors review evidence that need satisfaction promotes close relationships that are satisfying to partners (e.g., Patrick et al., 2007) and that lead to more secure attachment (e.g., La Guardia, Ryan, & Couchman, 2000). Chapter 7 argues that positive aspects of romantic relationships, including lower relationship-relevant defense, less conflict, and more perceived closeness lead to higher romantic relationship commitment. Expanding this to the context of client-therapist relationships in Chap. 14, Lynch reviews evidence that autonomy-support and need satisfaction in therapeutic relationships promotes more commitment to therapy and an alliance between the therapist and the client. This quality of relationship promotes more productive relationships in this professional context that supports client psychological growth.

A final theme evident in these chapters involves *well-being* outcomes of relating to others in an autonomous fashion. This sense of well-being is derived both from individual and contextual contributors: from the motivation that drives relationship engagement and from need supports offered in the relationship. These motivational qualities increase wellness, operationalized in terms of higher positive affect and self-esteem, and lower depression and anxiety, among other indicators. Research that distinguishes between need support and need thwarting indicates need supports promote well-being indicators such as positive affect and self-esteem, and, independently, need thwarting promote ill-being indicators such as depression and anxiety. Furthermore, need supports may be especially important for well-being when individuals feel vulnerable, for example, when self-disclosing stigmatized personally held identities, such as lesbian-gay-bisexual-transgender (LGBT) identities. In all cases, central figures—romantic partners, parents, and close friends—seem to be especially likely to influence well-being; these chapters indicate that as relationships are more central, they play an increasingly important role.

Conclusion

This chapter offers a basic model for understanding the nature of motivation in the context of human relationships. In it we have argued that relationships and motivational constructs have a cyclical relation that can over time foster growth and integration and lead to psychological well-being, or alternatively derail growth processes and undermine wellness. We have reviewed a body of work that suggests that both important relationships and daily interactions shape the qualities of human motivation that drive daily behavior and influence the way people understand and interpret their world. We have argued that, in turn, these motivational qualities shape the ways that individuals approach social contexts, for example in ways that are open, receptive, and responsive to social partners, or alternatively in defensive ways that increase interpersonal conflict and foster prejudice and aggression. Through the subsequent chapters in this book, each of these topics is discussed in greater detail and together they offer a diversified and thoughtful empirically based understanding of the role of human motivation in relationships.

References

Alberto, P., & Troutman, A. C. (1999). *Applied behavior analysis for teachers*. Upper Saddle River, NJ: Merrill.

Amabile, T. M. (1983). The social psychology of creativity: A componential conceptualization. *Journal of Personality and Social Psychology, 45*(2), 357–376. doi:10.1037/0022-3514.45.2.357.

Assor, A., Kaplan, H., & Roth, G. (2002). Choice is good, but relevance is excellent: Autonomy-enhancing and suppressing teacher behaviours predicting students' engagement in schoolwork. *British Journal of Educational Psychology, 72*(2), 261–278.

Baard, P. P., Deci, E. L., & Ryan, R. M. (2004). Intrinsic need satisfaction: A motivational basis of performance and well-being in two work settings. *Journal of Applied Social Psychology, 34*(10), 2045–2068. doi:10.1111/j.1559-1816.2004.tb02690.x.

Bandura, A., & McClelland, D. C. (1977). *Social learning theory*. Oxford, UK: Prentice-Hall.

Barber, B. K., Stolz, H. E., & Olsen, J. A. (2005). Parental support, psychological control, and behavioral control: Assessing relevance across time, culture and method. *Monographs of the Society for Research in Child Development, 70*(4), 1–147.

Bartholomew, K., Ntoumanis, N., Ryan, R. M., & Thøgersen-Ntoumani, C. (2011). Psychological need thwarting in the sport context: Assessing the darker side of Athletic experience. *Journal of Sport & Exercise Psychology, 33*, 75–102.

Benware, C. A., & Deci, E. L. (1984). Quality of learning with an active versus passive motivational set. *American Educational Research Journal, 21*(4), 755–765.

Black, A. E., & Deci, E. L. (2000). The effects of instructors' autonomy support and students' autonomous motivation on learning organic chemistry: A self-determination theory perspective. *Science Education, 84*(6), 740–756.

Brown, K. W., & Ryan, R. M. (2003). The benefits of being present: Mindfulness and its role in psychological well-being. *Journal of Personality and Social Psychology, 84*(4), 822–848. doi:10.1037/0022-3514.84.4.822.

Chirkov, V. I., & Ryan, R. M. (2001). Parent and teacher autonomy-support in Russian and U.S. adolescents. *Journal of Cross-Cultural Psychology, 32*, 618–635.

Chirkov, V. I., Ryan, R. M., Kim, Y., & Kaplan, U. (2003). Differentiating autonomy from individualism and independence: A self-determination theory perspective on internalization of cultural orientations and well-being. *Journal of Personality and Social Psychology, 84*(1), 97–110. doi:10.1037/0022-3514.84.1.97.

Deci, E. L. (1975). *Intrinsic motivation.* New York: Plenum Publishing Co. Japanese Edition, Tokyo: Seishin Shobo, 1980.

Deci, E. L., Driver, R. E., Hotchkiss, L., Robbins, R. J., & Wilson, I. M. (1993). The relation of mothers' controlling vocalizations to children's intrinsic motivation. *Journal of Experimental Child Psychology, 55*, 151–162.

Deci, E. L., Eghrari, H., Patrick, B. C., & Leone, D. R. (1994). Facilitating internalization: The self-determination theory perspective. *Journal of Personality, 62*(1), 119–142.

Deci, E. L., Koestner, R., & Ryan, R. M. (1999). A meta-analytic review of experiments examining the effects of extrinsic rewards on intrinsic motivation. *Psychological Bulletin, 125*(6), 627.

Deci, E. L., & Ryan, R. M. (1985). *Intrinsic motivation and self-determination in human behavior.* New York: Plenum Press.

Deci, E. L., & Ryan, R. M. (2000). The "what" and "why" of goal pursuits: Human needs and the self-determination of behavior. *Psychological Inquiry, 11*(4), 227–268. doi:10.1207/S15327965PLI1104_01.

Deci, E. L., & Ryan, R. M. (2002). The paradox of achievement: The harder you push, the worse it gets. In J. Aronson (Ed.), *Improving academic achievement: Impact of psychological factors on education* (1st ed.). Bingley, UK: Emerald Group Publishing.

Deci, E. L., & Ryan, R. M. (2012). Self-determination theory. In P. A. M. Van Lange, A. W. Kruglanski, & E. T. Higgins (Eds.), *Handbook of theories of social psychology: Vol. 1* (pp. 416–437). Thousand Oaks, CA: Sage.

Deci, E. L., Schwartz, A. J., Sheinman, L., & Ryan, R. M. (1981). An instrument to assess adults' orientations toward control versus autonomy with children: Reflections on intrinsic motivation and perceived competence. *Journal of Educational Psychology, 73*(5), 642.

Flavell, J. (1977). *Cognitive development.* Englewood Cliffs, NJ: Prentice-Hall.

Fortune, D. G., Richards, H. L., Main, C. J., & Griffiths, C. E. M. (2002). Patients' strategies for coping with psoriasis. *Clinical and Experimental Dermatology, 27*(3), 177–184. doi:10.1046/j.1365-2230.2002.01055.x.

Gagné, M. (2003). The role of autonomy support and autonomy orientation in prosocial behavior engagement. *Motivation and Emotion, 27*(3), 199–223.

Grolnick, W. S., & Ryan, R. M. (1987). Autonomy in children's learning: An experimental and individual difference investigation. *Journal of Personality and Social Psychology, 52*(5), 890–898.

Grolnick, W. S., & Ryan, R. M. (1989). Parent styles associated with children's self-regulation and competence in school. *Journal of Educational Psychology, 81*(2), 143–154.

Harlow, H. F. (1950). Learning and satiation of response in intrinsically motivated complex puzzle performance by monkeys. *Journal of Comparative and Physiological Psychology, 43*, 289–294. doi:10.1037/h0058114.

Hodgins, H. S. (2008). Motivation, threshold for threat, and quieting the ego. In H. A. Wayment & J. J. Bauer (Eds.), *Transcending self-interest: Psychological explorations of the quiet ego* (pp. 117–124). Washington, DC: American Psychological Association.

Hodgins, H. S., & Knee, C. R. (2002). The integrating self and conscious experience. In E. L. Deci & R. M. Ryan (Eds.), *Handbook of self-determination theory research* (pp. 87–100). Rochester, NY: University of Rochester Press.

Hodgins, H. S., & Liebeskind, E. (2003). Apology versus defense: Antecedents and consequences. *Journal of Experimental Social Psychology, 39*, 297–316.

Hodgins, H. S., Weisbust, K. S., Weinstein, N., Shiffman, S., Miller, A., Coombs, G., et al. (2010). The cost of self-protection: Threat response and performance as a function of autonomous and controlled motivations. *Personality and Social Psychology Bulletin, 36*, 1101–1114.

Jang, H., Reeve, J., & Deci, E. L. (2010). Engaging students in learning activities: It is not autonomy support or structure but autonomy support and structure. *Journal of Educational Psychology, 102*(3), 588–600.

Joussemet, M., Landry, R., & Koestner, R. (2008). A self-determination theory perspective on parenting. *Canadian Psychology/Psychologie Canadienne, 49*(3), 194–200. doi:10.1037/a0012754.
Kerr, M., & Stattin, H. (2000). What parents know, how they know it, and several forms of adolescent adjustment: Further support for a reinterpretation of monitoring. *Developmental Psychology, 36*, 366–380.
Kerr, M., Stattin, H., & Trost, K. (1999). To know you is to trust you: Parents' trust is rooted in child disclosure of information. *Journal of Adolescence, 22*, 737–752.
Knee, C. R., Lonsbary, C., & Canevello, A. (2005). Self-determination and conflict in romantic relationships. *Journal of Personality and Social Psychology, 89*, 997–1009.
Kochanska, G., & Aksan, N. (1995). Mother-child mutually positive affect, the quality of child compliance to requests and prohibitions, and maternal control as correlates of early internalization. *Child Development, 66*(1), 236–254.
Koestner, R., & Losier, G. F. (2002). Distinguishing three ways of being highly motivated: A closer look at introjection, identification, and intrinsic motivation. In E. L. Deci & R. M. Ryan (Eds.), *Handbook of self-determination theory research* (pp. 101–121). Rochester, NY: University of Rochester Press.
La Guardia, J. G., & Ryan, R. M. (2007). Why identities fluctuate: Variability in traits as a function of situational variations in autonomy support. *Journal of Personality, 75*, 1205–1228.
La Guardia, J. G., Ryan, R. M., & Couchman, C. E. (2000). Within-person variation in security of attachment: A self-determination theory perspective on attachment, need fulfillment, and well-being. *Journal of Personality and Social Psychology, 79*, 367–384.
Loevinger, J. (1976). *Ego development*. San Francisco: Jossey-Bass.
Lynch, M. F., Plant, R. W., & Ryan, R. M. (2005). Psychological needs and threat to safety: Implications for staff and patients in a psychiatric hospital for youth. *Professional Psychology: Research and Practice, 36*(4), 415–425. doi:10.1037/0735-7028.36.4.415.
Niemiec, C. P., & Deci, E. L. (2012). *The effects of provision and deprivation of autonomy on interaction quality between strangers*. Unpublished manuscript. Rochester, NY: University of Rochester.
Niemiec, C. P., Lynch, M. F., Vansteenkiste, M., Bernstein, J., Deci, E. L., & Ryan, R. M. (2006). The antecedents and consequences of autonomous self-regulation for college: A self-determination theory perspective on socialization. *Journal of Adolescence, 29*(5), 761–775. doi:10.1016/j.adolescence.2005.11.009.
Patrick, H., Knee, C. R., Canevello, A., & Lonsbary, C. (2007). The role of need fulfillment in relationship functioning and well-being: A self-determination theory perspective. *Journal of Personality and Social Psychology, 92*, 434–457.
Pelletier, L. G., Dion, S., & Lévesque, C. (2004). Can self-determination help protect women against sociocultural influences about body image and reduce their risk of experiencing bulimic symptoms. *Journal of Social and Clinical Psychology, 23*, 61–88.
Perls, F. S. (1973). *The gestalt approach & eye witness to therapy*. Ben Lomond, CA: Science and Behavior Books.
Reeve, J. (2009). Why teachers adopt a controlling motivating style toward students and how they can become more autonomy supportive. *Educational Psychologist, 44*, 159–178.
Reeve, J., Jang, H., Carrell, D., Jeon, S., & Barch, J. (2004). Enhancing students "engagement by increasing teachers" autonomy support. *Motivation and Emotion, 28*, 147–169.
Reinboth, M., Duda, J. L., & Ntoumanis, N. (2004). Dimensions of coaching behavior, need satisfaction, and the psychological and physical welfare of young athletes. *Motivation and Emotion, 28*(3), 297–313.
Reis, H. T., Sheldon, K. M., Gable, S. L., Roscoe, J., & Ryan, R. M. (2000). Daily well-being: The role of autonomy, competence, and relatedness. *Personality and Social Psychology Bulletin, 26*(4), 419–435.
Ricoeur, P. (1966). *Freedom and nature: The voluntary and the in- voluntary* (E. V. Kohak, Trans.). Chicago: Northwestern University Press.
Rogers, C. R. (1957). The necessary and sufficient conditions of therapeutic personality change. *Journal of Consulting Psychology, 21*, 95–103.

Roth, G., & Assor, A. (2010). Parental conditional regard as a predictor of deficiencies in young children's capacities to respond to sad feelings. *Infant and Child Development, 19*(5), 465–477.

Roth, S., & Cohen, L. J. (1986). Approach, avoidance, and coping with stress. *American Psychologist, 41*(7), 813–819. doi:10.1037/0003-066X.41.7.813.

Ryan, R. M. (1993). Agency and organization: Intrinsic motivation, autonomy, and the self in psychological development. In J. Jacobs (Ed.), *Nebraska symposium on motivation: Developmental perspectives on motivation* (Vol. 40, pp. 1–56). Lincoln, NE: University of Nebraska Press.

Ryan, R. M. (1995). Psychological needs and the facilitation of integrative processes. *Journal of Personality, 63*, 397–427.

Ryan, R. M., & Brown, K. W. (2003). Why we don't need self-esteem: On fundamental needs, contingent love, and mindfulness. *Psychological Inquiry, 14*(1), 71–76.

Ryan, R. M., & Connell, J. P. (1989). Perceived locus of causality and internalization: Examining reasons for acting in two domains. *Journal of Personality and Social Psychology, 57*(5), 749–761.

Ryan, R. M., & Deci, E. L. (2000a). Self-determination theory and the facilitation of intrinsic motivation, social development, and well-being. *American Psychologist, 55*, 68–78.

Ryan, R. M., & Deci, E. L. (2000b). When rewards compete with nature: The undermining of intrinsic motivation and self-regulation. In C. Sansone & J. M. Harackiewicz (Eds.), *Intrinsic and extrinsic motivation: The search for optimal motivation and performance* (pp. 14–54). San Francisco: Academic.

Ryan, R. M., & Deci, E. L. (2001). On happiness and human potentials: A review of research on hedonic and eudaimonic well-being. *Annual Review of Psychology, 52*, 141–166.

Ryan, R. M., & Deci, E. L. (2006). Self-regulation and the problem of human autonomy: Does psychology need choice, self-determination, and will? *Journal of Personality, 74*(6), 1557–1586.

Ryan, R. M., Deci, E. L., Grolnick, W. S., & La Guardia, J. G. (2006). The significance of autonomy and autonomy support in psychological development and psychopathology. In D. Cicchetti & D. J. Cohen (Eds.), *Developmental psychopathology: Theory and method* (2nd ed., Vol. 1, pp. 795–849). Hoboken, NJ: Wiley.

Ryan, R. M., & Frederick, C. (1997). On energy, personality, and health: Subjective vitality as a dynamic reflection of well-being. *Journal of Personality, 65*(3), 529–565.

Ryan, R. M., Kuhl, J., & Deci, E. L. (1997). Nature and autonomy: An organizational view of social and neurobiological aspects of self-regulation in behavior and development. *Development and Psychopathology, 9*, 701–728.

Ryan, R. M., La Guardia, J. G., Solky-Butzel, J. S., Chirkov, V. I., & Kim, Y. (2005). On the interpersonal regulation of emotions: Emotional reliance across gender, relationships, and cultures. *Personal Relationships, 12*, 145–163.

Ryan, R. M., Rigby, S., & King, K. (1993). Two types of religious internalization and their relations to religious orientations and mental health. *Journal of Personality and Social Psychology, 65*(3), 586–596.

Sheldon, K. M., Ryan, R. M., & Reis, H. T. (1996). What makes for a good day? Competence and autonomy in the day and in the person. *Personality and Social Psychology Bulletin, 22*, 1270–1279.

Shontz, F. C. (1975). *The psychological aspects of physical illness and disability*. New York: Macmillan College.

Shostrom, E. L. (1964). An inventory for the measurement of self-actualization. *Educational and Psychological Measurement, 24*(2), 207–218. doi:10.1177/001316446402400203.

Sierens, E., Vansteenkiste, M., Goossens, L., Soenens, B., & Dochy, F. (2007). *The interactive effect of perceived autonomy support and structure in the prediction of self-regulated learning*. Presented at the third international conference on self-determination theory, Toronto, Canada.

Soenens, B., Vansteenkiste, M., & Niemiec, C. P. (2009). Should parental prohibition of adolescents' peer relationships be prohibited? *Personal Relationships, 16*, 507–530.

Stowell, J. R., Kiecolt-Glaser, J. K., & Glaser, R. (2001). Perceived stress and cellular immunity: When coping counts. *Journal of Behavioral Medicine, 24*(4), 323–339.
Weinstein, N., Deci, E., & Ryan, R. M. (2011). Motivational determinants of integrating positive and negative past identities. *Journal of Personality and Social Psychology, 100*, 527–544.
Weinstein, N., & Hodgins, H. S. (2009). The moderating role of autonomy and control on the benefits of written emotion expression. *Personality and Social Psychology Bulletin, 35*(3), 351–364.
Weinstein, N., Hodgins, H. S., & Ryan, R. M. (2010). Autonomy and nondefense in dyads: The effect of primed motivation on interaction quality and joint creative performance. *Personality and Social Psychology Bulletin, 36*(12), 1603–1617.
Weinstein, N., Przybylski, A. K., & Ryan, R. M. (2012). The index of autonomous functioning: Development of a scale of human autonomy. *Journal of Research in Personality, 46*, 397–413.
White, R. W. (1959). Motivation reconsidered: The concept of competence. *Psychological Review, 66*(5), 297–333.
White, R. W. (1963). *Ego and reality in psychoanalytic theory* (G. S. Klein, Ed.) (Psychological issues, Vol. 3, No. 3, Monograph 11). New York: International Universities Press, Inc.
Zuroff, D. C., Koestner, R., Moskowitz, D. S., McBride, C., Bagby, M., & Marshall, M. (2007). Autonomous motivation for therapy: A new non-specific predictor of outcome in brief treatments of depression. *Psychotherapy Research, 17*, 137–148.

Chapter 2
The Universality of Psychological Autonomy Across Cultures: Arguments from Developmental and Social Psychology

Valery Chirkov

Psychological autonomy is one of the ancient concepts covering the exclusive human modes of living and behaving, which have been the objects of debates and arguments among philosophers and researchers for centuries (Augistine, 1968; Baer, Kaufman, & Baumeister, 2008; Erasmus-Luther, 1988; Murphy & Brown, 2007; Paul, Miller, & Paul, 2003; Schneewind, 1998). Are human autonomy and the psychological freedom that comes with it ever possible? What role do society and culture play in the emergence and functioning of psychological autonomy? How do autonomous individuals relate to other people and broader communities? These are only a few of the questions that scholars try to answer. The debates about the nature of human autonomy and its role in people's motivation, functioning, and well-being have arisen again in the recent decades because of the emergence of positive psychology and the economics of happiness, and because of the dissatisfaction scholars have with both behaviorist and cognitivist approaches to human behaviour and its motivation (Chirkov, 2011a; Chirkov, Ryan, & Sheldon, 2010; Jenkins, 2008; Pugno, 2010; Ryan & Deci, 2006). Neurophysiological studies have had a strong impact on the recent debates about human freedom of will and agency, giving rise to ideas which have been labelled 'brain determinism' – theorizing that considers brain rather than the active conscious self to be the ultimate determinant of individual's social actions and behaviours (Baumeister, Mele, & Vohs, 2010; Baumeister & Vohs, 2011; Lowe, 1999; Magni, 2009; Mele, 2009; Murphy & Brown, 2007; Pockett, Banks, &

To be published in Netta Weinstein (Ed). The Autonomous Personality in Interpersonal Interactions: Theory, Research, and Applications. Springer

Portions of this chapter are based on (Chirkov, 2010, 2011b).

This project was partially implemented in the framework of the Programme of Fundamental Studies of the Higher School of Economics in 2011 (project 63.0 "The role of sociocultural context and values in socio-economic behaviour in modern Russia").

V. Chirkov (✉)
University of Saskatchewan, Saskatoon, SK, Canada

Higher School of Economics - National Research University, Moscow, Russia
e-mail: v.chirkov@usask.ca

N. Weinstein (ed.), *Human Motivation and Interpersonal Relationships: Theory, Research, and Applications*, DOI 10.1007/978-94-017-8542-6_2,

Gallagher, 2009; Sternberg, 2010; Stillman, Baumeister, & Mele, 2011). Another area of intensive debates about human autonomy and agency is the cultural relativity of autonomy and the social construction of human agency (Becker & Marecek, 2008; Christopher & Hickinbottom, 2008; Ewing, 1991; Hollan, 1992; Kenwood, 1996; Mines, 1988). These debates are becoming more relevant as the issues of globalization, the intensive migration of thousands of people around the globe and the emerging problems of their health, well-being, and successful functioning move to the foreground of public and scientific debates (Chirkov, 2007, 2011a, 2011b, 2012; Chirkov & Lebedeva, 2011; Chirkov, Lebedeva, Molodtsova, & Tatarko, 2011; Kagitcibasi, 2003; Leung, Pe-Pua, & Karnilowicz, 2006; Rumbaut, 1991): To what extent are individuals autonomous in their course of actions within and among different cultural communities? Are cultural and societal prescriptions unavoidable frameworks for people's thinking, feeling, and behaving? Do individuals have the power to move beyond their cultural heritage and act autonomously and responsibly relatively independently of their social and cultural backgrounds?

Despite of the long history and crucial importance of psychological autonomy for people's efficient and happy living, this concept is still a marginal one in mainstream psychology and is not a frequent topic for theorizing or empirical research in different areas of psychology.[1] One area of argument and research is the domain of psychological autonomy and human relationships (Gaine & La Guardia, 2009; Jenkins, 2001; Martin, 2008). Networks of human connections are regarded both as the source and the outcome of a person's autonomous functioning, and thus the important questions here are: How do autonomous individuals emerge within the network of social, communal, and interpersonal relationships and how does their autonomous mode of functioning relate to and influence these relationships? Do different socio-cultural communities construct the meaning of psychological autonomy differently, and, as a result, treat autonomous people differently? In this chapter, I will try to elaborate on and provide some answers to these and related questions using philosophical, theoretical, and empirical arguments. The arguments here are driven by the idea of dialectical relations between human relationships considered at the different levels – interpersonal, communal, and cultural – and the psychological autonomy of individuals. This dialectics means that human autonomy emerges only within the context of meaningful, symbolic social interactions among human beings who belong to a particular cultural community; it also means that social communities and their intersubjective networks of meanings and practices are crucially important for maintaining and facilitating the functioning of autonomous individuals as well as for limiting or even destroying their autonomy if the conditions are not favourable. This dialectics also manifests itself in the ability of mature autonomous individuals to reflect on and either accept or reject the existing communal and cultural practices and, in the case of rejection, to be the source of culture change. Autonomous individuals who accept the existing cultural milieu serve

[1] For examples of autonomy research in social and personality psychology see the self-determination theory studies (Ryan & Niemiec, 2009); in developmental psychology see (Brandtstädter, 1999; Grolnick, 2003; Helwig, 2006; Kagitcibasi, 2007; Keller, 2007; Rogoff, 2003); in psychotherapy see (Gruen, 2007; Ryan & Deci, 2008; Shapiro, 1984).

as the major supporters and maintainers of it through mindful and reflective externalization of their own self-determined values and moral prescriptions in interactions with other members of their community.

This chapter will start with a short introduction of the concept of psychological autonomy and its components and levels of functioning. Then I will discuss the role of symbolic meaningful interactions in the emergence of autonomy from potentiality to actuality and will show that human autonomy is a universal human capability that may emerge in any cultural community as long as meaningful symbolic interactions among its members exist. The emergence of a sense of self as a fundamental condition for autonomous functioning will also be covered. Finally, I will discuss the major problems and confusions that accompany the study of psychological autonomy in different cultural contexts.

Introduction to the Concept of Psychological Autonomy

My impression is that philosophers from different times and countries, not psychologists, contributed the most to our understanding of nature of psychological autonomy.[2] Psychologists only recently started addressing this issue (Ryan & Deci, 2004; Ryan, Deci, Grolnick, & La Guardia, 2006). It is not surprising that, because of these dispersed opinions and articulations, there is confusion among scholars and lay people about the nature of this phenomenon. Summarizing the available interpretations and the author's reflections about human autonomy (Chirkov, 2010, 2011b), the following defining description of autonomy can be provided. It is important to distinguish personal and motivational forms of autonomy. *Personal autonomy* relates to an individual's life as a whole, which he or she wants to be *self-directed* (enacted according to his or her own goals and values) and *self-governed* (coordinated by the rules, norms, and laws which he or she prescribed to him or herself) (Oshana, 2003; Uyl, 2003). *Motivational autonomy* refers to particular actions or segments of a person's life where he or she acts autonomously or heteronomously. This form of autonomy may refer to academic activity, health-related behaviours, work performance, volunteering, helping others and many other forms of everyday. The conditions of self-directedness and self-governance are relevant here too, but in a more specific and particular manner, depending on the type of activities they apply to.

Psychological autonomy is a specific mode of functioning of human beings that includes: first, a set of self-generated life-goals and values accompanied by

[2] The main contributors to this endeavor are Stoic philosophers (Bobzien, 1998; Cooper, 2003; Hadot, 1995, 1998; Long, 2004), Spinoza (Spinoza, 2000; Uyl, 2003) and Kant (Guyer, 2000, 2003) with a strong input from existential, humanistic psychologists, and moral philosophers (Maslow, 1968; May, 1981; Oshana, 2003). Modern interpreters of Confucius and his followers tackle the problem of the Ancient Chinese interpretations of human self, self-determination and free will and demonstrated that they are similar to the Western understandings of the same phenomena (Chan, 2002; Cheng, 2004; Chong, 2003).

self-determined moral norms and rules which they use to attain these goals. These goals, values, and moral norms are the core of autonomous functioning because consciousness, which makes people free from animalistic instincts as the major regulators of their lives and behaviour, creates a condition of existential freedom for human beings (Fromm, 1955/1976) which requires guiding principles in order to navigate one's life in the sea of opportunities and possibilities of human actuality. Without them, humans' lives become aimless and meaningless (Bettelheim, 1960; Frankl, 1971). As such, life values and moral laws for one's life and behaviour serve as a 'compass', and the more self-determined this compass is the more stable is the course of the ship. These guiding principles should be built on the understanding of the nature of things and how the world, societies, and people's lives are actually run.[3] They have to incorporate people's understanding of their own needs, capacities, and skills, so that these goals work as realistic and achievable objectives. They also have to be based on insights about other people's needs and goals as well as the conditions and characteristics of the communities wherein they live. Second, autonomous functioning is comprised of awareness and reflections on various bodily, sensual, and affective impulses, urges, and desires that naturally happen in a course of every person's life. Autonomous persons have the power and skills to understand the origins, mechanisms, and consequences of these urges and impulses for their lives. Based on this knowledge and guided by the compass of their life-goals and moral laws, they may decide to follow them, or to postpone their gratification, or to reject them as detriments to their life course or actions (Solomon, 2003). People's struggles with their emotions and desires is probably one of the richest topics ever presented in religious and philosophical texts as well as in art and literature. In modern time this struggle is a main concern of clinical psychologists and psychotherapists in dealing with people's psychological problems and concerns.

Third, autonomous people are aware of and understand the cultural and societal demands and expectations that they, as members of a community, inevitably have to deal with. Autonomously functioning individuals comprehend the sources and dynamics of influences of these demands and expectations, and the effects these influences have on their lives. Similar to sensual desires, these people may decide to go along with these demands, postpone them, or reject as being detrimental to their life course or actions. The struggle of autonomous individual with different societal institutions – church, governments, educational institutions, etc. – is another highly explored topic in literature, cinematography, and theatre. These three elements of autonomous functioning – life goals and moral laws, affective and sensual demands, and social norms and expectations – constitute the essential components on which

[3] Starting with the Stoics and followed by many religions and philosophical doctrines, this proposition of following the nature of things has been associated with understanding the gods' divine script about the universe and human beings in it and acting in accordance with it (Cooper, 2003). This spiritual component of autonomous functioning has for the most part been neglected in modern thinking about autonomy. For atheists this proposition means that autonomous people have to acquire a high level of knowledge about the world, societies, and human beings so that their goals and values do not go against the ways in which the world functions.

psychological autonomy is built. In order for autonomy to function, each of these components has to go through three levels of processing: awareness/mindfulness, reflections, and rational decision making.

Awareness or mindfulness is a state of mind when individuals are fully aware of and focus their attention on a situation where they are, on their bodily sensations, emotional states, motivation, and societal demands (not necessarily all at once). Mindfulness has recently become an intensively studied topic and a factor of high importance in the treatment of emotional disorders and other aspects of human malfunctioning (Brown, Ryan, & Creswell, 2007; Segal, Williams, & Teasdale, 2002; Teasdale, Segal, & Williams, 1995). But mindfulness has never being considered as a prerequisite for autonomous functioning or the process through which psychological autonomy manifests itself. According to the understanding of autonomy presented here, in order to be autonomous an individual first must be aware and mindful of his or her own conditions and circumstances, goals and aims, of bodily sensations, emotions, and impulses that are occurring to him or her, as well as of the presence of other people, their concerns, and the demands that they and the current situation impose on a person. If a person is not mindful about these and many other aspects of his or her life situations, he or she cannot be considered ready for autonomous functioning. Recent studies on mindfulness (Brown & Ryan, 2003) demonstrated that this trait positively relates in day-to-day activities to the relative prevalence of autonomous motivation for engaging in these activities over controlled one. Another study (Levesque & Brown, 2007) also demonstrated that mindfulness is involved in the manifestations of autonomy in everyday activities. Mindfulness is beneficial because it is a constituent of psychological autonomy, which in turn brings benefits to people's lives.

To progress to mature psychological autonomy, mindfulness should be accompanied by reflection: the process of psychological distancing oneself from the objects of awareness and attention; first, from a person's thoughts, feelings, and intentions, second, from societal prescriptions and expectations, and, finally, proceeding to contemplations about them with regard to their origins, mechanisms, and consequences. If we were to function autonomously, "we are to subject our different beliefs and desires to a critical, normative evaluation, it is not sufficient simply to have first-personal experience of the states in question. It is not enough to be immediately and implicitly aware of them" (Gallagher & Zahavi, 2008, p. 65). These processes of mindful reflections constitute perhaps the most important component of psychological autonomy.

> Autonomy is defined *not* by the presence or absence of external influences but rather by one's consent or assent to such influences. ... Autonomy entails endorsement of one's actions at the *highest order of reflection*. Thus, people could reflect on motives that emerge from them, and they would be autonomous to the degree that they act in accord with the reflected appraisal of those motives. They might turn to evaluate their autonomy with regard to acting on that appraisal by again reflecting on it from yet a higher-order perspective. (Ryan & Deci, 2004, p. 453).

Recently a group of Israeli psychologists empirically addressed these processes of reflection and their relations to students' autonomy and other academic and well-being outcomes (Assor, 2012; Assor & Kaplan, 2001). These researchers differentiated educational and parenting practices of "supporting value examination" and "fostering inner directed valuing processes" from a psychological process of "reflective value/goal exploration" (Assor, 2012). The 'supporting value examination' practice "refers to acts that encourage youth to engage in activities, experiences and discussions that allow them to examine and reflect seriously and critically on their goals, values and interests" (Assor, 2012, p. 429). The 'fostering inner–directed valuing process' includes: "(a) enhancing students' ability to withstand confusion and take their time before they make serious decisions, (b) encouraging the examination of one's values and goals when faced with a difficult decision and/or social pressures, and (c) encouraging the consideration of alternatives and relevant information before making a decision" (Assor, 2012, p. 436). Empirical studies that assessed the role of supporting value examination in students' academic activity indicated that the utilization of this practice promotes students' sense of autonomy for academic behaviour which is accompanied by engaging in studying and a feeling of vitality while in school. Another study (Assor, Cohen-Malayev, Kaplan, & Friedman, 2005) tested the full model of the reflective internalization of religious beliefs of young Israeli Jews. The support for values examination that parents encourage in their children through critical religious thinking resulted in "the willingness to withhold judgment, to entertain uncertainty and paradox (…), to accept the coexistence of non complementary systems of explanation, and to engage in complex self-reflection and reasoning" (p. 117). A combination of these critical and reflective skills in young men and women supported a relatively harmonious integration both religion and modernity into their identity.

Another reflective practice: perspective taking – the active contemplation of others' psychological experiences – has been one an intensively studied techniques for improving social interactions (Galinsky, Maddux, Gilin, & White, 2008). As I will describe later, the ability to contemplate other people's perspectives and imagine oneself in the 'shoes' of another person constitutes one of the most fundamental human capacity that promotes social coordination as well as the development of mature and autonomous self (Mead, 1934/1962). This practice has recently received attention from social psychologists who study various forms of prejudice and stereotypes and has been empirically investigated with regard to fighting racial biases; its beneficial effects have been registered (Galinsky & Moskowitz, 2000; Todd, Bodenhause, Richeson, & Galinsky, 2011).

The third type of processing during autonomous functioning is a rational decision-making regarding the results of the reflections and contemplations. The essence of this process is comprised of deciding what to do with internal (emotional, motivational, and cognitive) and external (social and cultural) demands: either to follow them or to ignore them. These decisions may be deeply intimate and personal and may be concerned exclusively with reinterpreting and re-evaluating one's personal meaning of the events, other people, one's feelings and actions, or they may guide a person's actions and thus be publicly noticeable. The mindful reflections and decision making that happen deep inside a person's self constitutes what is called 'intra-psychic autonomy' (Ewing, 1991), or, following Rollo May's labelling, 'authentic inner freedom' (1981). Through the externalization in behavioural acts, psychological autonomy becomes a motivator of a person's actions and a driving force of people's autonomous agency and self-determined behaviours, and thus presents itself as behavioural autonomy/freedom (Chirkov, 2011b). Thus, autonomous functioning starts with awareness of and mindfulness about inner events, then moves to reflections and contemplations about them, and, finally, determines a person's decision making with regard to his or her life or actions. This is how Bettelheim (1960) described personal autonomy:

> (…) The concept of autonomy used here has little to do with what is sometimes called "rugged individualism," the cult of personality, or noisy self assertion. It has to do with man's inner ability to govern himself, and with a conscientious search for meaning despite the realization that, as we know, there is no purpose to one's life. It is concept that does not imply a revolt against authority qua authority, but rather a quiet acting out of inner conviction, not out of convenience or resentment, or because of external persuasion or controls. (…) The continuous balancing and resolving of opposing tendencies within oneself, and between self and society – the ability to do this in keeping with personal values, an enlightened self interest, and the interests of the society one lives in – all these lead to an increasing consciousness of freedom and form the basis for man's deepening sense of identity, self respect and inner freedom, in short his autonomy. (p. 75)

In his book, Bruno Bettelheim, a psychoanalyst and survivor of the Nazi concentration camps, provides one of the best accounts of the role psychological autonomy plays in prisoners' physical and psychological survival (see also (Marcus, 1999)). He extends his analysis into the role modern mass society plays in diminishing and reducing people's autonomy and what can be done to protect it.

The components and processing of psychological autonomy work universally across cultures – regardless of the specific contents of people's goals, emotions, and social demands, which are indeed culture dependent – the same way as human consciousness, language, and other higher mental functions work universally across all representatives of human species. Conversely, their contents are socially and culturally specific. Before I move to the topic of relationships of an autonomous person and his or her cultural milieu, it is important to introduce the concept of self as it is used in this chapter with regard to such processes as self-directions, self-governance, and self-determination.

The Role of the Self in Autonomous Functioning

It is natural to ask, who is actually aware and reflective of all the circumstances of a person's life and condition? Who is reflecting on bodily and emotional impulses? Who is making decisions? And who, finally, acts upon these decisions? In medieval times the scholiasts invented the idea of *'homunculus'* – a metaphorical minuscule individual who sits in a person's head, observes the world, and guides his or her actions. This invention of the homunculus metaphor, which inevitably failed because it required the explanation of the behaviour of a homunculus, was a result of the high complexity of the topics of self-consciousness, self-reflection, and self-determination that medieval scholars were trying to explain. The modern concept that addresses these and related phenomena is the notion of self or the sense of self that every healthy person develops during the course of his or her life. From the point of view of modern phenomenological cognitive psychology (Damasio, 1999, 2012; Gallagher, 2000; Gallagher & Zahavi, 2008), a person's sense of self consists of two aspects: a core experiential pre-reflective self and an autobiographical, narrative, and reflected self. Both these aspects of the self participate in and are crucially important for people's autonomous functioning. The experiential aspect of the self "possesses experiential reality, and is in fact identified with the first-personal *appearance* of the experiential phenomena" (Gallagher & Zahavi, 2008, p. 204). This means that all persons perceive their life-worlds, including their own bodies, mental functioning and actions, as *their own*. The functioning and actions are referred to and emanate from *them* and not from others, and they are given to *them* and not to others. It is *their* view of the world and it is *they* who act upon this world. Due to this the experiential-phenomenological self the "experiences that I live through in the first person perspective are *my* experiences" (p. 204). These experiences are pre-reflective and presented to us as implicitly given our first-hand subjective phenomena of different quality (visionary, auditory or pure mental) and delivered through different modalities. With regard to potential autonomy and agency there are two aspects of the experiential self that are relevant here. According to Gallagher (2000) these two aspects are: first, *a sense of ownership* of acts of living, "the sense that I am the one who is undergoing an experience. For example, the sense that my body is moving regardless of whether the movement is voluntary or involuntary" (2000, p. 15), and the second is *a sense of agency,* "the sense that I am the one who is causing or generating an action" (2000, p. 15). These are the building blocks of the phenomenology of psychological autonomy: to sense oneself owning and initiating one's own actions. In order to unfold into a mature autonomous functioning this pre-reflective first-person experience have to be reflected upon, verbally framed, referred to previous episodes of actions and non-actions as well as to the contextual conditions of acting, meaning that this experiential sense of self has to be transformed into the autobiographical/narrative and reflected self. Through "the narrative self – a self linked to sociality, memory, and language" (Gallagher & Zahavi, 2008, p. 205) a person articulates verbally and connects socially his or her experiential self to his or her history and to the social and cultural conditions of his or her life. The narrative self participates in organizing verbally and culturally the reflections and contemplations regarding the representations that an experiential self produces and encounters. Through this self individuals acquire their reflective and agentic powers that enable them to contemplate not only on the world but on themselves and their actions in this world. As soon as this type of self emerges, it, together with the never-ending experiences of the phenomenological self with its first-person perspective, becomes the major producer, regulator, and executioner of psychological autonomy. These are persons with elaborated narrative selves that are capable of adjusting themselves to different social environments by constructing different 'public' or 'social' selves that work as 'personas', or 'masks' to cover and protect their inner authentic self. Individuals with fully elaborated autobiographical selves are capable of initiating the actions that go in their determination beyond pure bodily or environmental pressures. This is where the power of self-direction, self-determination and, based on them, the possibility for autonomous and agentic actions come from. A fully developed autonomy is founded on complex interactions between the experiential first-person perspectival self (Martin, 2008) and the culturally and socially-shaped narrative self. An autonomous person has both aspects of his or her self fully developed and functional in the face of life and action decisions.

> This is a self understood as *an embodied first-person perspective (an 'I'), the worldly experience of which enable a constantly evolving self-understanding (a 'me') with sufficient stability and coherence to permit generally effective personal functioning in the biophysical and sociocultural world in which it develops* (Martin, Sugarman, & Hickinbottom, 2009, p. 110). (…) The reality of the *self* as a unified inner entity capable of exerting agentive influence that goes beyond relevant sociocultural determinants and practices. (p. 107)

The experience of a sense of self and the duality of this experience is a universal feature of any socialized human being across times and places. That is why it is not surprising that the contemplations and writings of Indian and Chinese philosophers are so relevant and complementary to the Western conceptualizations of the phenomenological self (Chong, 2003; Elvin, 1985; Lo, 2003; Sanderson, 1985). For example, Cheng (2004) identified in Confucius's and his followers' writings a similar dual-composite structure of a person's self. In particular, he stated that the Chinese notion of self is conceptualised as *ziji,* and consists of two parts: *zi* "the active and initiating aspect of self or the self that can take action upon oneself, whereas the use of *ji* suggests that it stands for the reflective aspect of self or the self that is the result of the reflective action on the self" (p. 126). "The human self is hence *[sic]* a union and unity of the reflective-substantive *ji* and the initiative-reflective *zi*, hence the resulting notion of *ziji*" (p. 127). As in the above contemplations about self-determination and autonomy, this Chinese understanding of self leads its followers logically to the conclusion that the self is capable of self-transformation and self-directedness: "Upon reflection, the self acquires an identity as well as a power for self-transformation" (p. 126) [and for self-determination and autonomy]. It was Mencius (1970), the principal interpreter of Confucius, who recognized the will of the human self and labelled it "the *zhi*, that is a choice and decision that self makes in view or in recognition of an ideal value or a potential reality that can be achieved through one's efforts" (p. 131). This is a definite formulation of the autonomous power of self similar to the Western one presented above. The ancient Chinese philosophers came to a similar understanding as modern Western scholars regarding the ideas of self-determination and autonomy (Cheng, 2004; Chong, 2003). Here is their conclusion: "Thus *zhi* is not a physical human desire, nor a mental wish, nor simply a recognition of a truth. It is nothing more and nothing less than an independent power of free choice that could choose a goal based on considerations, which could lead to the successful creation of a life-world" (Cheng, 2004, p. 132).

These cross-time and cross-cultural comparisons of the structure and functions of the sense of self reveal the fundamental universality of the experiential-phenomenological and narrative-reflective side of the human self, and its potential power for self-directedness, self-transformation, and self-determination – psychological autonomy.

The Socio-Cultural Origins of Psychological Autonomy

In this section I will address the topic of the origin of psychological autonomy and show that, as all the higher mental functions of human beings, psychological autonomy has socio-cultural origins that are enabled through a person's active interactions with members of their cultural community. The body, brain, and a socio-cultural community, combined together into a system by meaningful social actions and interactions of individuals, work together on the systemic level in producing human psychological autonomy (Chirkov, 2010).

The psychological basis for autonomy is constituted by the symbolic representations (Murphy & Brown, 2007) of the primary sensual, bodily, perceptual, affective, and cognitive presentations, which are given to us directly without linguistic or other symbolic transformations (Damasio, 1999). Symbolic representations, mostly in the linguistic forms, constitute the second layer of our apprehension of internal and external realities and the skilful and meaningful manipulation of these representations constitutes the backbone of any form of autonomy (Deacon, 1997). Another important developmental achievement that makes autonomy possible is the emergence of a person's autobiographical self (Snow, 1990), which is built upon the nascent or proto-self (Gallese & Sinigaglia, 2010; Stern, 1985), and emerges based on the experiential self. The autobiographical self has access to the symbolic representations and through their manipulation acquires its own power for self-transformation and self-determination. But how do they all come to life? This is the fundamental question for the psychology of human autonomy development.

Any socio-cultural community has a fundamental core of attributes that makes it "the species-typical and species-unique 'ontogenetic niche' for human development" (Tomasello, 1999, p. 79). These attributes are: a collective of people, who speak the same language, have an established way of life and practices that these people successfully utilise for their living; they create and share the meanings of different aspects of their physical and social reality and these shared intersubjective symbolic meanings constitute the milieu within which the socialization and enculturation of new members happens. The third component is the network of meaningful interactions among the members of the community and between its new members and their caregivers. Meaningful linguistically mediated social interactions are the medium of human development, which constitute the vehicle that make enculturation and socialization possible (Tomasello, 1999). These universal features of any cultural community make the development of healthy human being into mature and fully functioning adults achievable regardless of the specifics and idiosynchronicity of particular communities. These specifics, related to different values, practices, and meanings, constitute particular cultures, such as national cultures or sub-cultures of different ethnic and social groups. An important cultural particular for our analysis here is the meaning and value that these communities assign to personal autonomy in people's functioning, which can be either supportive and facilitating, or restrictive and diminishing.

According to modern theorizing on child development, in their first months of life infants play out the skills and capacities that they are equipped with from their birth: some perceptual, cognitive, and social skills as well as an inherently proactive way of engagement with the world (Tronick, 2007). Based on their first interactions with the world, infants start developing their proto-self or 'ecological-self (Cicchetti & Beeghly, 1990; Neisser, 1988; Stern, 1985), which becomes the cornerstone of their future more elaborated selfhood. "Of special importance, in directing behaviors at external entities infants experience their own behavioral goals as well as the outcomes of their actions on the environment as external entities accede to or resists their goal-directed activities" (Tomasello, 1999, p. 60). Their pre-reflective sense of self is a source of their own activity that is different from the external objects toward which it is directed. Through this experience, their experiential self starts developing (Stern, 1985). It becomes even more powerful as infants incorporate the sensations and schemas of their bodies into their proto-self (Gallese & Sinigaglia, 2010). The first fundamental breakthrough in children's development toward their future autonomy happens within their first 9–12 months of life. As Tomasello (1999) worded this breakthrough, infants "begin to understand other persons as intentional agents like the self. Intentional agents are animate beings who have goals and who make active choices among behavioral means for attending those goals, including active choices about what to pay attention to in pursuing those goals" (p. 68). This understanding emerges through the 'joint attentional behaviors' (Tomasello, 1999) that infants share with the adults who care for them. Joint attentional behaviors happen among the infant, the adult, and the object of their attention. When the child and the adult jointly attend to the object, when the child follows the attention of the adult toward the object and when the child directs the attention of the adult toward the object, he or she starts to develop his or her understanding of other persons' possessions of an intentional (directed toward external objects) capacity, and the realization that this capacity can be managed and manipulated by this person him or herself or externally. This understanding of others as intentional agents combined with the infants' sense of proto-self agency creates a new understanding that they are also intentional agents whose intentional activities can be managed either by them or by others. The discovery substantially complements their sense of proto-self first by acknowledging that they are similar to others in their intentionality and that they may become objects of the intentional activity of others (Meltzoff, 1990). This new and fundamental acquisition concerns the ability of children to look at themselves as others look at them; the proto-looking-glass sense of self lies at the basis of a crucial component of the future self-system, specifically the concept of 'Me'. In addition to these new understandings, infants "have come to differentiate the goals they are pursuing from the behavioral means they use to pursue that goal much more clearly than in their previous sensory-motor actions" (Tomasello, 1999, p. 73). These new revolutionary emergencies are universal and happen to the infants in all cultural communities at about the same age (Tomasello, 1999).

Due to infants' new capacity to understand others as intentional agents like their own selves,

> a whole new world of intersubjectively shared reality [culture – VC] begins to open up. It is a world populated by material and symbolic artefacts and social practices that members of their culture, both past and present, have created for the use of others. To be able to use these artefacts as they were meant to be used, and to participate in these social practices as they were meant to be participated in, children have to be able to imagine themselves in the position of the adult users and participants as they observe them. (Tomasello, 1999, p. 91)

Children themselves are part of their cultures and, when adults direct their culturally shaped intentional activities, the assigned meanings, and emotional attitudes toward them, children's own sense of self starts developing from the proto-self into the experiential and then into the autobiographical sense of self (Neisser, 1988).

Another breakthrough in developing the basis for psychological autonomy is the acquisition of language and the emergence of symbolic mental representations of children's internal and external worlds (Bates, 1990; Wolf, 1990). When linguistic symbols are applied to children's experiencing and imaginary objects, actions, events, feeling, intentions, thoughts and other physical and mental events and phenomena, this opens a unique opportunity to manage these phenomena not physically but mentally by distancing oneself from them, by applying different perspectives to seeing them, reinterpreting their meanings and either accepting or rejecting them (Fonagy & Target, 2002). Language and other symbols of any cultural community "embody the myriad ways of construing the world intersubjectively that have accumulated in a culture over historical time, and the process of acquiring the conventional use of these symbolic artefacts, and so internalizing these construals, fundamentally transforms the nature of children's cognitive representations" (Tomasello, 1999, pp. 95–96). The nature of this transformation lies in the transition of a child's cognition from non-symbolic sensory-motor representations into symbolic ones. This is how Tomasello described this process:

> (…) Today's child is faced with a panoply of different linguistic symbols and constructions that embody many different attentional construals of any given situation. Consequently, as the child internalizes a linguistic symbol – as she learns the human perspectives embodied in a linguistic symbol – she cognitively represents not just the perceptual or motor aspects of a situation but also one way, among other ways of which she is aware, that the current situation may be attentionally construed by 'us,' the users of that symbol. (p. 126)

Symbolic representations open the opportunity of a 'perspectival' view of the world, people in this world, and the self. As soon as a person becomes capable of voluntarily manipulating these different perspectives, he or she actually becomes capable of psychological autonomy with regard to the existing and future conditions of living. Therefore, it is possible to say that psychologically autonomy is rooted in the intentional and perspectival manipulation and regulation of the symbolic representations (Chirkov, 2010). "The way that human beings use linguistic symbols thus creates a clear break with straightforward perceptual or sensory-motor representations, and it is due entirely to the social nature of linguistic symbols" (Tomasello, 1999, p. 126). The benefits of these symbolic representations for knowing the world and regulating one's own activities in it are enormous (Damasio, 1999). They allow a person to create abstract concepts and to think about events in a psychologically distancing way; they serve as the basis for a person's theory of others' minds and, based on this theory, together with the ability of 'other persons' perspective taking to manage his or her social interactions with people in very sophisticated ways, they allow people to plan their future actions and entertain different courses of actions without necessarily executing them; they open up practically unlimited opportunities for self-reflections and self-transformations that are impossible to do based on sensory-motor presentations. Finally, they allow a person to start constructing his or her own autobiographical/narrative self as well as his or her personal and social identities. This narrative self, together with the identities, constitute the centre of a person's social and cultural experiences as well as of their experiences of his or her life and actions ownership, self-determination, and autonomy. At approximately the same time children become involved in the development of moral reasoning based on "reflective discourses in which children make comments or ask questions involving the beliefs and desires of others or themselves" (Tomasello, 1999, p. 181; see also, (Cicchetti & Beeghly, 1990)).

The emerging capacities for self-determined action as well as for moral and other forms of psychological autonomy are built upon the skills that developmental cognitive psychologists have labelled 'metacognition', self-regulation, reflective and representational redistribution capabilities (Cicchetti & Beeghly, 1990; Fonagy & Target, 2002; Tomasello, 1999). The first step to the development of these skills is the internalization by children of instructions, rules, and regulations that adults use to manage children's behaviour. This management happens through dialogs between the adult and the child. By the means of internalization these dialogs move from the interpersonal domain to the intrapersonal sphere of a child's self. The child applies the same rules and instructions to him- or herself that adults direct to him or her and starts practicing self-regulation of his or her own behaviours. They acquire the skills of not only self-regulating own behaviour but the capacity to consider their own thinking and thus, self-regulate their mental activities as well. These metacognitive mental self-regulation skills give rise to what Karmiloff-Smith (1992) labelled 'representational redistribution': "My claim is that a specifically human way to gain knowledge is for the mind to exploit internally the information it has already stored (both innate and acquired), by redescribing its representations or, more precisely, by iteratively re-presenting in different representational formats what is internal representations represent" (p. 15). Children all over the world acquire these skills as long as they are born into cultural communities and have adults who care about them (Rogoff, 2003). These skills create a cognitive basis for psychological autonomy – behavioural, moral, emotional, motivational, and personal.

One of the arguments toward the universality of psychological autonomy has been the thesis about the evolutionary basis and adaptation advantages of autonomous functioning (Waller, 1998). Although there are no doubts that psychological autonomy is built upon universal evolution-based mechanisms of the human brain, some scholars argued that autonomy could be an exaptation of other more fundamental evolutionary adjustments (Tomasello, 1999). According to Panksepp and Panksepp (2000), "At present, it remains possible that most of the higher aspects of the human brain/mind arise largely from the interaction between general-purpose neural systems of the multimodal cortical association areas and the very basic life experiences encoded by more ancestral emotional/mind systems that all mammals share" (p. 112). These evolutionary supported cortical associations lay at the basis of the "general-purpose representational abilities (e.g., internal imaginary and language)" (p. 115) which sustains humans' higher mental capacities. Tomasello (1999) speculated that "the ability of human beings to reflect on their own behaviour" [the cognitive basis of autonomy – VC] may be an "ontogenetic elaboration" [or exaptation – VC] of the primary "evolutionary adaptations, aimed at the ability of human beings to coordinate their social behavior with one another – to understand one another as intentional beings" (p. 197). This means that the capacity toward autonomy emerged as a consequence of the adaptation to the social life of human groups; specifically, of people's necessity to understand each other and coordinate each other's activities. This fundamental mental advantage of understanding others' minds is built on the general-purpose representational abilities that became specialized for this social regulation purpose. Psychological autonomy has probably emerged as a consequence of this adaptation.

This collection of skills: understanding others as intentional agents, seeing the world from others' perspectives, developing symbolic mental representations and being able to do their redistribution and reformatting, in addition to metacognitive and reflectivity skills and the skills for self-regulation and self-transformation forms the cognitive basis for psychological autonomy and are acquired by all children around the world, but of course to the different extent. In order for autonomy to become a fully pledged transformative capacity, individuals have to undergo other important developments.

Autonomy, as it is presented here, is not a mere collection of specific cognitive skills, rather it is a state of mind and a mode of being that a person chooses for him or herself; it is a specific motivation to live one's life and act as one decides to do. Thus, in addition to described cognitive skills a person has to have a well-articulated and reflected autobiographical self which is equipped with elaborated personal and social identities. An autonomous person has to have knowledge about the world, society, other people and oneself, so that he or she is not swamped in illusions, unjustified expectations, and superficial knowledge. He or she has to develop a system of values and life-goals that will work as a higher-level organizer for all the reflections, representations, and intentions that a person develops in his of her life. All these components of autonomy can be developed only within cultural communities through meaningful interactions with their members. In the next section I will address some of the problems and confusions with regard to the understanding of the interaction of culture and autonomous persons.

Individualism and Collectivism, Cultural Models of Self, and Psychological Autonomy Across Cultures

Every cultural community develops a set of ideas about what a person and his or her elements (self, motivation, intelligence, etc.) mean to its members. This set of ideas is known in the literature as the cultural models/theories of a person and self (Hollan, 1992). The most known cultural models used to understand a person are individualism and collectivism (Triandis, 1995) and independent and interdependent self-construals of personal selves (Markus & Kitayama, 1991). These are cultural and ideological constructions created either by lay members of a community and which constitutes a part of the community's folk psychology or by academics who are reflecting on the social and cultural arrangements of a particular society (Morris, 1994).

Psychological autonomy, on the other hand, is based on an individual's first-person perspective on the world, awareness of his or her situation, reflection on all the demands that he or she has to deal with and then making a decision about either reinterpreting the situation or changing his or her actions within it. Autonomy is an experiential, cognitive, and motivational phenomenon that belongs exclusively to the subjectivity of an individual. Autonomous individuals act and function within the existing cultural models and theories of the world, community, person and self, but they are in no way a mirror reflection of these models. The lack of differentiation of cultural models of self from the experiential selves of particular members of a community is one of the most widely spread confusions of cross-cultural and cultural psychologists. In his treatise of a category of person, Mauss (1985) devised these two aspects:

> Nor shall I speak to you of psychology, ... I shall leave aside everything which relates to the 'self' (*moi*), the conscious personality as such. Let me merely say that it is plain, particularly to us, that there has never existed a human being who has not been aware, not only of his body, but also at the same time of his individuality, both spiritual and physical. ... My subject is entirely different, and independent of this. It is one relating to social history. Over the centuries, in numerous societies, how has it slowly evolved – not the sense of 'self (*moi*) – but the notion or concept that men in different ages have formed of it? (p. 3)

This confusion has led to the conflating of individualism with psychological autonomy, the independent self-construals with agency and the interdependent ones with a lack of it (Markus & Kitayama, 1991, 2003). In addition, it has led to an idea that members of collectivist cultures are more responsible toward their close ones and members of individualist cultures strive for independence from social obligations (Miller, Das, & Chakravarty, 2011).

Hollan (1992) continued elaborating this distinction:

> (...) 'Cultural models', [is] the presupposed, taken-for-granted, commonsensical, and widely shared assumptions which a groups of people hold about the world and its objects. Cultural models (of selves or anything else) present a simplified and often idealized conception of objects and processes in which much of the blooming, buzzing complexity of phenomena is either suppressed or ignored.... If cultural models of the self, like most of other types of cultural models, are simplified and/or idealized, then we should not mistakenly assume that they encompass all aspects of the experiential self or that they alone should serve as the basis for a comparison of the self. (pp. 285–286)

Many anthropologists as well as cultural and social psychologists, according to his opinion, "too readily assume a close correspondence, or even identity, between cultural model or theories [of self – VC] and subjective experience" (p. 284);

> just as one cannot assume that cultural models of the self are merely projections of individual phenomenology, one cannot assume that the individual's experiential self can be reduced to the concepts and terms which are used to talk about it. While the two are no doubt intimately and dynamically related, the extent to which they influence and shape one another should remain an empirical question. (p. 287)

If, according to Hollan, anthropologists and psychologists want to work with the sense of self related to the subjective experience of oneself and others as subjects and objects of intentional actions, (which is similar to the notion of self presented in this chapter with regard to psychological autonomy and self-determination), they have to ask questions about the origins of this self and the role cultural models and ideologies about the self play in shaping and formatting personal experiential and narrative selves. The theorists who emphasize a close match between theories of self and experiential/narrative individual selves practically leave no space for the idiosyncratic, perspectival, particularistic and, finally, autonomous shaping of one's self through self-reflections, self-transformations, and self-development.

> (…) By emphasising a one-to-one correspondence between cultural models and the experiential self, one underplays the extent to which aspects of subjective experience are also a product of psychobiological propensities (Hallowell, 1955, 1959) and social encounters (Mead, 1934; Cooley, 1922; Blumer, 1969) which may actually run counter to, or contradict, ideal cultural representations. (p. 286)

In the empirical part of his article, Hollan (1992) provides vivid examples of strongly relational aspects in the Americans' experiential/narrative selves, which are considered by the cultural model to be highly independent and autonomous, as well as examples of autonomy and self-determination of the experiential/narrative selves of the members of a highly sociocentric tribe in Indonesia.

The same arguments about the differentiation from and non-equivalency of the experiential selves of Indian persons with the socio-centric and highly prescriptive cultural model of self in Indian culture is provided by Mines (1988). His conclusion, which is based on interviews with various representatives of this culture, is that Indians, just as other people around the world, have their own first-person perspectives on the realities around them, can freely identify their self-interests and exercise mastery and ownership over life-important decisions, and are capable of practicing and getting satisfaction from their psychological autonomy. Indeed, we need to accept that the dynamics of the development of autonomy in communities with different cultural models of self may take different trajectories, but neither the presence of individualism nor collectivism prevent people from developing their autonomous experiential selves.

An important condition for the development of psychological autonomy is the communities' attitudes, norms, and practices toward people who demonstrate autonomous functioning. As Benson (2001) commented, "Some societies value the individual as a responsible co-creator of her own life and work to give her the skills and values to do this, thereby building in her powers of autonomy and choice. Others require and produce selves that largely reproduce what they have become without the sense of need or the ability to change the model" (p. 92). This statement means that cultural communities construct systems of ideas regarding the value, meaning, and cultivation of psychological autonomy. These systems are embedded in the more general cultural models of a person. Many social scientists confuse the cultural valuing of autonomy with the ideology of individualism as well as with the conditions of independence or interdependence of individuals within their groups.

Cultural valuing of autonomy means that communities recognize and respect an individual's first-person perspective on the world which is based on their needs, values, and goals. The communities take them into consideration and provide conditions for exercising these attributes. Such communities deem the meaning of autonomy and self-determination as a valuable commodity of any human being, a commodity that needs to be respected and cared for. This valuing may happen within the ideologies of either collectivism (interdependence) or individualism (independence) and can easily be observed through different parenting practices (Rogoff, 2003). One example of the conflict between the ideology of individualism and the value for autonomy is the Western practice of infants' independent sleeping. "Folk wisdom in European American middle-class communities has portrayed nighttime separation of infants from their parents as essential for healthy psychological development, to develop a spirit of independence" (Rogoff, pp. 196–197). This is the ideology of individualism and the cultural model for the development of independent individuals. On the other hand, an infant has his or her fears and a need to have a secure haven for a comfortable sleep. If parents are to respect infants' autonomy they have to respect this need and help them gratify it. But this does not happen in the strict culture of individualism: "Infants and parents in this community frequently engage in conflicts over independent nighttime sleeping, in which parents and infants often act as adversaries in a battle of wills" (p. 197). This battle of wills is a direct indication of disrespect for the infants' autonomy for the sake of the culturally prescribed development of independence and individualism. Another example of an attack on human autonomy within Western cultural traditions may be found in the recommendations of John Wesley, the founder of Methodism, with regard to upbringing children: "Break their will betimes, begin this work before they can run alone, before they can speak plain, perhaps before they can speak at all. Whatever pains it costs, break their will, if you would not damn the child" (Rogoff, p. 206). Thus, the ideology of individualism may pretty brutally go against valuing and practicing autonomy.

Rogoff (2003) also provides ample examples of respect for children's autonomy and freedom of choice within various, so-called, collectivist communities, the communities that highly emphasize coordination among members of groups, an orientation toward the collective and the ability to smoothly function within various social roles and obligations. The respect for autonomy in such highly 'interdependent' communities means that there is a belief that "people can both coordinate with others and act autonomously' (p. 202). In this case "people in many communities have the responsibility to coordinate with the group but the freedom to do otherwise" (p. 202). For instance, "'Inviolability of the individual is a central value widespread among North and Central American Indians. … At any age, people have the right to make their own decisions about their own actions; it is inappropriate to force others to do something against their will" (p. 202); and further, "individual autonomy is respected with Mayan infants because it is inappropriate to go against people's self-determination, even if they themselves do not understand how to act in a responsible interdependent way" (p. 203). She also provides examples of autonomy valuing in such traditionally collectivistic communities as Mexican and Japanese families. Her conclusion is: valuing personal autonomy can peacefully coexist with the collectivistic and interdependent prescriptions for communal life and can be antagonistic to the demands of the ideology of individualism and independence.

Confusion with regard to the understanding the role motivational autonomy plays in different communities also arises with regard to the autonomous versus controlled execution of socially prescribed prosocial behaviours. This problem with autonomy, interpersonal relations, and culture can be summarized as follows: In many cultural communities the behaviour of its members is frequently driven by traditions and a strong feeling of obligation to perform one's duties within the range of assigned social roles and related expectations. Some examples of such behaviours are: helping the poor, filial piety, helping family members, friends and strangers, respecting elders and authorities. It is not surprising that these interpersonal relations have become strongly socially regulated because they maintain the fabric of societal harmony, cohesiveness, and structure, without which the mere survival of these communities could be jeopardized. Different cultural communities endorse and require the execution of these obligations to different degrees, thus leading to the identification of 'tight' and 'loose' cultures (Gelfand et al., 2011; Triandis, 2004). What role does psychological autonomy play in these conditions? Are people in 'tight' cultures less autonomous in executing their social obligations than people in 'loose' cultures? These questions may be elaborated further: Do, for example, Indians or Chinese people choose their prosocial actions exclusively on societal norms or can they exercise their own deliberations in choosing their own course of prosocial actions? Can they critically evaluate the existing normative prescriptions regarding prosocial behaviour and reason their own course of actions? Although a reader may find these questions confusing with regard to their counter-intuitive nature (of course, Indian or Chinese nationals are capable of autonomous and self-determined actions!), they are still legitimate for many social psychologists who are addressing helping behaviour in different cultural settings: "(…) Do people from a Hindu Indian cultural background, which tends to emphasize collectivist cultural values and role-related obligations, feel a reduced sense of agency when they meet their role-related obligations, just like North American folk psychology suggests people do?" (Miller et al., 2011, p. 46).

Self-determination theory (SDT) clearly differentiates these and similar aspects of cultural ideologies and personal functioning by acknowledging that practices of individualism and collectivism as well as practices of socially prescribed prosocial actions may be executed due to different motivation: people may be autonomously collectivistic or be controlled individualists, meaning that peoples' personal motivation behind executing cultural prescriptions and prosocial behaviour may vary strongly along the continuum from external to highly autonomous (Chirkov, Ryan, Kim, & Kaplan, 2003; Chirkov, Ryan, & Willness, 2005; Weinstein & Ryan, 2010).

In their recent study Miller et al. (2011) decided to challenge this conclusion of the self-determination research by investigating different motivation for helping family members and strangers among American and Indian students and studying the relations of this motivation to students' satisfaction, feeling of choice, and autonomy. The initial hypotheses of this study were that

> among the Indian respondents, but not the U.S. respondents, duty/responsibility to help family and friends would be positively associated with autonomous reasons for action as well as with satisfaction and choice. We also hypothesized that only among the U.S. respondents and not among the Indian respondents the presence of strong compared with weak social expectations to help family and friends would be linked with less autonomous reasons for actions and with a lesser sense of satisfaction and choice. (pp. 48–49)

It is clear that both of these hypotheses are built on a flawed confusion of cultural models of self (in India – duties and obligations driven interdependent selves; and in the U.S. – obligation-free independent selves) and the actual behaviour of individuals based on their experiential/narrative selves, which determines the levels of their personal endorsements of the helping behaviours. SDT predicts that in both cultures the execution of family duties may be perceived either as external coercion or as freely chosen prosocial actions. Not surprisingly, the actual results of this study confirm the SDT prediction and not the 'cultural models' hypotheses.

> The results of the present studies are congruent with the claims made in SDT that choice is central to agency universally. ... The results imply that in a collectivist cultural context involving strong social expectations to in-group members, normative obligation to be responsive to the needs of family and friends may come to be internalized so that individuals experience a sense of agency that involves choice in meeting them.... In sum, the present results challenge certain earlier assertions of some theorists within cultural psychology and support the claims of SDT that choice entailed universally in the internalization of social expectations. (p. 58)

This study and its related theorizing invite social and cross-cultural psychologists to pay more attention to the nature of autonomous motivation with regard to its execution in different cultural contexts. The confusion of cultural models of self with the experiential and phenomenological self of an acting person should be clearly addressed.

Conclusion

The goal of this chapter was to clarify some propositions about the nature of psychological autonomy, its socio-cultural origin and dialectical relations of autonomous people with their cultural environment. These clarifications can be summarized as follows.

Psychological autonomy is a fundamental and universal capacity of all human beings, and is a derivate of their sociality, consciousness, and language. It has a sociocultural origin that is based on the presence of cultural, linguistic, and moral communities, in which members interact meaningfully with newly born children and care for them. The development of the cognitive prerequisites for psychological autonomy goes through a relatively universal sequence of stages by the mediation of meaningful symbolic interactions with adult caregivers. Cultural values systems including the valuing of psychological autonomy play an important role in shaping people's capability for autonomous functioning. Autonomous people are able to reflect on their culture and be the agents of its change. Many cross-cultural studies of and theorizing about psychological autonomy, both personal and motivational, are contaminated by several confusions: equating autonomy with individualism and independence and thus denying the value of autonomy in, so-called, collectivistic and interdependent cultures; as well as confusing cultural theories of self with a first-person experience of the ownership of one's actions, which is executed through a person's narrative autobiographical self. These confusions need to be theoretically and empirically clarified and resolved in order to provide a more conceptually refined understanding of the psychological autonomy functioning in different cultural settings.

References

Assor, A. (2012). Allowing choice and nurturing an inner compass: Educational practices supporting students' need for autonomy. In S. L. Christenson, A. L. Reschly, & C. Wylie (Eds.), *The handbook of research on student engagement* (pp. 421–440). New York: Springer.

Assor, A., Cohen-Malayev, M., Kaplan, A., & Friedman, D. (2005). Choosing to stay religious in a modern world: Socialization and exploration processes leading to an integrated internalization of religion among Israeli Jewish youth. In S. Karabenchick & T. C. Urdan (Eds.), *Advances in motivation and achievement: Motivation and religion* (Vol. 14, pp. 105–150). Bingley, UK: Emerald Books.

Assor, A., & Kaplan, H. (2001). Mapping the domain of autonomy support: Five important ways to enhance or undermine students' experience of autonomy in learning. In A. Efklides, J. Kuhl, & R. M. Sorrentino (Eds.), *Trends and prospects in motivation research* (pp. 101–120). Boston, MA: Kluwer Academic Publishers.

Augistine, S. (1968). *The teacher, the free choice of the will, grace and free will* (R. P. Russel, Trans., Vol. 59). Washington, DC: The Catholic University of America Press.

Baer, J., Kaufman, J. C., & Baumeister, R. F. (Eds.). (2008). *Are we free? Psychology and free will.* Oxford, NY: Oxford University Press.

Bates, E. (1990). Language about me and you: Pronominal reference and the emerging concept of self. In D. Cicchetti & M. Beeghly (Eds.), *The self in transition: Infancy to childhood* (pp. 165–182). Chicago: University of Chicago Press.

Baumeister, R. F., Mele, A. R., & Vohs, K. D. (Eds.). (2010). *Free will and consciousness: How might they work?* Oxford, NY: Oxford University Press.

Baumeister, R. F., & Vohs, K. D. (2011). Do conscious thoughts cause behavior? *Annual Review of Psychology, 62*, 331–361.

Becker, D., & Marecek, J. (2008). Dreaming the American dream: Individualism and positive psychology. *Social and Personality Psychology Compass, 2*(5), 1768–1780.

Benson, C. (2001). *The cultural psychology of self: Place, morality and art in human worlds*. London: Routledge.

Bettelheim, B. (1960). *The informed heart: Autonomy in a mass age*. New York: Avon Books.

Bobzien, S. (1998). *Determinism and freedom in Stoic philosophy*. Oxford, NY: Oxford University Press.

Brandtstädter, J. (1999). The self in action and development: Cultural, biosocial, and ontogenetic bases of intentional self-development. In J. Brandtstädter & R. M. Lerner (Eds.), *Action and self-development: Theory and research through the life span* (pp. 37–65). Thousand Oaks, CA: Sage.

Brown, K. W., & Ryan, R. M. (2003). The benefits of being present: Mindfulness and its role in psychological well-being. *Journal of Personality and Social Psychology, 84*, 822–848.

Brown, K. W., Ryan, R. M., & Creswell, J. D. (2007). Mindfulness: Theoretical foundations and evidence for its salutary effects. *Psychological Inquiry, 18*(4), 211–237.

Chan, J. (2002). Moral autonomy, civil liberties, and Confucianism. *Philosophy East and West, 52*(3), 281–310.

Cheng, C.-y. (2004). A theory of Confucian selfhood: Self-cultivation and free will in Confucian philosophy. In K.-l. Shun & D. B. Wong (Eds.), *Confucian ethics: A comparative study of self, autonomy, and community* (pp. 124–142). New York: Cambridge University Press.

Chirkov, V. (2007). Culture, personal autonomy and individualism: Their relationships and implications for personal growth and well-being. In G. Zheng, K. Leung, & J. G. Adair (Eds.), *Perspectives and progress in contemporary cross-cultural psychology* (pp. 247–263). Beijing, China: China Light Industry Press.

Chirkov, V. (2010). Dialectical relationships among human autonomy, the brain, and culture. In V. I. Chirkov, R. M. Ryan, & K. M. Sheldon (Eds.), *Human autonomy in cross-cultural contexts: Perspectives on the psychology of agency, freedom, and well-being* (pp. 65–92). Dordrecht, The Netherlands: Springer.

Chirkov, V. (2011a). *Enculturation, acquisition of autonomy, and acculturation: A phenomenological perspective on the analysis of immigrants' life-worlds*. Paper presented at the regional conference of the international association for cross-cultural psychology, Istanbul, Turkey.

Chirkov, V. (2011b). Human psychological autonomy: Reflections on the debates about its understanding in modern psychology. *Social and Personality Psychology Compass, 5*(9), 609–620.

Chirkov, V. (2012). The motivational nature of good living: Human autonomy and why it is good for people and societies. In D. A. Leontiev (Ed.), *Motivation, consciousness and self-regulation* (pp. 105–126). New York: Nova.

Chirkov, V., & Lebedeva, N. (2011). *Psychological autonomy, human happiness and socio-economic relations: A search for humanistic criteria for market evaluations*. Paper presented at the conference "Market and happiness: Do economic interactions crowd out civic virtues and human capabilities?", Milan, Italy.

Chirkov, V., Lebedeva, N., Molodtsova, I., & Tatarko, A. (2011). Social capital, motivational autonomy, and health behavior in Canadian and Russian youth. In D. Chadee & A. Kostic (Eds.), *Social psychological dynamics* (pp. 211–241). Trinidad, WI: University of West Indies Press.

Chirkov, V., Ryan, R. M., Kim, Y., & Kaplan, U. (2003). Differentiating autonomy from individualism and independence: A self-determination theory perspective on internalization of cultural orientations and well-being. *Journal of Personality and Social Psychology, 84*(1), 97–110.

Chirkov, V., Ryan, R. M., & Sheldon, K. M. (Eds.). (2010). *Human autonomy in cross-cultural contexts: Perspectives on the psychology of agency, freedom, and well-being*. Dordrecht, The Netherlands: Springer.

Chirkov, V., Ryan, R. M., & Willness, C. (2005). Cultural context and psychological needs in Canada and Brazil: Testing a self-determination approach to internalization of cultural practices, identity and well-being. *Journal of Cross-Cultural Psychology, 36*(4), 425–443.

Chong, K.-c. (2003). Autonomy in the analects. In K. Chong, S. Tan, & C. L. Ten (Eds.), *The moral circle and the self: Chinese and western approaches* (pp. 269–282). Chicago: Open Court.

Christopher, J. C., & Hickinbottom, S. (2008). Positive psychology, ethnocentrism, and the disguised ideology of individualism. *Theory & Psychology, 18*(5), 563–589.

Cicchetti, D., & Beeghly, M. (1990). *The self in transition: Infancy to childhood.* Chicago: University of Chicago Press.
Cooper, J. M. (2003). Stoic autonomy. In E. F. Paul, F. D. Miller Jr., & J. Paul (Eds.), *Autonomy* (pp. 1–29). Cambridge, UK: Cambridge University Press.
Damasio, A. R. (1999). *The feeling of what happens: Body and emotion in the making of consciousness* (1st ed.). New York: Harcourt Brace.
Damasio, A. R. (2012). *Self comes to mind: Constructing the conscious brain* (1st ed.). New York: Vintage Books.
Deacon, T. W. (1997). *The symbolic species: The co-evolution of language and the brain.* New York: Norton.
Elvin, M. (1985). Between the earth and haven: Conceptions of the self in China. In M. Carrithers, S. Collins, & S. Lukes (Eds.), *The category of the person: Anthropology, philosophy, history* (pp. 156–189). Cambridge, UK: Cambridge University Press.
Erasmus-Luther (1988). *Discourse on free will.* New York: Continuum.
Ewing, K. P. (1991). Can psychoanalytic theories explain the Pakistani woman? Intrapsychic autonomy and interpersonal engagement in the extended family. *Ethos, 19*(2), 131–160.
Fonagy, P., & Target, M. (2002). Early intervention and the development of self-regulation. *Psychoanalytic Inquiry, 22*(3), 307–335.
Frankl, V. (1971). *Man's search for meaning: An introduction to logotherapy.* New York: Pocket Books.
Fromm, E. (1955/1976). *The sane society.* New York: Holt, Rinehart and Winston.
Gaine, G. S., & La Guardia, J. G. (2009). The unique contributions of motivations to maintain a relationship and motivations toward relational activities to relationship well-being. *Motivation and Emotion, 33*, 184–202.
Galinsky, A. D., Maddux, W. W., Gilin, D., & White, J. B. (2008). Why it pays to get inside the head of your opponent: The differential effects of perspective-taking and empathy in strategic interactions. *Psychological Science, 19*, 378–384.
Galinsky, A. D., & Moskowitz, G. B. (2000). Perspective-taking: Decreasing stereotype expression, stereotype accessibility, and intergroup favouritism. *Journal of Personality and Social Psychology, 78*, 708–724.
Gallagher, S. (2000). Philosophical conceptions of the self: Implications for cognitive science. *Trends in Cognitive Sciences, 4*(1), 14–21.
Gallagher, S., & Zahavi, D. (2008). *The phenomenological mind: An introduction to philosophy of mind and cognitive science.* London: Routledge.
Gallese, V., & Sinigaglia, C. (2010). The bodily self as power for action. *Neuropsychologia, 48*(3), 746–755.
Gelfand, M. J., Raver, J. L., Nishii, L., Leslie, L. M., Lun, J., Lim, B. C., et al. (2011). Difference between tight and loose cultures: A 33-nation study. *Science, 332*, 1100–1104.
Grolnick, W. S. (2003). *The psychology of parental control: How well-meant parenting backfires.* Mahwah, NJ: Lawrence Erlbaum Associates.
Gruen, A. (2007). *The betrayal of the self: The fear of autonomy in men and women.* Berkeley, CA: Human Development Books.
Guyer, P. (2000). *Kant on freedom, law, and happiness.* Cambridge, UK: Cambridge University Press.
Guyer, P. (2003). Kant on theory and practice of autonomy. In E. F. Paul, F. D. Miller, & J. Paul (Eds.), *Autonomy* (pp. 70–98). Cambridge, UK: Cambridge University Press.
Hadot, P. (1995). *Philosophy as a way of life: Spiritual exercises from Socrates to Foucault.* Malden, MA: Blackwell Publishing.
Hadot, P. (1998). *The inner citadel: The meditations of Marcus Aurelius.* Cambridge, MA: Harvard University Press.
Helwig, C. C. (2006). The development of personal autonomy throughout cultures. *Cognitive Development, 21*, 458–473.
Hollan, D. (1992). Cross-cultural differences in the self. *Journal of Anthropological Research, 48*(4), 283–300.

Jenkins, A. H. (2001). Individuality in cultural context: The case of psychological agency. *Theory and Psychology, 11*(3), 347–362.

Jenkins, A. H. (2008). Psychological agency: A necessarily human concept. In R. Frie (Ed.), *Psychological agency: Theory, practice, and culture* (pp. 177–200). Cambridge, MA: The MIT Press.

Kagitcibasi, C. (2003). Autonomy, embeddedness and adaptability in immigration contexts. *Human Development, 46*, 145–150.

Kagitcibasi, C. (2007). *Family, self, and human development across cultures* (2nd ed.). Mahwah, NJ: Lawrence Erlbaum.

Karmiloff-Smith, A. (1992). *Beyond modularity: A developmental perspective on cognitive science*. Cambridge, MA: MIT Press.

Keller, H. (2007). *Cultures of infancy*. Mahwah, NJ: Lawrence Erlbaum.

Kenwood, C. (1996). Does volition need social constructionism? *Theory & Psychology, 6*(3), 533–538.

Leung, C., Pe-Pua, R., & Karnilowicz, W. (2006). Psychological adaptation and autonomy among adolescents in Australia: A comparison of Anglo-Celtic and three Asian groups. *International Journal of Intercultural Relations, 30*(1), 99–118.

Levesque, C. S., & Brown, K. W. (2007). Mindfulness as a moderator of the effect of implicit motivational self-concept on day-to-day behavioral motivation. *Motivation and Emotion, 31*, 284–299.

Lo, Y. K. (2003). Finding the self in the analects: A philological approach. In K. Chong, S. Tan, & C. L. Ten (Eds.), *The moral circle and the self: Chinese and western approaches* (pp. 250–267). Chicago: Open Court.

Long, A. A. (2004). *Epictetus: A Stoic and Socratic guide to life*. Oxford, NY: Oxford University Press.

Lowe, E. J. (1999). Self, agency, and mental causation. In B. Libet, A. Freeman, & K. Sutherland (Eds.), *The volitional brain: Towards a neuroscience of free will* (pp. 225–239). Thorverton, UK: Imprint Academic.

Magni, S. F. (2009). Brain determinism and free will. *Etica & Politica, XI*(2), 57–67.

Marcus, P. (1999). *Autonomy in the extreme situation: Bruno Bettelheim, the Nazi concentration camps and the mass society*. Westport, CT: Praeger.

Markus, H. R., & Kitayama, S. (1991). Culture and the self: Implications for cognitions, emotion, and motivation. *Psychological Review, 98*, 224–253.

Markus, H. R., & Kitayama, S. (2003). Models of agency: Sociocultural diversity in the construction of action. *Nebraska Symposium on Motivation, 49*, 1–57.

Martin, J. (2008). Perspectival selves and agents: Agency within sociality. In R. Frie (Ed.), *Psychological agency: Theory, practice, and culture* (pp. 97–116). Cambridge, MA: The MIT Press.

Martin, J., Sugarman, J., & Hickinbottom, S. (2009). *Persons: Understanding psychological selfhood and agency*. New York: Springer.

Maslow, A. (1968). *Toward a psychology of being* (2nd ed.). Princeton, NJ: Van Nostrand.

Mauss, M. (1985). A category of human mind: The notion of person; the notion of self. In M. Carrithers, S. Collins, & S. Lukes (Eds.), *The category of the person: Anthropology, philosophy, history* (pp. 1–25). Cambridge, UK: Cambridge University Press.

May, R. (1981). *Freedom and destiny* (1st ed.). New York: Norton.

Mele, A. R. (2009). *Effective intentions: The power of conscious will*. Oxford, NY: Oxford University Press.

Meltzoff, A. N. (1990). Foundations for developing a concept of self: The role of imitation in relating self to other, and the value of social mirroring, social modeling, self-practice in infancy. In D. Cicchetti & M. Beeghly (Eds.), *The self in transition: Infancy to childhood* (pp. 139–164). Chicago: University of Chicago Press.

Mencius. (1970). *Mencius* (D. C. Lau, Trans.). London: Penguin Classics.

Miller, J. G., Das, R., & Chakravarty, S. (2011). Culture and the role of choice in agency. *Journal of Personal and Social Psychology, 101*(1), 46–61.

Mines, M. (1988). Conceptualizing the person: Hierarchical society and individual autonomy in India. *American Anthropologist, 90*(3), 568–579.
Morris, B. (1994). *Anthropology of the self: The individual in cultural perspective*. London: Pluto Press.
Murphy, N. C., & Brown, W. S. (2007). *Did my neurons make me do it? Philosophical and neurobiological perspectives on moral responsibility and free will*. Oxford, NY: Oxford University Press.
Neisser, U. (1988). Five kind of self-knowledge. *Philosophical Psychology, 1*, 35–59.
Oshana, M. (2003). How much should we values autonomy? In E. F. Paul, F. D. Miller, & J. Paul (Eds.), *Autonomy* (pp. 99–126). Cambridge, UK: Cambridge University Press.
Panksepp, J., & Panksepp, J. B. (2000). Seven sins of evolutionary psychology. *Evolution and Cognition, 6*(2), 108–131.
Paul, E. F., Miller, F. D., & Paul, J. (Eds.). (2003). *Autonomy*. Cambridge, UK: Cambridge University Press.
Pockett, S., Banks, P. W., & Gallagher, S. (Eds.). (2009). *Does consciousness cause behavior?* Cambridge, MA: MIT Press.
Pugno, M. (2010). Economy, people's personal autonomy, and well-being. In V. I. Chirkov, R. M. Ryan, & K. M. Sheldon (Eds.), *Human autonomy in cross-cultural contexts: Perspectives on the psychology of agency, freedom, and well-being* (pp. 207–239). Dordrecht, The Netherlands: Springer.
Rogoff, B. (2003). *The cultural nature of human development*. New York: Oxford University Press.
Rumbaut, R. G. (1991). The agony of exile: A study of the migration and adaptation of Indochinese refugee adults and children. In J. Frederick, L. Ahearn, & J. L. Athey (Eds.), *Refugee children: Theory, research, and services* (pp. 53–91). Baltimore, MD: Johns Hopkins University Press.
Ryan, R. M., & Deci, E. L. (2004). Autonomy is no illusion: Self-determination theory and the empirical study of authenticity, awareness, and will. In J. Greenberg, S. L. Koole, & T. Pyszczynski (Eds.), *Handbook of experimental existential psychology*. New York: The Guilford Press.
Ryan, R. M., & Deci, E. L. (2006). Self-regulation and the problem of human autonomy: Does psychology need choice, self-determination, and will? *Journal of Personality, 71*(6), 1557–1585.
Ryan, R. M., & Deci, E. L. (2008). A self-determination theory approach to psychotherapy: The motivational basis for effective change. *Canadian Psychology, 49*(3), 186–193.
Ryan, R. M., Deci, E. L., Grolnick, W. S., & La Guardia, J. G. (2006). The significance of autonomy and autonomy support in psychological development and psychopathology. In D. Cicchetti & D. J. Cohen (Eds.), *Developmental psychopathology* (2nd ed., Vol. 1, pp. 795–849). New York: Wiley.
Ryan, R., & Niemiec, C. (Eds.). (2009). Symposium on self-determination theory. *Theory and Research in Education, 7*(2).
Sanderson, A. (1985). Purity and power among the Brahmans of Kashmir. In M. Carrithers, S. Collins, & S. Lukes (Eds.), *The category of the person: Anthropology, philosophy, history* (pp. 190–216). Cambridge, UK: Cambridge University Press.
Schneewind, J. B. (1998). *The invention of autonomy: A history of modern moral philosophy*. Cambridge, UK: Cambridge University Press.
Segal, Z. V., Williams, J. M. G., & Teasdale, J. D. (2002). *Mindfulness-based cognitive therapy for depression: A new approach to preventing relapse*. New York: Guilford Press.
Shapiro, D. (1984). *Autonomy and rigid character*. New York: Basic Books, Inc.
Snow, C. E. (1990). Building memories: The ontogeny of autobiography. In D. Cicchetti & M. Beeghly (Eds.), *The self in transition: Infancy to childhood* (pp. 213–242). Chicago: University of Chicago Press.
Solomon, R. C. (2003). *Not passion's slave: Emotions and choice*. Oxford, NY: Oxford University Press.
Spinoza, B. (2000). *Ethics* (G. H. R. Parkinson, Trans.). Oxford, UK: Oxford University Press.

Stern, D. N. (1985). *The interpersonal world of the infant: A view from psychoanalysis and developmental psychology*. New York: Basic Books.

Sternberg, E. J. (2010). *My brain made me do it: The rise of neuroscience and the threat to moral responsibility*. Amherst, NY: Prometheus Books.

Stillman, T. F., Baumeister, R. F., & Mele, A. R. (2011). Free will in everyday life: Autobiographical accounts of free and unfree actions. *Philosophical Psychology, 24*(3), 381–394.

Teasdale, J. D., Segal, Z., & Williams, J. M. G. (1995). How does cognitive therapy prevent depressive relapse and why should attentional control (mindfulness) training help? *Behaviour Research and Therapy, 33*(1), 25–39.

Todd, A. R., Bodenhause, G. V., Richeson, J. A., & Galinsky, A. D. (2011). Perspective taking combats automatic expression of racial bias. *Journal of Personality and Social Psychology, 100*(6), 1027–1042.

Tomasello, M. (1999). *The cultural origins of human cognition*. Cambridge, MA: Harvard University Press.

Triandis, H. C. (1995). *Individualism and collectivism*. Coulder, CO: Westview Press.

Triandis, H. C. (2004). Dimensions of culture beyond Hofstede. In H. Vinken, J. Soeters, & P. Ester (Eds.), *Comparing cultures: Dimensions of culture in a comparative perspective* (pp. 28–42). Leiden, The Netherlands: Brill.

Tronick, E. (2007). *The neurobehavioral and social-emotional development of infants and children*. New York: Norton.

Uyl, D. D. (2003). Autonomous autonomy: Spinoza on autonomy, perfectionism, and politics. In E. F. Paul, F. D. Miller, & J. Paul (Eds.), *Autonomy* (pp. 30–69). Cambridge, UK: Cambridge University Press.

Waller, B. N. (1998). *The natural selection of autonomy*. Albany, NY: State University of New York.

Weinstein, N., & Ryan, R. M. (2010). When helping helps: Autonomous motivation for prosocial behavior and its influence on well-being for the helper and recipient. *Journal of Personality and Social Psychology, 98*(2), 222–244.

Wolf, D. P. (1990). Being of several minds: Voices and versions of the self in early childhood. In D. Cicchetti & M. Beeghly (Eds.), *The self in transition: Infancy to childhood* (pp. 183–212). Chicago: University of Chicago Press.

Chapter 3
Autonomy and Need Satisfaction in Close Relationships: Relationships Motivation Theory

Edward L. Deci and Richard M. Ryan

Among the most important values and motives of people around the world is to feel connected and meaningfully related to others (e.g., La Guardia & Patrick, 2008; Reis, 2011). Yet not all social interactions yield a true sense of relatedness. Although in some social situations people can feel cared for and acknowledged and experience a sense of belongingness, in other situations they can feel isolated or misunderstood, instrumentally used, or in other ways frustrated in their desire of connection or relatedness. It is thus important to distinguish those elements within social interactions, affiliations, and relationships that truly foster a sense of relatedness and connection from those elements and dynamics that thwart that experience.

According to self-determination theory (SDT; Ryan & Deci, 2000), all human beings have a fundamental psychological need to experience *relatedness*—that is, to feel personally accepted by and significant to others, and to feel cared for by others and caring of them (e.g., Deci & Ryan, 2000; Lavigne, Vallerand, & Crevier-Braud, 2011). Although some theories view relationship motivation as derived from other instrumental outcomes such as drive gratifications (e.g., Freud, 1925), physical security (Bowlby, 1969), or resource exchanges (Thibaut & Kelley, 1959), SDT posits that relatedness is an evolved psychological need in its own right, which, although associated with adaptive advantages, takes on an intrinsic character in human nature. That is, people find relatedness to be inherently satisfying, independent of instrumental advantages. Indeed, individuals often value and maintain connections that afford a sense of relatedness to their distinct material disadvantage.

A basic or inherent need for relatedness thus underlies people's motivated tendencies to make interpersonal contacts, and to adopt identities and join groups that socially connect them with others. The concept of a *need*, however, is distinct from that of motivation. People can fail to be motivated for that which they actually need. Thus the idea of a relatedness need goes beyond the suggestion that relatedness

E.L. Deci (✉) • R.M. Ryan
Department of Psychology, University of Rochester, Rochester, NY, USA
e-mail: deci@psych.rochester.edu

N. Weinstein (ed.), *Human Motivation and Interpersonal Relationships: Theory, Research, and Applications*, DOI 10.1007/978-94-017-8542-6_3,

is something merely preferred, desired, or considered important, for SDT argues that relatedness is essential to human wellness. That is, people require relatedness to be vital and to thrive. Even people who say and, indeed, believe, that they do not want to connect with others will nonetheless suffer ill effects if they do not experience relatedness or belonging. Similarly, even within organizations or cultures that do not give primacy to relatedness and collectivity, people suffer if they lack a sense of relatedness (e.g., Ryan, Bernstein, & Brown, 2010). Human nature thus declares interpersonal relatedness to have primacy, and families, institutions, and cultures must provide the pathways for this need to be satisfied if their constituents are to be well.

SDT is not the only psychological theory to emphasize that belonging and feeling personally close to others promote human flourishing. In social psychology for example, a number of researchers have vigorously investigated a wide range of phenomena among people who are personally close, finding many benefits that accrue from acceptance and interpersonal support (e.g., Baumeister & Leary, 1995; Shaver & Mikulincer, 2011). Clinicians in the object relations theoretical tradition have written extensively about the necessity of close relationships, initially with primary caregivers but also with peers as individuals progress through the lifespan (e.g., Winnicott, 1965). Even in research with nonhumans, Harlow (1958) showed convincingly that close personal contact was necessary for healthy development among rhesus monkeys. These as well as various other researchers have accepted, either implicitly or explicitly, that relatedness or belongingness is a fundamental psychological need, although few contemporary empirical approaches have made the concept of need a central concept within their theorizing.

SDT and Basic Psychological Needs

SDT is a contemporary, research-based psychological theory that has specified, highlighted, and emphasized the importance of the concept of universal psychological needs in order to make predictions and provide interpretations of empirical phenomena (e.g., Deci & Ryan, 2000; Ryan, 1995). As we will discuss below, SDT posits three basic psychological needs—competence and autonomy, in addition to relatedness. In general, a central prediction made by the theory is that, when people experience greater satisfaction of the relatedness need, they will evidence higher levels of psychological wellness; whereas when satisfaction of this need has been thwarted, they will display signs of ill-being (e.g., Bartholomew, Ntoumanis, Ryan, Bosch, & Thogersen-Ntoumani, 2011). SDT's need theory thus supplies a dynamic model, because it suggests both that needs explain behavior and outcomes independently of conscious expectancies and values, and moreover that people respond predictably when needs are satisfied versus thwarted. As we will see in what follows, numerous phenomena can also be interpreted in ways that are derived from and are congruent with this general proposition.

Different Definitions of Needs

Although the concept of psychological needs appears in several theories within social-personality psychology (e.g., McClelland, 1985; Murray, 1938), most researchers treat the concept as an individual difference variable, reflecting the varying strengths of individuals' motives. In other words, assessment of a need provides an index of how important or strong that desire or attribute is for the person. In personality psychology, for example, the need for achievement (Atkinson, 1958) and the need for intimacy (McAdams, 1989) are assessed for individuals and then used to predict behaviors, affects, and outcomes in the corresponding domains. In social psychology, needs such as the *need for cognition* (Cacioppo, Petty, & Kao, 1984) and the *need for closure* (Webster & Kruglanski, 1994) are used to make predictions, often in conjunction with experimental manipulations concerning whether being high versus low on the strength of some need moderates various outcomes.

In SDT, in contrast, our primary concern is the main effects. SDT has specified fundamental psychological needs for relatedness, competence, and autonomy, and proposed that satisfaction of each of these psychological needs is necessary in an ongoing way for people to function optimally and to display a high level of psychological health, regardless of individual differences in motives or preferences. *Competence* refers to feeling effective and confident with respect to some behavior or goal (e.g., White, 1959), and *autonomy* concerns the feeling of volition, willingness, concurrence, and choice with respect to a behavior or experience one is engaged in (e.g., de Charms, 1968). SDT proposes that if satisfaction of any of the three psychological needs is deprived or thwarted, some type of negative consequence will ensue.

SDT does recognize individual differences in motives related to these basic psychological needs, as well as in motivational orientations (Deci & Ryan, 1985; Weinstein, Przybylski, & Ryan, 2012b), but it suggests nonetheless that the most important predictors of psychological health, well-being, and social functioning are variables assessing need satisfaction versus thwarting. In fact, SDT sees differences in need strength or importance as often being reflective of dynamic reactions, or attempts to cope with, past need deprivation or thwarting.

SDT further highlights that under optimal conditions there are positive interrelations among the three basic needs. At the general level, people who get one of these needs well satisfied often also get the others satisfied. For example, if people were afforded opportunities for autonomy, they would more likely feel psychologically free and able to find or create opportunities to also get their needs for relatedness and competence satisfied. Reciprocally, if they felt deep satisfaction of their relatedness need through connections with accepting others, they would likely experience the interpersonal support necessary to take risks and enact their own autonomous motives. Indeed, it is thus the case that correlations among satisfaction of the three needs, at the global or general level, across situations is relatively and expectably high.

Relationships Motivation Theory (RMT)

RMT is one of the six mini-theories contained within SDT. Its central proposition is that, although satisfaction of the need for relatedness predicts people's experiences of relationship satisfaction or relational well-being, relatedness need satisfaction alone is not enough to ensure high-quality relationships. Flourishing relationships also require that people experience satisfaction of the need for autonomy, as well as the need for competence, within the relationships. Indeed, research has shown that satisfaction of the latter two needs also contribute independently to positive relationship outcomes (e.g., La Guardia, Ryan, Couchman, & Deci, 2000). In other words, the theory, as well as the data, suggest that all three of these basic psychological needs, which are essential for optimal wellness and flourishing and which mutually support one another, must be satisfied in order for people to experience the highest quality close relationships.

Need Satisfaction, Well-Being, and Relationship Outcomes

Experience sampling studies in which participants recorded the degree to which they experienced satisfaction of each of the basic psychological needs have demonstrated strong relations among the three basic need satisfactions, and between these satisfactions and wellness. For example, in a daily dairy study of students, Reis, Sheldon, Gable, Roscoe, and Ryan (2000) used a multi-level modeling strategy to confirm the SDT hypothesis that, at both the between-person (i.e., individual-difference) and within-person (i.e., across-time) levels of analysis, satisfaction of each of the three basic needs predicted independent variance in people's psychological wellness. In other words, people who in general felt more satisfaction of each of the three needs (i.e., the between-person level) also felt more psychological well-being. Further, on any given day, the amount of satisfaction people felt for each need independently contributed to well-being on that day (controlling for well-being on the prior day).

More recently, Ryan et al. (2010) assessed the three basic need satisfactions multiple times a day in a heterogeneous sample of adult workers. Similar to Reis et al. (2000) they found that each of the needs was independently associated with variations in wellness, measured with multiple variables, including variables tapping positive and negative affect, vitality, and physical symptoms. There was also a large and predicted "weekend effect," in which workers on average had substantially higher physical and psychological wellness on weekends. This effect was fully mediated by the needs for autonomy and relatedness. Indeed, the multiple daily assessments revealed that it was largely in their work environments that people felt thwarted in their autonomy and relatedness, which in turn negatively affected wellness. In workplaces where relatedness was higher, wellness was higher, and for those workers the weekend effect was less pronounced. One implication of this study for organizations was the high costs in terms of daily employee wellness of low workplace relatedness.

Satisfaction of each need is also important within close relationships. Patrick, Knee, Canavello, and Lonsbury (2007) did a group of studies in which they assessed participants' satisfaction of each of the basic psychological needs within a close relationship. They found that each need contributed to all of the important outcomes they examined, including personal well-being, relationship quality, and effectively managing conflict within the relationship. In one of the studies these investigators also showed that if an individual's partner were feeling greater satisfaction of the basic psychological needs, this also independently contributed to the individual perceiving the relationship to be of greater quality.

Need Satisfaction and Attachment Security

Ainsworth and colleagues (e.g., Ainsworth, Blehar, Waters, & Wall, 1978) developed a paradigm for empirically studying the concept of attachment (Bowlby, 1969) between infants and their caregivers. Considerable research has shown that when caregivers are sensitive and responsive, infants and caregivers develop more secure attachments, evidenced in part by the infants being engaged and interested even when the caregivers are absent. These secure attachments are considered to be the basis for what are called *working models* (e.g., Bretherton, 1987), which implies that, as individuals grow up, their experience of others (e.g., romantic partners and best friends) will tend to mirror the attachments they developed with their primary caregiver. In other words, attachment security is considered an individual difference aspect of people's personalities, which then get applied in future close relationships, especially romantic relationships (e.g., Shaver & Mikulincer, 2011).

Research by La Guardia et al. (2000) investigated the attachment security of young adults across multiple partners. They began by examining the degree to which attachment security is in fact consistent across relationships. In three studies, analyses indicated that about one-third of the variance in attachment security was at the between-person level, suggesting that attachment security is, to this extent, an individual difference, and providing support for the working-model aspect of attachment theory. Yet, the finding also means that a preponderance of variance is not accounted for at the individual-difference level, but varies within person. La Guardia et al. argued that this within-person variance across relationships is a function of the basic need-related dynamics between the person and each of his or her partners. Specifically, the researchers suggested that people experience different levels of basic psychological need satisfaction in their interactions with different relational partners, and that the level of need satisfaction a person experiences with a particular partner should predict the person's security of attachment with that partner. La Guardia et al. found that, indeed, within each close relationship, the need satisfaction that was unique to that partner also predicted the unique security of attachment with that partner.

Of the three needs, satisfaction of the relatedness need explained the greatest amount of within-person variance in attachment security, which of course makes sense, and is essentially tautological. Thus, La Guardia et al. controlled for relatedness satisfaction and found that autonomy satisfaction remained a significant and, moreover, substantial predictor of attachment security for every relationship type, including parental and peer. Further, competence satisfaction also predicted security of attachment, although, as expected, that relation was somewhat weaker.

Summary

A growing number of studies, only some of which were reviewed here, have indicated that when people experience satisfaction of autonomy and competence needs within relationships, they experience higher quality relationships, including a more secure sense of attachment, as well as greater psychological well-being. These results hold up at the general, between-person level, as well as at the within-person level when considering individuals' experiences across days and also across partners. They also hold up across varied ages and cultural groups. Such results both attest to the interdependence of basic psychological needs and to the notion that relatedness satisfaction is a product of only certain relationships, namely those that beyond being warm and positive also convey respect and support for autonomy.

Autonomous Motivation for Being in a Close Relationship

We have frequently argued that when people are autonomously motivated in some situation or for a particular behavior or class of behaviors, they will typically feel satisfaction of all three of the basic psychological needs, because autonomous motivation yields direct satisfaction of the autonomy need and provides people the psychological freedom to find satisfaction of the relatedness and competence needs for themselves. Accordingly, we have hypothesized that when people enter, commit to, and persist at close relationships autonomously they will likely experience the relationships to be of higher quality than when their motivation for the relationship is more controlled.

Both questionnaire and experimental studies have tested this hypothesis. In the first such study, Blais, Sabourin, Boucher, and Vallerand (1990) examined married or cohabiting couples, assessing the degree to which their reasons for maintaining their relationships were more versus less autonomous. The results indicated that the more autonomous the partners' motivation for maintaining the relationship, the greater was the relationship satisfaction and dyadic adjustment. A structural model indicated that when the partners were more autonomous, they experienced more positive relational behaviors, which led to greater personal happiness and satisfaction in the dyad.

In other research Knee, Lonsbury, Canevello, and Patrick (2005) showed that, when partners who were more autonomously motivated to be in their relationships encountered a disagreement, they were less defensive and more understanding of their partners' point of view. The research showed not only that a target person's autonomy predicts his or her being more effective in handling relationship conflict, but also when the target person's partner was more autonomously motivated for the relationship, the target person handled the conflict in an even more effective, non-defensive way. Gaine and La Guardia (2009) further found that if they assessed individuals' autonomous motivation for specific relational behaviors, in addition to autonomous motivation for being in the relationship more generally, the relationship-specific autonomy explained additional variance in relationship well-being.

Recent work by Niemiec and Deci (2014) used an experimental paradigm to examine the importance of autonomous motivation in developing relationships between new acquaintances. In one such study, autonomous versus controlled motivation was primed within pairs of participants who did not know each other, using the scrambled-sentence priming method. Then, the two participants spent their time mutually self-disclosing to the other and in so doing developing a "new relationship." The researchers found that the pairs who were primed with autonomous motivation felt more satisfaction within their new relationship, more positive affect, more relatedness need satisfaction, and greater well-being than was the case for the pairs that were primed with controlled motivation. Because, in this study, the type of motivation was manipulated experimentally rather than simply assessed with a questionnaire format, the results allowed for a causal interpretation. In other words, this study showed that autonomous, relative to controlled, motivation promoted higher-quality, more-satisfying interactions with the acquaintances, which likely also means that it would facilitate longer-term relationships as well.

Another study also primed autonomous and controlled motivation among participants who had not known each other but were working together on creative activities (Weinstein, Hodgins, & Ryan, 2010). In this study trained observers rated videotaped interactions of partners working together on creative tasks. Results indicated that the autonomously primed pairs were more attuned to one another both emotionally and cognitively, and were more encouraging and empathic with one another than was the case with pairs who were primed with controlled motivation. The autonomous pairs, relative to the controlled pairs, were also more effective in doing the activities and reported greater closeness with each other.

To summarize, several studies, including experiments, have confirmed that when people are more autonomously engaged in relationships, they experience greater relationship satisfaction and well-being, a phenomenon that applies across both close relationships and new encounters.

When Social Contexts Support Need Satisfaction

We have thus far seen that when people were either autonomously motivated for a relationship or felt satisfaction of their basic psychological needs within a relationship they evidenced various positive outcomes, including greater relationship satisfaction and positive affect, in addition to enhanced psychological wellness. It was a logical extension to hypothesize that, when others provided target individuals with autonomy support or, more broadly, support for satisfaction of all of the basic psychological needs, the individuals would experience both personal and relational well-being, because numerous studies have confirmed that autonomy-supportive and need-supportive interpersonal contexts enhance autonomous motivation and basic-need satisfaction (see, e.g., Deci & Ryan, 2000; Ryan & Deci, 2008 for reviews). These studies have been of two sorts: some have examined developmental trends of children becoming more autonomous or more stably need satisfied as a function of need support, and some have examined concurrent need support relating to more autonomous motivation and more basic need satisfaction in a current situation.

Developmental research has shown for example that, when children grow up in social environments that are supportive of basic psychological needs, they tend not only to have more secure and satisfying relationships with parents but they also tend to become more autonomously motivated for many tasks and activities in their lives. Their intrinsic motivation tends to be maintained or enhanced over time (see, Deci & Ryan, 1980) and they tend to more fully internalize extrinsic motivation (Grolnick & Ryan, 1989) thus acting more autonomously even for uninteresting activities that are deemed important for their development and effectiveness.

Typically, social contexts have one or more key individuals within them, often in a position of authority. For example, social contexts in youth sports have coaches as the key authorities; social contexts in schools have teachers; and the contexts in homes have parents as authorities. For social contexts to be need-supportive for the target persons who are acting within them (e.g., athletes, students, or children) the authorities can best begin by appreciating and acknowledging the perspectives and frame of reference of those they would motivate at times of both setbacks and successes. These contexts also involve the authorities providing support for trying new things and making choices, providing warmth and respect, providing rationales when asking target individuals to do something, and refraining from using controlling language and controlling rewards or threats of punishment.

Much research has shown that, within these need-supportive interpersonal environments, individuals tend to become more autonomously motivated (e.g., Grolnick & Ryan, 1987; Niemiec, Lynch, Vansteenkiste, Bernstein, Deci, & Ryan, 2006; Roth, Assor, Niemiec, Ryan, & Deci, 2009). Need-supportive environments have been found to not only facilitate autonomous motivation, but also to foster, in turn, more effective performance and well-being (e.g., Deci, Eghrari, Patrick, & Leone, 1994; Vansteenkiste, Simons, Lens, Sheldon, & Deci, 2004). Further, studies have shown that, in current situations such as schools or workplaces, when the environment is autonomy supportive, people report higher levels of psychological need satisfaction, which has positive links to engagement, performance, and psychological well-being (Baard, Deci, & Ryan, 2004; Deci, Ryan, Gagné, Leone, Usunov, & Kornazheva, 2001).

Need Support in Peer Relationships

Recent studies of peer relationships have shown that when one person receives need support from a partner, the person will also evidence various benefits such as increased autonomy, more personal well-being, and greater relationship satisfaction. The difference between these studies and the need-support studies discussed in the previous few paragraphs is that these studies involve relationships that do not have differentials in authority (at least structurally) but instead involve two people who, by the nature of their relationships, are more equal or mutual in their interactions.

In one program of research, Ryan, La Guardia, Solky-Butzel, Chirkov, and Kim (2005) examined the interpersonal phenomenon of people turning to others to share experiences or gain support when they were having strong emotional experiences, whether positive or negative. Some of the studies examined *emotional reliance* as an individual difference—that is, they explored whether individuals who were more likely to turn to others during emotional experiences would show positive benefits relative to individuals who were less likely to rely on others. In fact, the research did indicate that those who were more inclined to volitionally depend on others did show less anxiety and depression and more vitality, suggesting that, when people feel they can turn to close friends, romantic partners, and family members during very moving emotional times, they tend generally to be psychologically healthier. Thus, this finding represents an example of how being independent of others, which is often touted in our culture as being an important indicator of well-being, is not as important as some have argued (e.g., Steinberg & Silverberg, 1986) and is not a basic need. Indeed, being volitionally dependent on one's close relational partners seems to be a meaningful antecedent of optimal psychological functioning, which would also, of course, involve some amount of volitional independence.

Some of the studies done by Ryan et al. (2005) followed up on the above by examining mediation of the positive relations between emotional reliance and psychological wellness. Specifically, the researchers hypothesized that the reason emotional reliance is a positive predictor of well-being is that people tend to experience need satisfaction when they are willingly relying on others—that is, they will tend to feel close and cared for, to feel volitional, and to feel support for their own competence in relation to the situation. Indeed, the results of the research indicated that basic need satisfaction mediated the relation between emotional reliance and psychological well-being. That is, emotional reliance led significantly to basic need support, which in turn led significantly to more well-being and less ill-being.

Importantly, other studies in the Ryan et al. (2005) research program investigated emotional reliance in terms not of individual differences but rather in terms of whom people tended to rely on when they were emotionally charged. That is, the researchers hypothesized and found that people had multiple important relationships but that they emotionally relied on their different relational partners to differing degrees. For example, in one study the researchers assessed the degree to which college students relied on their mothers or fathers, and they found that, although in general students tended to rely more on mothers in times of emotional upheaval, reliance on either of their parents was a function of that parent's perceived need supportiveness. The researchers also examined people's reliance on best friends and romantic partners, and as with parents, the findings showed that people were likely to rely on such others during times of upset, conflict, or elation, but only to the degree that each of those relational partners provided need support. In a final study, Ryan et al. collected data in Russia, Korea, Turkey, and the United States and found that the measure of emotional reliance was psychometrically comparable across cultures. Further, although the amount of emotional reliance people reported varied somewhat from culture to culture, emotional reliance was associated with greater well-being across the countries. In short, volitionally turning to close others when people are experiencing strong emotions, especially turning to those close others who tend to be supportive of their psychological needs, appears to be important for well-being across cultures.

In short, theses studies indicated that people benefited from turning to others when they were having strong emotions and that the others to whom they were most likely to turn were those people in their lives who, in general, provided the most basic psychological need support.

Extending cross-cultural research in this area, Lynch, La Guardia, and Ryan (2009) did a study of within-person differences in relationship quality that involved samples from China, the U.S., and Russia. They predicted and found that across all three nations people reported their highest relationship quality as occurring with the social partners whom they experienced as most autonomy supportive. Moreover across countries they reported being more authentic with autonomy-supportive others, and as being able, themselves, to act more in accord with their own ideal ways of being. In other words, the quality of relationships was a function of autonomy support, and people saw themselves as functioning most optimally when they were with others who were autonomy supportive.

Experiments on Autonomy Support in Close Relationships

Niemiec and Deci (2014) did a series of experiments examining how support for autonomy or lack thereof would affect people's experiences of interaction quality when they engaged in a mutual self-disclosure activity (Aron, Melinat, Aron, Vallone, & Bator, 1997). In these studies participants interacted with an experimental accomplice who posed as a second participant, and support versus deprivation of autonomy was manipulated by introducing one of the various experimental induction that had previously been shown to either decrease or enhance autonomy. Specifically, in two experiments, the participant was paid for engaging in the self-disclosure activity and in one the participant was induced to be ego-involved in the activity. Both of these manipulations had been shown previously to diminish people's autonomy (Deci, Koestner, & Ryan, 1999; Ryan, 1982). In yet another experiment participants were given an autonomy-supportive induction, in which choice was provided and their feelings were acknowledged (Deci et al., 1994).

In the studies in which a true participant was paid for interacting with the other "participant," the participants reported finding the interaction *per se* less satisfying, being less emotionally reliant on the other, and having less positive affect than the control-group participants who were not paid. In one of the studies that included a behavioral measure, the paid participants also displayed less behavioral closeness with the partner. In the study of ego-involvement the pattern of results was very similar to that from the reward studies. Finally, in the experiment in which autonomy support was provided, participants reported finding the interaction to be of higher quality than the participants in the control group.

To summarize, in four experiments, when participants' autonomy was manipulated with contextual inductions, those inductions that had previously been found to decrease autonomy were found to lead to the experience of lower-quality interactions, whereas inductions that had previously been found to enhance autonomy led to higher quality interpersonal interactions.

Mutuality in Relationships

Relationships involving close friends and romantic partners tend to be characterized by consent and mutuality, lacking in the element of authority differentials that are present in so many relationships in life. Yet friends too can be more or less need supportive toward each other; they can be more or less controlling (vs. autonomy supportive), more or less cold or rejecting (vs. relationally supportive), more or less critical, negative, or condescending (vs. competence supportive). Friendship quality, then, is a function not only of the experienced support with the relationship but also by the characteristic mutuality of support and caring that defines close friendships.

Two studies by Deci, La Guardia, Moller, Scheiner, and Ryan (2006) with best-friend pairs focused on the amount of autonomy support that each partner provided to the other. Because each partner provided data, it was necessary to use a multi-level approach to analyses, with individuals nested within pairs (Griffin & Gonzales, 1995). First, the analyses showed that the amounts of autonomy support each individual provided to his or her partner was significantly related. This highlights how in close friendships there is mutuality in this type of support; the level that one person provides tends to be mirrored in the level that the other provides. Interestingly, there were several indicators of relationship quality in this research, and analyses also indicated that each of these indicators was also significantly mutual; that is, the partners tended to agree on how healthy and satisfying their friendships tended to be. Further, analyses also showed that the amount of mutuality that the pairs experienced on autonomy support also predicted the amount of mutuality experienced on the various relationship-quality variables.

It was also the case that in this research, analyses at the individual level tended to replicate results of many prior studies showing that the amount of autonomy support that an individual received from another person predicted the target individual's relationship satisfaction and general well-being, although, as already mentioned, much of that prior research involved the target individual being in a relationship with an authority figure. In the Deci et al. (2006) research, individuals who perceived more autonomy support from their best friends also reported more relationship satisfaction, attachment security with their partners, emotional reliance on the partners, dyadic adjustment, and inclusion of their friends in their own sense of self. Those analyses were done after controlling for pair-level relations, and the results did apply to each partner individually. Thus, as would be expected, when a person receives autonomy support from a close friend, the person tends to benefit meaningfully in terms of both relational and individual well-being.

We have seen then that autonomy support was important in relationships for each individual who received it, and we have also seen that there tended to be mutuality in the level of autonomy support as well as the levels of relationship-quality indicators. What we have not yet seen is whether the degree of mutuality in autonomy support would predict the level of relationship quality and well-being; that is whether individuals' giving autonomy support to their partners helps those who give it beyond the help they get from receiving autonomy support from the friends. If it did, it would mean that both giving and receiving autonomy support had positive effects, thus confirming the importance of mutuality in friendships.

Deci et al. (2006) addressed this question using structural equation modeling in which both partners were included in the model, with four independent variables and two dependent variables. The autonomy support received by the first person and the autonomy support given by that same person were used to predict a relationship quality indicator as that person perceived it, and further the autonomy support received by the second person and the autonomy support given by that person were used to predict the same dependent variable but this time as the second person perceived it. Finally, each of the four independent variables was linked to one another within the model. As for results, both giving and receiving autonomy support for each partner correspondingly predicted basic psychological need satisfaction for each, thus confirming that giving as well as receiving autonomy support was need satisfying for people. Then, when the relationship-quality variables were examined, both the giving and receiving of each partner predicted each of those outcome variables. Thus, it is clear that mutuality of autonomy support in close relationships does signify that the relationships will be experienced as high quality. Additionally, psychological well-being was used as an outcome variable in this same type of analysis, and it was interesting that the giving of autonomy support was more strongly linked to well-being than was receiving autonomy support when the two variables competed for variance.

As a final set of analyses, Deci et al. separated dyads consisting of two females from those consisting of two males. This allowed the researchers to analyze female and male data separately to determine whether giving and receiving autonomy support is important for both genders. The data confirmed that the giving and receiving of autonomy support were both significant predictors of relationship quality whether the dyads consisted of males or females. This indicated that autonomy and relatedness are not antagonist for either males or females within relationships; rather, high-quality relationships for each gender require autonomy to be present within the relationship, in a mutual way, which is facilitated by each partner giving as well as receiving autonomy support.

Turning Autonomy and Relatedness Against Each Other

Considerable research has shown that satisfaction of all three psychological needs is necessary for psychological health and well-being; that optimal relationships require all three needs to be satisfied; and that autonomy and relatedness, rather than being inherently antagonist, are instead quite complimentary. Nonetheless, other research has shown that it is possible for social environments to be structured in ways that turn the needs against each other. In particular, the autonomy and relatedness needs, although inherently synergistic, have been found to be antagonistic under conditions with various interpersonal elements. One example of this that has been explored in several studies is the commonly used socializing practice of parental conditional regard (Assor, Roth, & Deci, 2004). *Conditional regard* involves parents providing additional love, attention, and approval when their children do as the parents want, and withdrawing love, attention, and approval when the children do not. This approach is derived from the behaviorist tradition in that the provision of additional attention and affection is considered a reinforcer, the withdrawal of those elements is a punishment, and the avoidance of the withdrawal would serve as a negative reinforcement. Yet, one could also view both the provision and withdrawal of these interpersonal rewards as subtle forms of control, because the message is essentially that, to receive the "reward" of attention and affection, the children would have to do what their parents value or support, regardless of their own feelings of volition. Simply stated, to get relatedness from their parents, the children have to relinquish their autonomy.

In one of the first SDT studies of parental conditional regard (PCR), Assor et al. found that when college students perceived their parents as having been conditionally regarding, the students did engage in the behaviors that were instrumental to the PCR, but the behavioral engagement was controlled—that is, it was regulated by introjects—and the students felt little sense of choice about doing the behavior. Further, the students felt only short-lived positive affect when they succeeded but felt longer-lived guilt and shame when they failed. They also evidenced contingent, unstable self-esteem. Interestingly, another study showed that the use of PCR was generationally transmitted. That is, evidence showed that mothers who themselves paid costs for their parents' conditional regard nonetheless tended to use that same socializing strategy with their own children.

Even more interestingly, Assor et al. found that the more the parents of the college students used PCR, the more their children felt rejected by the parents and the more resentful they were toward their parents. In other words, the use of PCR not only had negative effects on the children's well-being, but it also had unfortunate consequences for the parent-child relationships. A follow up study by Roth et al. (2009) showed further that PCR interfered with children's emotional self-regulation. Whereas autonomy supportive parenting led to integrated regulation within their children, PCR led to a mix of suppression and dysregulation of the emotions. That is, when the children experienced PCR, they attempted to suppress the emotions to get the parents' affection, but the emotions tended to leak out in unregulated ways.

PCR and Close Relationships

Together these initial studies suggested that parental conditional regard tended to have negative consequences for close personal relationships, which led Moller,

Roth, Niemiec, and Deci (2014) to perform a series of studies in which they related the degree of conditional regard used by the parents of college students to the degree that the students perceived their best friends and romantic partners as conditionally regarding. The general expectation was that the level of conditional regard of each parent would relate significantly negatively to the children's relationship satisfaction with that parent and perhaps with others close relationships as well, and also that these relations between PCR and relationship satisfaction would be mediated by within-relationship need satisfaction. In a first study Moller et al. found that students' perceptions of their mothers' conditional regard was negatively related to the students' relationship satisfaction and security of attachment with their mothers, and that both of these relations were mediated by need satisfaction with the mothers. A very similar set of relations was found for fathers. Even more important for our current discussion, both mothers' and fathers' conditional regard negatively predicted relationship satisfaction and security of attachment with the students' romantic partners, and these relations were mediated by the students' within-relationship need satisfaction with their romantic partners.

The next study in the Moller et al. series examined this issue at the between- and within-person levels of analysis with students' perceptions of the degrees to which their mothers, fathers, best friends, and romantic partners were conditionally regarding of them. First, analyses indicated that the correlation of perceived conditional regard for each of the six pairs of partners (e.g., mom and best friend, romantic partner and dad, etc.) was significantly positive, with the lowest being .26 between best friends and romantic partners and the highest being .63 between moms and dads. Second, using multi-level modeling, analyses showed at the between-person (i.e., individual difference) level that, in general, perceptions of parental conditional regard negatively predicted security of attachment within the peer relationships. That is, when young-adult children viewed their parents as more conditionally regarding, they also tended to have peer relationships that were lower in security of attachment. At the within-person level, both the students' experiences of receiving conditional regard from their peer partners, and also the students' experiences of relationship-specific satisfaction of the basic psychological needs with these partners, predicted security of attachment with the partners.

The primary message from these studies was that young adults who perceived their parents as having been conditionally regarding of them while they were growing up tended also to perceive both their best friends and their romantic partners as being conditionally regarding. These findings raise two interesting questions. First, might these young adults have selected best friends and romantic partners who reminded them of their parents in that their relational partners were similarly conditionally regarding? Second, might these young adults have internalized from their parents the mental representation that close others are conditionally regarding of them and then essentially projected that representation onto their two closest peers? Two more studies in the Moller et al. (2014) series addressed these issues, recognizing that the answer might be both.

In the first of the studies, participants were assessed regarding the conditional regard they get from their mothers, fathers, and romantic partners, as well as their security of attachment to each of these important others, their need satisfaction with each, and other relevant variables. The romantic partners also completed questionnaires assessing the degree to which they were conditionally regarding of their participant partners. Notably, participants' perceptions of their parents being conditionally regarding of them were significantly related to their perceptions of their romantic partners' being conditionally regarding, replicating results from the two previous studies. Most importantly, the target participants' perceptions of each of their parents being conditionally regarding was significantly related to the amount of conditional regard that their romantic partners reported giving to them—the target participants. In other words, the young adults who were the target individuals for this research appeared to have picked romantic partners who were similar to their parents in terms of being conditionally regarding.

In a final study, Moller et al. had participants interact with an experimental accomplice who posed as another participant. The two individuals, who had not known each other, interacted in a mutual self-disclosure activity intended to build closeness in the interaction. Subsequently, the participant completed questionnaires, one of which assessed the degree to which he or she perceived the "partner" (i.e., the experimental accomplice) to be conditionally regarding. Having had no prior interactions with the "partner" and having in the experiment interacted in a very structured way with the "partner" who had been trained to treat all participants the same way, the participants had no basis for knowing the degree to which the "partner" was being conditionally regarding. Hence, the ratings the participants made of the partners being conditionally regarding would have been primarily projections, very likely of the relationships they had with their parents. Results showed that indeed there were significant relations between perceptions of the conditional regard of parents and perceptions of conditional regard of the peer "partners," indicating that the participants were projecting the conditional regard onto the people with whom they were "building a relationship." In sum, results of these last two studies showed that people tend to select romantic partners who are like their own parents in being conditionally regarding, and that they also tend to develop a perceptual bias, projecting conditional regard onto their peer partners if that is what they experienced from parents.

Partners as Objects

Mutuality of autonomy support implies that each partner in a relationship is acting in caring and responsive ways that are respecting of the self of the other. As we have seen, this leads to more satisfying relationships for both partners. Yet many peer relationships do not evidence this mutuality, with one partner (and perhaps both) being either actively or passively aggressive or controlling rather than sensitive and supportive. One partner may be treating the other as an object to be controlled or used. Stated differently, some individuals in relationships relate to their partners not for who they are but for what they possess or represent. Perhaps the first partner has financial resources and the second partner relates to the first one's wealth rather than to a person who has his or her own needs, emotions, and attributes (e.g., Kasser & Ryan, 1996; McHoskey, 1999). Perhaps the second partner relates to the first as someone over whom he or she can wield power, or as someone whose attractiveness enhances, in the eyes of other people, the second partner's worth (Ryan, Sheldon, Kasser, & Deci, 1996). In all these cases the partner is not intrinsically valued, but instead valued for some instrumental reason.

SDT-based data show in fact that attribution manipulations that have others thinking that one is relating to them for extrinsic reasons lowers their sense of engagement, trust, and interest in relating (e.g., Wild, Enzle, Nix, & Deci, 1997). Furthermore, even when somebody else objectively helps an individual, the individual is not likely to feel good or to appreciate the help unless the other did it willingly or autonomously (Weinstein & Ryan, 2010). That is, people only feel positively related to by others when the others are willingly giving. After all, if someone helps an individual for an extrinsic reason the helper has not conveyed care for the recipient, but instead for a contingent outcome.

RMT similarly hypothesizes that people who place high importance on extrinsic goals such as wealth, fame, and image are more likely to view their partners less as individuals to be related to in a mutual fashion, but instead as instruments for attaining extrinsic goals or aspirations (Kasser & Ryan, 1996). Such relationships would accordingly be more superficial and less deeply satisfying. In fact, research has shown that both holding and attaining strong extrinsic, relative to intrinsic, life goals was associated not only with poorer well-being but also with poorer-quality romantic relationships and less-satisfying friendships (Kasser & Ryan, 2001). Further, individuals' development of stronger extrinsic aspirations has been shown to result from being in relationships with parents and other authority figures who were controlling and rejecting—relationships that essentially treated the individuals as objects rather than developing organisms (Kasser, Ryan, Zax, & Sameroff, 1995; Williams, Cox, Hedberg, & Deci, 2000).

More recently Weinstein, Law, and Ryan (2012a) did a series of studies in which they tested the hypothesis that the salience of extrinsic goals for financial wealth encourages an instrumental orientation toward others, and is negatively associated with seeing others as inherently worthwhile (i.e., with having a valuing orientation). Eight studies using varied methods, both experimental and cross-sectional, yielded evidence supporting this hypothesis, across varied relationship foci including strangers, friends, and romantic partners. These relations of wealth goals to more instrumental or objectifying social orientations suggest again that only when others are non-contingently valued, or cared for in their own right, are interpersonal relationships of the highest quality.

Conclusions

Relationships Motivation Theory, which is one of the six mini-theories of SDT, is concerned with high-quality close relationships. Central to the theory is that, out of a need for relatedness, people will, when fully functioning, seek out contact and belongingness with others, and attempt to develop intimate relationships. RMT also holds, however, that not all social encounters provide true relationship satisfaction. In fact, considerable research confirms that for social interactions to promote personal and relational well-being, people must experience not only relatedness satisfaction but also autonomy support and autonomy satisfaction within the relationships. As well, competence need satisfaction within relationships also contributes to the quality of the relationships. The more need satisfaction people experience in a relationship the more satisfied they will be with the relationship and the better they will be in dealing with the inevitable conflicts in the relationship.

RMT also proposes and research has found that if people are autonomously motivated to be in relationships, they will experience them as being of higher quality, and if they feel like their partners are supporting their basic psychological needs they will also feel like the relationships are more satisfying. Further, RMT proposes that the highest quality relationships require not only that the people are autonomous and experience autonomy support from their partners, but also that there is mutuality of autonomy and autonomy support within them such that each person not only receives support for the basic needs from his or her partner but also gives need support to the partner. Indeed, research has confirmed that giving as well as receiving autonomy support in a relationship both contribute to the partners' experiencing the relationship as being of high quality.

Further, research has shown that people must experience satisfaction of each of the basic needs within relationships for the relationships to be optimal, and yet the social context—in which a person's partner is often the key element—may turn satisfaction of basic needs against each other. For example, one partner may provide conditional regard to the other, in which case the first partner is essentially conveying that the second partner would have to relinquish autonomy, doing what the first partner wants, in order to receive relatedness, attention, and affection from that first partner. This has been associated with the experience of low quality relationships. Finally, some low quality relationships result from one partner treating the other as an object rather than a person. Such objectification, which is sometimes mutual in relationships, interferes with basic need satisfaction and leaves people with bad feelings about the relationship. For example, when people have high aspirations to be wealthy and attractive, or to be with partners who are wealthy and attractive, those people may be relating to the partners as objects—that is, as the bearers of wealth and beauty—rather than as human beings with their own needs, desires, and inclinations toward mutually satisfying relationships.

A central point of RMT is therefore that there is much more to good, high-quality, relationships than merely warmth or tangible supports. Instead people have a deep need to experience relatedness, or the sense that they are valued and cared for. Relatedness however only results when another cares for and supports one's self. It is when we feel non-contingently valued, or loved for our own sake, and supported in our autonomy, that relatedness is most fulfilled. In contrast instrumental use of others, treating them like objects or vehicles to outcomes, undermines the sense of connection people so naturally desire to feel.

References

Ainsworth, M. D. S., Blehar, M. C., Waters, E., & Wall, S. (1978). *Patterns of attachment*. Hillsdale, NJ: Erlbaum.

Aron, A., Melinat, E., Aron, E. N., Vallone, R. D., & Bator, R. J. (1997). The experimental generation of interpersonal closeness: A procedure and some preliminary findings. *Personality and Social Psychology Bulletin, 23*, 363–377. doi: 10.1177/0146167297234003.

Assor, A., Roth, G., & Deci, E. L. (2004). The emotional costs of perceived parental conditional regard: A self-determination theory analysis. *Journal of Personality, 72*, 47–87. doi: 10.1111/j.0022-3506.2004.00256.x.

Atkinson, J. W. (1958). *Motives in fantasy, action and society*. Princeton, NJ: Van Nostrand.

Baard, P. P., Deci, E. L., & Ryan, R. M. (2004). Intrinsic need satisfaction: A motivational basis of performance and well-being in two work settings. *Journal of Applied Social Psychology, 34*, 2045–2068. doi: 10.1111/j.1559-1816.2004.tb02690.x.

Bartholomew, K. J., Ntoumanis, N., Ryan, R. M., Bosch, J., & Thogersen-Ntoumani, C. (2011). Self-determination theory and diminished functioning: The role of interpersonal control and psychological need thwarting. *Personality and Social Psychology Bulletin, 37*, 1459–1473. doi: 10.1177/0146167211413125.

Baumeister, R., & Leary, M. R. (1995). The need to belong: Desire for interpersonal attachments as a fundamental human motivation. *Psychological Bulletin, 117*, 497–529. doi: 10.1037/0033-2909.117.3.497.

Blais, M. R., Sabourin, S., Boucher, C., & Vallerand, R. (1990). Toward a motivational model of couple happiness. *Journal of Personality and Social Psychology, 59*, 1021–1031. doi: 10.1037/0022-3514.59.5.1021.

Bowlby, J. (1969). *Attachment*. New York: Basic Books.

Bretherton, I. (1987). New perspectives on attachment relations: Security, communication and internal working models. In J. Osofsky (Ed.), *Handbook of infant development* (pp. 1061–1100). New York: Wiley.

Cacioppo, J. T., Petty, R. E., & Kao, C. F. (1984). The efficient assessment of need for cognition. *Journal of Personality Assessment, 48*, 306–307. doi: 10.1207/s15327752jpa4803_13.

de Charms, R. (1968). *Personal causation: The internal affective determinants of behavior*. New York: Academic.

Deci, E. L., Eghrari, H., Patrick, B. C., & Leone, D. R. (1994). Facilitating internalization: The self-determination theory perspective. *Journal of Personality, 62*, 119–142. doi: 10.1111/j.1467-6494.1994.tb00797.x.

Deci, E. L., Koestner, R., & Ryan, R. M. (1999). A meta-analytic review of experiments examining the effects of extrinsic rewards on intrinsic motivation. *Psychological Bulletin, 125*, 627–668. doi: 10.1037/0033-2909.125.6.627.

Deci, E. L., La Guardia, J. G., Moller, A. C., Scheiner, M. J., & Ryan, R. M. (2006). On the benefits of giving as well as receiving autonomy support: Mutuality in close friendships. *Personality and Social Psychology Bulletin, 32*, 313–327. doi: 10.1177/0146167205282148.

Deci, E. L., & Ryan, R. M. (1980). The empirical exploration of intrinsic motivational processes. In L. Berkowitz (Ed.), *Advances in experimental social psychology* (Vol. 13, pp. 39–80). New York: Academic.

Deci, E. L., & Ryan, R. M. (1985). *Intrinsic motivation and self-determination in human behavior*. New York: Plenum.

Deci, E. L., & Ryan, R. M. (2000). The "what" and "why" of goal pursuits: Human needs and the self-determination of behavior. *Psychological Inquiry, 11*, 227–268. doi: 10.1207/S15327965PLI1104_01.

Deci, E. L., Ryan, R. M., Gagné, M., Leone, D. R., Usunov, J., & Kornazheva, B. P. (2001). Need satisfaction, motivation, and well-being in the work organizations of a former Eastern Bloc country. *Personality and Social Psychology Bulletin, 27*, 930–942. doi: 10.1177/0146167201278002.

Freud, S. (1925). Instincts and their vicissitudes. In *Collected papers* (Vol. 4, pp. 60–83). London: Hogarth. (Originally published in 1915).

Gaine, G. S., & La Guardia, J. G. (2009). The unique contributions of motivations to maintain a relationships and motivations toward relational activities to relationship well-being. *Motivation and Emotion, 33*, 184–202. doi: 10.1007/s11031-009-9120-x.

Griffin, D., & Gonzales, R. (1995). Correlational analysis of dyad-level data in the exchangeable case. *Psychological Bulletin, 118*, 430–439. doi: 10.1037/0033-2909.118.3.430.

Grolnick, W. S., & Ryan, R. M. (1987). Autonomy in children's learning: An experimental and individual difference investigation. *Journal of Personality and Social Psychology, 52*, 890–898. doi: 10.1037/0022-3514.52.5.890.

Grolnick, W. S., & Ryan, R. M. (1989). Parent styles associated with children's self-regulation and competence in school. *Journal of Educational Psychology, 81*, 143–154. doi: 10.1037/0022-0663.81.2.143.

Harlow, H. F. (1958). The nature of love. *American Psychologist, 13*, 673–685. doi: 10.1037/h0047884.

Kasser, T., & Ryan, R. M. (1996). Further examining the American dream: Differential correlates of intrinsic and extrinsic goals. *Personality and Social Psychology Bulletin, 22*, 80–87. doi: 10.1177/0146167296223006.

Kasser, T., & Ryan, R. M. (2001). Be careful what you wish for: Optimal functioning and the relative attainment of intrinsic and extrinsic goals. In P. Schmuck & K. M. Sheldon (Eds.), *Life goals and well-being: Towards a positive psychology of human striving* (pp. 115–129). Goettingen, Germany: Hogrefe & Huber Publishers.

Kasser, T., Ryan, R. M., Zax, M., & Sameroff, A. J. (1995). The relations of maternal and social environments to late adolescents' materialistic and prosocial values. *Developmental Psychology, 31*, 907–914. doi: 10.1037/0012-1649.31.6.907.

Knee, C. R., Lonsbary, C., Canevello, A., & Patrick, H. (2005). Self-determination and conflict in romantic relationships. *Journal of Personality and Social Psychology, 89*, 997–1009. doi: 10.1037/0022-3514.89.6.997.

La Guardia, J. G., & Patrick, H. (2008). Self-determination theory as a fundamental theory of close relationships. *Canadian Psychology, 49*, 201–209. doi: 10.1037/a0012760.

La Guardia, J. G., Ryan, R. M., Couchman, C. E., & Deci, E. L. (2000). Within-person variation in security of attachment: A self-determination theory perspective on attachment, need fulfillment, and well-being. *Journal of Personality and Social Psychology, 79*, 367–384. doi: 10.1037/0022-3514.79.3.367.

Lavigne, G. L., Vallerand, R. J., & Crevier-Braud, L. (2011). The fundamental need to belong: On the distinction between growth and deficit-reduction orientations. *Personality and Social Psychology Bulletin, 37*, 1185–1201. doi: 10.1177/0146167211405995.

Lynch, M. F., La Guardia, J. G., & Ryan, R. M. (2009). On being yourself in different cultures: Ideal and actual self-concept, autonomy support, and well-being in China, Russia, and the United States. *Journal of Positive Psychology, 4*, 290–304. doi: 10.1080/17439760902933765.

McAdams, D. P. (1989). *Intimacy: The need to be close*. New York: Doubleday.

McClelland, D. C. (1985). *Human motivation*. Glenview, IL: Scott, Foresman.

McHoskey, J. W. (1999). Machiavellianism, intrinsic versus extrinsic goals, and social interest: A self-determination theory analysis. *Motivation and Emotion, 23*, 267–283. doi: 10.1023/A:1021338809469.

Moller, A. C., Roth, G., Niemiec, C. P., & Deci, E. L. (2014). *Perceiving, selecting, and projecting: The effects of parental conditional regard on the best-friend and romantic relationships of their children*. Unpublished manuscript, University of Rochester.

Murray, H. A. (1938). *Explorations in personality*. New York: Oxford University Press.

Niemiec, C. P., & Deci, E. L. (2014). *Contextual supports for autonomy and the development of high-quality relationships following mutual self-disclosure*. Unpublished manuscript, University of Rochester.

Niemiec, C. P., Lynch, M. F., Vansteenkiste, M., Bernstein, J., Deci, E. L., & Ryan, R. M. (2006). The antecedents and consequences of autonomous self-regulation for college: A self-determination theory perspective on socialization. *Journal of Adolescence, 29*, 761–775. doi: 10.1016/j.adolescence.2005.11.009.

Patrick, H., Knee, C. R., Canevello, A., & Lonsbary, C. (2007). The role of need fulfillment in relationship functioning and well-being: A self-determination theory perspective. *Journal of Personality and Social Psychology, 92*, 434–457. doi: 10.1037/0022-3514.92.3.434.

Reis, H. T. (2011). Perceived partner responsiveness as an organizing theme for the study of relationships and well-being. In L. Campbell & T. J. Loving (Eds.), *Close relationships: An interdisciplinary integration*. Washington, DC: APA Books.

Reis, H. T., Sheldon, K. M., Gable, S. L., Roscoe, J., & Ryan, R. M. (2000). Daily well-being: The role of autonomy, competence, and relatedness. *Personality and Social Psychology Bulletin, 26*, 419–435. doi: 10.1177/0146167200266002.

Roth, G., Assor, A., Niemiec, C. P., Ryan, R. M., & Deci, E. L. (2009). The emotional and academic consequences of parental conditional regard: Comparing conditional positive regard, conditional negative regard, and autonomy support as parenting practices. *Developmental Psychology, 45*, 1119–1142. doi: 10.1037/a0015272.

Ryan, R. M. (1982). Control and information in the intrapersonal sphere: An extension of cognitive evaluation theory. *Journal of Personality and Social Psychology, 43*, 450–461. doi: 10.1037/0022-3514.43.3.450.

Ryan, R. M. (1995). Psychological needs and the facilitation of integrative processes. *Journal of Personality, 63*, 397–427. doi: 10.1111/j.1467-6494.1995.tb00501.x.

Ryan, R. M., Bernstein, J. H., & Brown, K. W. (2010). Weekends, work, and wellbeing: Psychological need satisfactions and day of the week effects on mood, vitality, and physical symptoms. *Journal of Social and Clinical Psychology, 29*, 95–122. doi: 10.1521/jscp.2010.29.1.95.

Ryan, R. M., & Deci, E. L. (2000). Self-determination theory and the facilitation of intrinsic motivation, social development, and well-being. *American Psychologist, 55*, 68–78. doi: 10.1037/0003-066X.55.1.68.

Ryan, R. M., & Deci, E. L. (2008). Self-determination theory and the role of basic psychological needs in personality and the organization of behavior. In O. P. John, R. W. Robbins, & L. A. Pervin (Eds.), *Handbook of personality: Theory and research* (pp. 654–678). New York: Guilford.

Ryan, R. M., La Guardia, J. G., Solky-Butzel, J., Chirkov, V., & Kim, Y. (2005). On the interpersonal regulation of emotions: Emotional reliance across gender, relationships, and cultures. *Personal Relationships, 12*, 145–163. doi: 10.1111/j.1350-4126.2005.00106.x.

Ryan, R. M., Sheldon, K. M., Kasser, T., & Deci, E. L. (1996). All goals are not created equal: An organismic perspective on the nature of goals and their regulation. In P. M. Gollwitzer & J. A. Bargh (Eds.), *The psychology of action: Linking cognition and motivation to behavior* (pp. 7–26). New York: Guilford.

Shaver, P. R., & Mikulincer, M. (2011). Attachment Theory. In P. A. M. Van Lange, A. W. Kruglanski, & E. T. Higgins (Eds.), *Handbook of theories of social psychology* (Vol. 2, pp. 160–179). Thousand Oaks, CA: Sage.

Steinberg, L., & Silverberg, S. (1986). The vicissitudes of autonomy in adolescence. *Child Development, 57*, 841–851. doi: 10.2307/1130361.

Thibaut, J. W., & Kelley, H. H. (1959). *The social psychology of groups*. New York: Wiley.

Vansteenkiste, M., Simons, J., Lens, W., Sheldon, K. M., & Deci, E. L. (2004). Motivating learning, performance, and persistence: The synergistic effects of intrinsic goal contents and autonomy-supportive contexts. *Journal of Personality and Social Psychology, 87*, 246–260. doi: 10.1037/0022-3514.87.2.246.

Webster, D. M., & Kruglanski, A. W. (1994). Individual differences in need for cognitive closure. *Journal of Personality and Social Psychology, 67*, 1049–1062. doi: 10.1037/0022-3514.67.6.1049.

Weinstein, N., Hodgins, H. S., & Ryan, R. M. (2010). Autonomy and control in dyads: Effects on interaction quality and joint creative performance. *Personality and Social Psychology Bulletin, 36*, 1603–1617. doi: 10.1177/0146167210386385.

Weinstein, N., Law, W., & Ryan, R. M. (2012a). *When money matters, people don't: Wealth goals promote an instrumental orientation towards others*. Manuscript under review.

Weinstein, N., Przybylski, A. K., & Ryan, R. M. (2012b). The index of autonomous functioning: Development of a scale of human autonomy. *Journal of Research in Personality, 46*, 397–413.

Weinstein, N., & Ryan, R. M. (2010). When helping helps: Autonomous motivation for prosocial behavior and its influence on well-being for the helper and recipient. *Journal of Personality and Social Psychology, 98*, 222–244. doi: 10.1037/a0016984.
White, R. W. (1959). Motivation reconsidered: The concept of competence. *Psychological Review, 66*, 297–333. doi: 10.1037/h0040934.
Wild, T. C., Enzle, M. E., Nix, G., & Deci, E. L. (1997). Perceiving others as intrinsically or extrinsically motivated: Effects on expectancy formation and task engagement. *Personality and Social Psychology Bulletin, 23*, 837–848. doi: 10.1177/0146167297238005.
Williams, G. C., Cox, E. M., Hedberg, V., & Deci, E. L. (2000). Extrinsic life goals and health risk behaviors in adolescents. *Journal of Applied Social Psychology, 30*, 1756–1771. doi: 10.1111/j.1559-1816.2000.tb02466.x.
Winnicott, D. W. (1965). *The maturational process and the facilitating environment*. New York: International Universities Press.

Part II
Mechanisms and Outcomes of Motivation: The 'Dark Side' and 'Bright Side' of Relationships

Chapter 4
Is Relatedness Enough? On the Importance of Need Support in Different Types of Social Experiences

Christopher P. Niemiec, Bart Soenens, and Maarten Vansteenkiste

Self-determination theory (SDT; Deci & Ryan, 2000, 2008; Niemiec, Ryan, & Deci, 2010; Ryan & Deci, 2000; Vansteenkiste, Niemiec, & Soenens, 2010) is an empirical approach to human motivation, emotion, and personality in social contexts. As with other developmental (Bowlby, 1969), clinical (Maslow, 1968), and social (Baumeister & Leary, 1995) perspectives in psychology, SDT recognizes the central importance of interpersonal relationships in the human experience and is deeply interested in how social dynamics can influence individuals' thoughts, feelings, and behaviors (La Guardia & Patrick, 2008). Humans are social beings, and therefore it is important to consider whether the sense of relatedness that can be derived from interpersonal experiences is enough to facilitate personal wellness and healthy social functioning.

According to SDT, all individuals require satisfaction of three basic psychological needs for autonomy, competence, and relatedness. Thus, in response to the question that was posed in the title, this chapter reviews recent research on the importance of need support—and especially support for autonomy—in different types of social experiences. Indeed, the importance of need support will be examined in non-reciprocal relationships, which are characterized by a clear and defined differential in authority between dyad members; in reciprocal relationships, which are characterized by the lack of a clear and defined differential in authority between dyad members; and in brief interactions, which involve two previously unacquainted individuals who engage in a mutual activity for a small amount of time. As will be discussed below, SDT assumes a universal perspective on the importance and compatibility of autonomy, competence, and relatedness. As a result, support

C.P. Niemiec (✉)
Department of Clinical and Social Sciences in Psychology, University of Rochester, Rochester, NY, USA
e-mail: niemiec@psych.rochester.edu

B. Soenens • M. Vansteenkiste
Department of Developmental, Social, and Personality Psychology, Gent University, Ghent, Belgium

N. Weinstein (ed.), *Human Motivation and Interpersonal Relationships: Theory, Research, and Applications*, DOI 10.1007/978-94-017-8542-6_4,

for basic psychological need satisfaction can be expected to confer benefits for personal wellness and healthy social functioning across a variety of types of social experiences.

The Meta-theoretical Underpinnings of Self-Determination Theory

The philosophical starting point for SDT is its organismic-dialectic meta-theory (Deci & Vansteenkiste, 2004; Ryan & Deci, 2002), which posits a specific set of assumptions about the nature of human beings that is used to guide subsequent theorizing about how social contexts can affect the natural developmental processes that promote full functioning and organismic wellness (cf. Niemiec & Ryan, 2013). From this perspective, humans are proactive (rather than passive) organisms who are oriented toward integration at the intrapersonal (autonomy) and interpersonal (homonomy) levels (Angyal, 1965). Such an organismic perspective on human nature is found in other psychological traditions, including psychoanalytic (Freud, 1923/1960; Loevinger, 1976), humanistic (Rogers, 1963), and developmental (Piaget, 1971) theories, and is echoed by thinkers from a wide range of other academic disciplines (Goldstein, 1963; Gottlieb, 2003; Kauffman & Clayton, 2006). Yet SDT builds on these meta-theoretical views with its assertion that the natural developmental tendencies toward psychological growth and adaptation to the environment are supported by social contexts that afford opportunities for volition, mastery, and connection with others. It follows, then, that humans are vulnerable to passivity and control, incompetence, and alienation, particularly when social conditions do not support (or actively thwart) their inherent propensities toward development and synthesis. Hence, SDT assumes an organismic-dialectic perspective on the nature of human beings.

The Psychological Content of Human Nature: Autonomy, Competence, and Relatedness

This set of meta-theoretical considerations suggests that there is specific and identifiable psychological content to human nature, which contrasts with the standard social science model (Barkow, Cosmides, & Tooby, 1992) view that humans are born *tabula rasa* and thus may take multiple, idiosyncratic routes to attain wellness. From the perspective of SDT, all individuals require satisfaction of the basic psychological needs for autonomy, competence, and relatedness to function in a healthy, integrated way. These needs, which are defined as "innate psychological nutriments that are essential for ongoing psychological growth, integrity, and well-being" (Deci & Ryan, 2000, p. 229), specify the psychological content of human nature and are used within SDT to understand how personal experiences and social interactions affect psychological, social, and physical well-being. The need for autonomy (de Charms, 1968) refers to the experience of behavior as choiceful, owned, volitional, and self-endorsed at a high level of personal reflection. It is important to note that the opposite of autonomy is not dependence but rather is heteronomy (Ryan & Deci, 2006), or the experience of behavior as pressured and controlled. The need for competence (White, 1959) refers to the experience of behavior as effective when interacting with the physical and social environment. The need for relatedness (Baumeister & Leary, 1995; Ryan, 1995) refers to the experience of close, caring, and mutually supportive connections with others.

In line with its organismic-dialectic meta-theory, SDT assumes a universal perspective on the importance of satisfaction of the basic psychological needs. In other words, satisfaction of autonomy, competence, and relatedness is theorized to confer benefits for the health and well-being of all individuals, regardless of gender, age, culture, social status, or any other delimiting factor. Indeed, research supports this theoretical tenet. For instance, Ryan, La Guardia, Solky-Butzel, Chirkov, and Kim (2005) found that the relation of need satisfaction to a composite index of well-being (indicated by subjective vitality, life satisfaction, self-esteem, and the reverse of depressive symptoms and anxiety) was not moderated by gender, suggesting that satisfaction of autonomy, competence, and relatedness is equally beneficial for the psychological health of men and women. Need satisfaction has been shown to predict psychological and social functioning across the lifespan, including among adolescents (Curran, Hill, & Niemiec, 2013; Thøgersen-Ntoumani, Ntoumanis, & Nikitaras, 2010), young adults (Niemiec, Ryan, & Deci, 2009; Sheldon & Niemiec, 2006), and working adults (Van den Broeck, Vansteenkiste, De Witte, Soenens, & Lens, 2010; Vansteenkiste et al., 2007), as well as across cultures, including in Bulgaria (Deci et al., 2001) and China (Vansteenkiste, Lens, Soenens, & Luyckx, 2006). Finally, the relevance of need support for physical and psychological health has been shown even in a sample of primarily poor and working-class Americans (Niemiec, Ryan, Patrick, Deci, & Williams, 2010; Williams, Niemiec, Patrick, Ryan, & Deci, 2009).

The specification of basic psychological needs as universal requirements for wellness and optimal functioning follows directly from the organismic-dialectic meta-theory of SDT, and data have supported this claim in a variety of life domains and cultures (Deci & Ryan, 2008). Yet the idea that satisfaction of the basic psychological needs would facilitate psychological, social, and physical health among all individuals is not without critics. Such debates have tended to focus on the importance of autonomy (rather than competence or relatedness) across several demographic groups. Speaking from a perspective of cultural relativism, Markus and Kitayama (1991, 2003) have suggested that autonomy is a value that is prominent in Western (but not Eastern) cultures and thus have questioned its relevance for individuals from Eastern societies. Iyengar and DeVoe (2003) have made similar arguments. Speaking from a feminist perspective, Jordan (1997) has suggested that autonomy is primarily a male value and thus has questioned its importance for women. Stephens, Markus, and Townsend (2007) have suggested that choice and agency are considered to be important among individuals from higher socio-economic strata and thus have questioned their relevance to the lives of the working class. The common theme that underlies such criticisms is that autonomy is expected to have importance only for groups of individuals that espouse its value. Yet from the perspective of SDT, autonomy does not refer to a culture-, gender-, or class-specific value but rather reflects the inner endorsement of cognitive, affective, and behavioral experiences and expressions. Accordingly, satisfaction of autonomy (as well as competence and relatedness), regardless of whether it is valued, is expected to promote personal and interpersonal wellness across demographic groups.

Another debate has focused on the dynamics among the basic psychological needs rather than on their universal importance, and specifically has addressed the compatibility of autonomy and relatedness. Indeed, some scholars outside SDT have suggested that these experiences may be antagonistic rather than complementary. For instance, Peterson and Taylor (1980) argued that children's progression toward autonomy during adolescence requires that they sever ties with parents. More recently, and with a focus on romantic relationships, Murray et al. (2009) asserted that interdependence imposes inevitable costs on autonomy. Such criticisms of autonomy, which focus on its universal importance and compatibility with relatedness, may stem from the specific definition given to autonomy by scholars outside SDT. As an example, within the developmental literature some theorists (Blos, 1979; Levy-Warren, 1999) maintain that autonomy development involves both the emotional and physical detachment from parents and the assumption of more personal responsibility without reliance on parents. When defined as a process of separation and individuation, autonomy may be viewed as antagonistic to a sense of relatedness and, indeed, the aforementioned criticisms have conceptualized autonomy as independence and distinction from others. It is interesting to note, though, that both emotional separation and independence have been associated with lower levels of adolescent functioning (Beyers & Goossens, 1999; Lopez, Campbell, & Watkins, 1988; Ryan & Lynch, 1989). As well, Soenens et al. (2007) reported that parental promotion of independence is empirically distinguishable from promotion of volitional functioning, and only the latter conceptualization of autonomy (which is aligned with SDT) was shown to predict unique variance in adolescents' psychosocial functioning. Again, within SDT the concept of autonomy (versus heteronomy) refers to an experience of self-governance that is based on personally endorsed interests, values, and goals, and is a construct that is distinct from independence (versus dependence).

From the perspective of SDT, the basic psychological needs for autonomy, competence, and relatedness are evolved experiential nutriments that are complementary and necessary for healthy functioning and wellness, and data have supported this theoretical proposition. Using structural equation modeling, Niemiec et al. (2006) demonstrated that supports for autonomy and relatedness from mothers and fathers loaded onto common latent factors, thus underscoring the compatibility of these two needs. Moreover, need support from both parents was found to predict composite indexes of well-being (indicated by life satisfaction and positive affect) and ill-being (indicated by depressive symptoms and negative affect) in theoretically consistent ways. Further highlighting the complementary nature of autonomy and relatedness, Ryan, Stiller, and Lynch (1994) found that adolescents who had stronger connections with their parents reported higher levels of volition and well-being. Using a cluster-analytic approach, Soenens, Vansteenkiste, and Sierens (2009) reported that parents can support their children's volitional functioning in a way that is perceived as promoting either independence from or dependence on the parents. Indeed, ratings of self-esteem and depressive symptoms did not differ between children who belonged to the *volitional independence* cluster and those who belonged to the *volitional dependence* cluster. These results speak to the compatibility of autonomy and relatedness, as volitional dependence on parents did not have an adverse effect on children's well-being. Taken together, this set of findings stands in opposition to the suggestions of Peterson and Taylor (1980) and Murray et al. (2009) that the experience of autonomy is antagonistic to interdependence in close relationships and reliance on others.

It is interesting to note, as well, that the dynamic between these two needs is such that their satisfaction can be pitted against one another. To illustrate, parental conditional regard is a common socialization technique in which children must forgo satisfaction of autonomy in order to gain the attention, affection, and approval of their parent(s). The message that parents who use this strategy communicate to their children is, "I will love you more if you do as I say" and/or "I will love you less if you do not do as I say." Of course, the conditional nature of their support for relatedness is rarely communicated by parents in such explicit terms, yet children's perception of this need conflict has been shown to yield deleterious consequences for their self-regulation and well-being (Assor, Roth, & Deci, 2004; Roth, Assor, Niemiec, Ryan, & Deci, 2009). In sum, the needs for autonomy and relatedness appear to be complementary (Ryan & Powelson, 1991), yet their satisfaction can be placed into conflict by controlling social contexts. This underscores the importance of an experience of relatedness that is marked by an absence of pressure and coercion for the promotion of healthy relationships (Ryan, 1991).

The Tenets of Need Support: Autonomy, Competence, and Relatedness in a Social Context

So far, the focus of this chapter has been on the definition and compatibility of autonomy, competence, and relatedness. Indeed, for more than 40 years research conducted within SDT has shown that experiences of need satisfaction are at the very heart of what it means to live well and in accord with one's nature (Ryan & Deci, 2001; Ryan, Huta, & Deci, 2008). That being said, humans are social beings (Baumeister & Leary, 1995) and, as a result, need satisfaction often occurs in a social context. Accordingly, it is important to consider some specific ways in which others in the social surround can provide support for satisfaction of autonomy, competence, and relatedness. This integration of human motivation and interpersonal relationships, in turn, will provide a context for a review of research on the importance of need support in different types of social experiences.

Support for basic psychological need satisfaction begins with an authority figure (parent, teacher, manager, and so on) or peer (friend, romantic partner, colleague,

Table 4.1 Strategies that can be used to provide support for autonomy, competence, and relatedness

Support for autonomy	1. Elicit, acknowledge, and accept the person's thoughts and feelings 2. Explore values and how they relate to the situation being discussed 3. Encourage self-initiation and provide a desired amount of choice 4. Provide a meaningful rationale when limits are set and for other relevant requests 5. Minimize use of controlling language ("should", "must", "ought", and "have to")
Support for competence	1. Maintain a positive attitude toward success 2. Initiate a conversation to identify barriers to success 3. Create optimal challenges in a context of autonomy support 4. Assist the person with skills building and problem solving 5. Provide immediate, accurate, and effectance-relevant feedback 6. Provide structure through the communication of clear, consistent, and reasonable guidelines
Support for relatedness	1. Assume a warm, empathic, and non-judgmental stance toward the person 2. Provide a sense of unconditional positive regard 3. Communicate genuine care, interest, focus, and non-contingent support toward the person

and so on) who takes the perspective of another person. Table 4.1 provides a brief overview of several strategies that can be used to provide support for autonomy, competence, and relatedness. Consider the following two hypothetical individuals for the purpose of illustration. Marie is in her late-30s and is the mother of Juliette, a young girl who recently has been having difficulties at school.

Support for Autonomy

To provide support for her daughter's autonomy, Marie starts by eliciting and acknowledging Juliette's thoughts about her experiences at school. In doing so, it is important for Marie to interact with Juliette in a direct, respectful, and non-confrontational way. For instance, Marie may say, "There seems to be some difficulty at school. How do you see the situation?" At the same time, Marie takes interest in Juliette's feelings around her experiences at school. Indeed, it is important for Marie to remain non-judgmental toward and accepting of Juliette's emotions, regardless of their valence. Having a clear understanding of Juliette's point of view affords Marie an opportunity to begin to encourage active problem solving. Thus, one component of autonomy support is to elicit, acknowledge, and accept all of the person's thoughts and feelings on a particular matter.

Another component of autonomy support is to explore values and how they relate to the situation being discussed. Accordingly, Marie initiates a conversation about the types of goals or aspirations that Juliette considers to be personally important. This may involve a consideration of intrinsic values such as personal growth, meaningful affiliation, community involvement, and physical health, and extrinsic values such as wealth, popularity, power, and an appealing image (Kasser & Ryan, 1996; Ryan et al., 1999). In doing so, it is important that Juliette be encouraged to reflect on her values and to consider how what she does at school may help and/or hinder her attaining those goals. Interestingly, Niemiec, Ryan, Deci, and Williams (2009) demonstrated that a similar values exploration in the health care domain predicted maintenance of health-behavior change over 2 years.

Another set of strategies that can be used to support autonomy focuses on self-initiation and self-direction of behavior. With an understanding of Juliette's perspective, Marie begins to encourage self-initiation around how Juliette might address her difficulties at school, and is sure to provide a desired amount of choice. Some scholars outside SDT have questioned the utility of choice and self-determination, suggesting they may be demotivating (Iyengar & Lepper, 2000) or even tyrannical (Schwartz, 2000). In contrast to such views, Patall, Cooper, and Robinson (2008) conducted a meta-analysis on 42 studies and found that choice is associated with higher levels of intrinsic motivation, which is an exemplar of volitional functioning (Niemiec & Ryan, 2009). Of course, Marie may find it useful to establish limits around Juliette's school-related activities and, if so, then Marie is sure to provide a meaningful rationale for those limits and for other relevant requests. In support of this practice, Koestner, Ryan, Bernieri, and Holt (1984) demonstrated that children's intrinsic motivation is maintained when limits are set in an autonomy-supportive way. As well, Marie minimizes her use of controlling language ("should", "must", "ought", and "have to") while interacting with her daughter, as such language has been shown to undermine intrinsic motivation (Ryan, 1982; Ryan, Mims, & Koestner, 1983), depth of processing, performance, and persistence (Vansteenkiste, Simons, Lens, Sheldon, & Deci, 2004).

Support for Competence

To provide support for her daughter's competence, Marie starts with a positive attitude toward Juliette's success at school and initiates a conversation to identify barriers to success, which is particularly important given her recent difficulties at school. Another element of competence support is to create optimal challenges, or experiences that are interesting and require resourcefulness for successful completion (Deci & Ryan, 1985). A core feature of optimal challenges is that the experience is neither too easy nor too difficult, which is conceptually similar to the state of flow (Csikszentmihalyi, 1990) in which personal skills are matched to situational demands. It is interesting to note that such preference has been observed even among infants at 7 and 8 months of age, who were found to allocate attention selectively to visual sequences that are neither too simple nor too complex, but rather allow for an intermediate rate of information absorption (Kidd, Piantadosi, & Aslin, 2012). It is also important that optimal challenges are pursued in a context of autonomy support, as research has shown that children (Danner & Lonky, 1981) and adults (Shapira, 1976) naturally select activities that stretch their capacities but that contingent rewards undermine their preference for such challenges.

Marie also attempts to assist her daughter with skills building and problem solving, and gives Juliette immediate, accurate, and effectance-relevant feedback along the way. Past research has shown that positive verbal feedback is conducive to optimal experience (Deci, 1971) and that negative feedback is antithetical to such experiences (Vallerand & Reid, 1984). Indeed, support for competence is aligned with provision of structure, another important feature of need support that involves the communication of clear, consistent, and reasonable guidelines to others (Reeve, 2002). It is interesting to note, as well, that structure has been associated with satisfaction of all three needs (Taylor & Ntoumanis, 2007), and that the benefits of structure are amplified under conditions of autonomy support (Jang, Reeve, & Deci, 2010; Sierens, Vansteenkiste, Goossens, Soenens, & Dochy, 2009).

Support for Relatedness

To provide support for her daughter's relatedness, Marie is sure to assume a warm, empathic, and non-judgmental stance toward Juliette in their interactions. Marie also provides a sense of unconditional positive regard for her daughter (Rogers, 1957), especially when confronting additional setbacks and difficulties. Such an interpersonal style is antagonistic to parental conditional regard and has been shown to yield positive consequences for children's self-regulation, emotion regulation, and interest-focused engagement at school (Roth et al., 2009). Overall, then, support for relatedness involves a genuine communication of care, interest, focus, and non-contingent support toward another person (La Guardia & Patrick, 2008).

A Call for Additional Research

Most, if not all, of these strategies have received either direct or indirect validation from previous research within SDT. That being said, some of these strategies have received no empirical attention in the domain of interpersonal relationships. Thus, it is important for additional research to examine these strategies systematically in different types of social contexts and interpersonal experiences.

On the Importance of Need Support in Different Types of Social Experiences

From the perspective of SDT, social contexts and relational partners can either support or thwart satisfaction of the basic psychological needs. Attesting to the benefits of need support for social wellness, relationship-specific levels of need satisfaction have been systematically linked to within-person variations in attachment security

(La Guardia, Ryan, Couchman, & Deci, 2000) and emotional reliance (Ryan et al., 2005) across those relationships. Accordingly, it is important to consider the importance of need support across various types of social experiences, namely, in non-reciprocal relationships, in reciprocal relationships, and in brief interactions.

Evidence in Non-reciprocal Relationships

In non-reciprocal relationships, such as those that occur between parents and children, managers and employees, teachers and students, doctors and patients, coaches and athletes, or even God and believers (see Soenens et al., 2012), there is a clear and defined differential in authority between dyad members. Indeed, most of the research within SDT on the importance of need support has examined social interactions that involve an authority differential, and several of the chapters in this volume have addressed these dynamics. To avoid too much overlap, this brief review of evidence in non-reciprocal relationships focuses on the importance of need support in parent-child interactions.

Interactions between parents and children have a central role in the human experience (van IJzendoorn, 1995), and thus it is useful to consider the correlates of need support in this type of non-reciprocal relationship. In fact, the importance of parental support for satisfaction of children's basic psychological needs has been noted almost from the start of life, and has been observed in childhood, adolescence, and early adulthood. For instance, controlling vocalization from mothers has been shown to undermine the mastery motivation of infants at 12 months of age (Grolnick, Frodi, & Bridges, 1984) and at 20 months of age (Frodi, Bridges, & Grolnick, 1985), and has been shown to undermine the intrinsic motivation of children at 6 and 7 years of age (Deci, Driver, Hotchkiss, Robbins, & Wilson, 1993). Controlling parenting has been shown to be a risk factor for physical aggression among children in day care (Hart, Nelson, Robinson, Olsen, & McNeilly-Choque, 1998) and during childhood from 6 to 12 years of age (Joussemet et al., 2008). Such a parenting style is antithetical to need support (Soenens & Vansteenkiste, 2010) and, indeed, provision of autonomy support from parents has been associated with higher levels of executive functioning among infants at 18 months and at 26 months of age (Bernier, Carlson, & Whipple, 2010), as well as higher levels of self-regulation and adjustment among 8- to 12-year olds (Grolnick & Ryan, 1989). The results of these studies suggest that parental support for basic psychological need satisfaction is conducive to intrinsic motivation, executive functioning, self-regulation, and adjustment in infancy and throughout childhood.

Parental support for children's satisfaction of autonomy, competence, and relatedness has been shown to promote psychological well-being, physical health, and social functioning among adolescents and young adults as well. For instance, provision of autonomy support from parents has been associated with lower levels of alcohol use among adolescents (Wong, 2008), as well as higher levels of a composite index of well-being (indicated by life satisfaction, self-esteem, self-actualization, and the reverse of depressive symptoms) among adolescents from Russia and the United States (Chirkov & Ryan, 2001). This latter finding is particularly noteworthy in that the importance of autonomy support was equivalent across these two nations, even though Russian adolescents perceived lower levels of need support than their counterparts in the United States. Addressing the importance of parental need support for healthy social functioning among adolescents, Soenens, Vansteenkiste, and Niemiec (2009) proposed that parents can prohibit their children's affiliation with deviant peers either in an autonomy-supportive or in a controlling way. Indeed, results suggested that autonomy-supportive prohibition is associated with lower levels of deviant peer affiliation and involvement in problem behaviors, whereas controlling prohibition is associated with higher levels of deviant peer affiliation and involvement in problem behaviors. Among young adults, Kanat-Maymon and Assor (2010) found that perceived maternal control is associated with lower levels of empathic concern and empathic support, as well as higher levels of personal distress. Indeed, the adverse consequences of maternal control were amplified under conditions of maternal responsiveness to distress, which again underscores the importance of an experience of relatedness (represented by maternal responsiveness) that is marked by an absence of pressure and coercion (Ryan, 1991).

Another line of research that is relevant to SDT has examined the influence of parental psychological control on adolescents' psychosocial functioning. Psychological control involves the excessive use of parenting strategies that intrude upon the child's psychological experience (Barber & Harmon, 2002; Soenens & Vansteenkiste, 2010), including guilt induction, shaming, instilling anxiety, invalidation, and love withdrawal. Such manipulative tactics are theorized to thwart the child's natural developmental tendencies toward volitional functioning and wellness. Indeed, past research has shown that psychological control from parents is associated with lower levels of commitment making, identification with commitment (Luyckx, Soenens, Vansteenkiste, Goossens, & Berzonsky, 2007), and self-esteem (Soenens, Vansteenkiste, Luyten, Duriez, & Goossens, 2005), as well as higher levels of depressive symptoms (Soenens et al., 2005), eating disorder symptoms and maladaptive perfectionism (Soenens et al., 2008), and relational aggression and loneliness (Soenens, Vansteenkiste, Goossens, Duriez, & Niemiec, 2008). Together, the findings from these studies speak to the importance of parental need support for their children's psychological, physical, and social wellness.

Evidence in Reciprocal Relationships

In reciprocal (or peer) relationships, such as those that occur between close friends, romantic partners, colleagues, or classmates, there is no clear and defined differential in authority between dyad members. Rather, these types of relationships are more likely to involve a mutual sense of care, concern, and support. Although there is a paucity of research on the importance of support for basic psychological needs in reciprocal relationships, it is reasonable to posit a similar set of dynamics due to the universal importance of autonomy, competence, and relatedness for interpersonal wellness. In fact, two sets of studies have examined the correlates of need support and need satisfaction in peer relationships.

Deci, La Guardia, Moller, Scheiner, and Ryan (2006) conducted two studies to examine mutuality of need support in close friendships. In a first study, results suggested that the amount of need support received from a friend is associated with higher levels of basic psychological need satisfaction, emotional reliance, security of attachment, dyadic adjustment, and inclusion of the friend in the self. In a second study, results suggested that the benefits of need support extend to indexes of psychological health, including higher levels of self-esteem, vitality, positive affect, and perceived ability to express positive and negative affect, as well as lower levels of depressive symptoms, anxiety, and negative affect. Moreover, the amount of need support given to a friend predicted independent variance in need satisfaction, relationship quality, and psychological well-being after controlling for the amount of need support received from the friend. Indeed, a similar set of correlates was observed among male-male and female-female dyads, thus highlighting the importance of need support in close friendships.

Patrick, Knee, Canevello, and Lonsbary (2007) conducted three studies to examine the role of need satisfaction in romantic relationship functioning and psychological health. In a first study, results of a meta-analysis conducted on eight samples suggested that basic psychological need satisfaction in romantic relationships is associated with higher levels of personal and dyadic well-being. In a second study, results suggested that need satisfaction is associated with higher levels of satisfaction and commitment to the relationship, as well as lower levels of perceived conflict and defensive responding to conflict. Of course, individuals in close relationships often exert mutual influence on each other (Kelley & Thibaut, 1978). Bespeaking the interdependent influence of autonomy, competence, and relatedness in romantic relationships, one's own need satisfaction predicted higher levels of satisfaction, as well as lower levels of perceived conflict and defensive responding to conflict, in the partner as well. In a third study, participants were tracked for 10 days and completed a diary record after each disagreement that they had with their romantic partner during that time. In line with the previous findings, results suggested that need satisfaction is associated with higher levels of post-disagreement satisfaction and commitment to the relationship. Therefore, given that need satisfaction is likely to be experienced with relational partners who are need supportive (Deci et al., 2006; see Ryan, 1995), the results of these studies underscore the importance of need support in romantic relationships.

Evidence in Brief Interactions

Although the vicissitudes of need support are likely to be most salient and readily apparent among individuals in established relationships, it is reasonable to posit a similar set of dynamics between strangers at the beginning of a new interaction.

In fact, two sets of experiments have examined the effects of contextual support for need satisfaction on the interaction quality of previously unacquainted dyads.

Using several manipulations that previously have been shown to be autonomy supportive or controlling, Niemiec and Deci (2012) conducted a set of five experiments on the causal role of contextual support for autonomy in facilitating interaction quality between strangers. In each of the studies, one naïve participant and confederate (Experiments 1–4) or two naïve participants (Experiment 5) were told that the study examined how personality styles affect the development of closeness between strangers and then completed a task designed to generate self-disclosure (see Aron, Melinat, Aron, Vallone, & Bator, 1997). After spending 20 min responding to the closeness-generating questions, the two individuals were moved to separate rooms and the naïve participants completed a series of dependent measures that assessed their experiences during the self-disclosure task.

In Experiment 1, deprivation of autonomy was operationalized as receipt of a monetary reward for engagement in the self-disclosure task. Past research has demonstrated that contingent rewards undermine the experiences of autonomy (Houlfort, Koestner, Joussemet, Nantel-Vivier, & Lekes, 2002) and intrinsic motivation (Deci, Koestner, & Ryan, 1999) in children and adults, and that reminders of money prime a self-sufficient orientation (Vohs, Mead, & Goode, 2006). In line with hypotheses, participants in the reward condition reported lower levels of autonomy and relatedness, emotional reliance, relationship satisfaction, and positive affect (marginal) compared to those in the no-reward condition. In Experiment 2, provision of autonomy was operationalized as autonomy support for engagement in the self-disclosure task. Previous research has shown that elements of autonomy support such as choice, a meaningful rationale, and acknowledgement of feelings are conducive to the experience of autonomy (Deci, Eghrari, Patrick, & Leone, 1994; Zuckerman, Porac, Lathin, Smith, & Deci, 1978). Participants in the autonomy-support condition reported higher levels of autonomy, emotional reliance, relationship satisfaction, positive affect, and vitality (marginal) compared to those in the no-support condition.

In Experiment 3, deprivation of autonomy was operationalized as ego-involvement and objective self-awareness, as both have been shown to undermine intrinsic motivation (Plant & Ryan, 1985; Ryan, 1982). Also, a behavioral measure of closeness was collected in this study, which was operationalized as the amount of distance that participants placed between two chairs for a presumed final interaction with the confederate (see Vohs et al., 2006). In parallel with the findings from the previous experiments, participants in the ego-involvement condition reported lower levels of autonomy and relatedness, emotional reliance, relationship satisfaction, positive affect, and vitality, as well as higher levels of negative affect, compared to those in the task-involvement condition. It is interesting to note that those in the ego-involvement condition put more distance between their chairs for a presumed final interaction. In Experiment 4, deprivation of autonomy was again operationalized as receipt of a monetary reward for engagement in the self-disclosure task, and results were comparable to those of Experiment 1. As well, data that assessed confederates' experiences during the self-disclosure task were collected to determine whether the adverse effect of contingent rewards would radiate to the confederates, even though they were kept blind to experimental condition. Confederates who interacted with participants in the reward condition reported lower levels of autonomy and relatedness, relationship satisfaction, positive affect, and vitality.

In Experiment 5, dyads that consisted of two naïve participants completed a scrambled sentence task (Hodgins, Brown, & Carver, 2007) intended to prime an autonomy orientation, a controlled orientation, or a neutral orientation. Past research has suggested that the autonomy orientation is associated with more positive social experiences (Hodgins, Koestner, & Duncan, 1996). Aligned with the results of the previous experiments, autonomy-primed dyads reported higher levels autonomy and relatedness, emotional reliance, relationship satisfaction, positive affect, and vitality compared to neutral-primed dyads. As well, autonomy-primed dyads put less distance between their chairs for a presumed final interaction (the contrast between autonomy- and control-primed dyads was not tested, although the means and standard deviations for control-primed dyads were similar to the descriptive statistics for neutral-primed dyads). Taken together, the results of these experiments underscore the importance of social contexts that afford choice and minimize control for an experience of interaction quality in new, brief encounters.

Weinstein, Hodgins, and Ryan (2010) conducted two experiments to examine the causal role of primed motivation orientations on interaction quality and joint creative task performance. In a first study, previously unacquainted dyads received either an autonomy orientation prime, a controlled orientation prime, or an orientation-free neutral prime. Dyad members then completed the Remote Associates Task, a task that requires verbal creativity for success. Results suggested that autonomy-primed dyads reported higher levels of closeness, empathy, and positive affect, as well as lower levels of negative affect, compared to neutral-primed dyads. The autonomy-primed dyads also reported higher levels of engagement in the task and actually solved more problems correctly than the neutral-primed dyads. Control-primed dyads showed the opposite pattern. In a second study, previously unacquainted dyads received either an autonomy orientation prime or a controlled orientation prime, and then completed the Remote Associates Task and played a game of charades, which requires non-verbal creativity for success. Results suggested that autonomy-primed dyads exhibited higher levels of observer-coded closeness behavior, encouragement, and engagement. The autonomy-primed dyads also reported higher levels of emotional and cognitive attunement, empathy, and positive affect, as well as lower levels of negative affect, and showed a higher level of performance on each task. Together, the findings from these experiments suggest that contextual support for need satisfaction is conducive both to interaction quality and to task performance in novel interactions.

Concluding Remarks

The concept of basic psychological needs is a unifying principle within SDT. Autonomy, competence, and relatedness specify the psychological content of human nature and can be used to understand how personal experiences and social interactions affect the natural developmental processes that promote full functioning and organismic wellness. The purpose of this review was to highlight recent research on the importance of support for basic psychological needs across a variety of types of social experiences. Such evidence was noted in non-reciprocal relationships, in reciprocal relationships, and in brief interactions, which underscores the universal importance of need support for the promotion of psychological, physical, and social wellness.

This prompts the question of why socializers and other relational partners may, at times, be controlling, especially in light of the adverse consequences of such an interpersonal style. Of course, some endorse attitudes toward controlling others' behavior (Grolnick, Benjet, Kurowski, & Apostoleris, 1997), and these types of attitudes can be transmitted intergenerationally (Assor et al., 2004). Yet it is also important to note that experiences of pressure can induce controlling attitudes and behaviors in socializers and other relational partners, as Grolnick (2003) suggested that need support requires adequate time and psychological resources. For instance, Grolnick, Gurland, DeCourcey, and Jacob (2002) found that mothers in an ego-involving condition, which is marked by a high level of pressure, were more controlling toward their children and, in fact, their children were shown to be less creative on an experimental task.

As an alternative to a controlling style, socializers and other relational partners may adopt an attitude of trust in organismic development (Landry et al., 2008), which is marked by a belief that the natural developmental tendencies toward integration and adaptation to the environment will operate most effectively in the absence of pressure and coercion. Indeed, Landry et al. found that mothers who report higher levels of trust make fewer social comparisons about their children and have more relaxed expectations for developmental milestones. As well, these mothers were observed to be more autonomy supportive of their 1-year old child, as indicated by higher levels of flexibility, perspective taking, and following the infant's pace. Such trust was associated with fewer behavior problems over time. It would be quite interesting for future research to examine the correlates of trust in organismic development in other interpersonal domains, such as work, education, romantic relationships, health care, and athletics.

Is relatedness enough? In other words, is the sense of relatedness that can be derived from interpersonal experiences enough to facilitate personal wellness and healthy social functioning? As made clear within this review, the importance of need support—and especially support for autonomy—for the promotion of intrapersonal and interpersonal well-being is quite apparent.

References

Angyal, A. (1965). *Neurosis and treatment: A holistic theory*. New York: Wiley.

Aron, A., Melinat, E., Aron, E. N., Vallone, R. D., & Bator, R. J. (1997). The experimental generation of interpersonal closeness: A procedure and some preliminary findings. *Personality and Social Psychology Bulletin, 23*, 363–377.

Assor, A., Roth, G., & Deci, E. L. (2004). The emotional costs of parents' conditional regard: A self-determination theory analysis. *Journal of Personality, 72*, 47–88.

Barber, B. K., & Harmon, E. L. (2002). Violating the self: Parental psychological control of children and adolescents. In B. K. Barber (Ed.), *Intrusive parenting: How psychological control affects children and adolescents* (pp. 15–52). Washington, DC: APA.

Barkow, J. H., Cosmides, L., & Tooby, J. (1992). *The adapted mind: Evolutionary psychology and the generation of culture*. New York: Oxford University Press.

Baumeister, R. F., & Leary, M. R. (1995). The need to belong: Desire for interpersonal attachments as a fundamental human motivation. *Psychological Bulletin, 117*, 497–529.

Bernier, A., Carlson, S. M., & Whipple, N. (2010). From external regulation to self-regulation: Early parenting precursors of young children's executive functioning. *Child Development, 81*, 326–339.

Beyers, W., & Goossens, L. (1999). Emotional autonomy, psychosocial adjustment, and parenting: Interactions, moderating and mediating effects. *Journal of Adolescence, 22*, 753–769.

Blos, P. (1979). *The adolescent passage*. Madison, CT: International Universities Press.

Bowlby, J. (1969). *Attachment and loss: Vol. 1. Attachment*. New York: Basic Books.

Chirkov, V. I., & Ryan, R. M. (2001). Parent and teacher autonomy-support in Russian and U.S. adolescents: Common effects on well-being and academic motivation. *Journal of Cross Cultural Psychology, 32*, 618–635.

Csikszentmihalyi, M. (1990). *Flow: The psychology of optimal experience*. New York: HarperCollins Publishers.

Curran, T., Hill, A. P., & Niemiec, C. P. (2013). A conditional process model of children's behavioural engagement and behavioural disaffection in sport based on self-determination theory. *Journal of Sport & Exercise Psychology, 35*, 30–43.

Danner, F. W., & Lonky, E. (1981). A cognitive-developmental approach to the effects of rewards on intrinsic motivation. *Child Development, 52*, 1043–1052.

de Charms, R. (1968). *Personal causation*. New York: Academic.

Deci, E. L. (1971). Effects of externally mediated rewards on intrinsic motivation. *Journal of Personality and Social Psychology, 18*, 105–115.

Deci, E. L., Driver, R. E., Hotchkiss, L., Robbins, R. J., & Wilson, I. M. (1993). The relation of mothers' controlling vocalizations to children's intrinsic motivation. *Journal of Experimental Child Psychology, 55*, 151–162.

Deci, E. L., Eghrari, H., Patrick, B. C., & Leone, D. R. (1994). Facilitating internalization: The self-determination theory perspective. *Journal of Personality, 62*, 119–142.

Deci, E. L., Koestner, R., & Ryan, R. M. (1999). A meta-analytic review of experiments examining the effects of extrinsic rewards on intrinsic motivation. *Psychological Bulletin, 125*, 627–668.

Deci, E. L., La Guardia, J. G., Moller, A. C., Scheiner, M. J., & Ryan, R. M. (2006). On the benefits of giving as well as receiving autonomy support: Mutuality in close friendships. *Personality and Social Psychology Bulletin, 32*, 313–327.

Deci, E. L., & Ryan, R. M. (1985). *Intrinsic motivation and self-determination in human behavior*. New York: Plenum.

Deci, E. L., & Ryan, R. M. (2000). The "what" and "why" of goal pursuits: Human needs and the self-determination of behavior. *Psychological Inquiry, 11*, 227–268.

Deci, E. L., & Ryan, R. M. (2008). Facilitating optimal motivation and psychological well-being across life's domains. *Canadian Psychology, 49*, 14–23.

Deci, E. L., Ryan, R. M., Gagné, M., Leone, D. R., Usunov, J., & Kornazheva, B. P. (2001). Need satisfaction, motivation, and well-being in the work organizations of a former Eastern Bloc country. *Personality and Social Psychology Bulletin, 27*, 930–942.

Deci, E. L., & Vansteenkiste, M. (2004). Self-determination theory and basic need satisfaction: Understanding human development in positive psychology. *Ricerche di Psicologia, 27*, 23–40.

Freud, S. (1960). *The ego and the id*. New York: Norton. (Original work published 1923).

Frodi, A., Bridges, L., & Grolnick, W. S. (1985). Correlates of mastery-related behavior: A short-term longitudinal study of infants in their second year. *Child Development, 56*, 1291–1298.

Goldstein, K. (1963). *The organism*. Boston: Beacon.

Gottlieb, G. (2003). Probabilistic epigenesis of development. In J. Valsiner & K. J. Connolly (Eds.), *Handbook of developmental psychology* (pp. 3–17). London: Sage.

Grolnick, W. S. (2003). *The psychology of parental control: How well-meant parenting backfires*. Mahwah, NJ: Erlbaum.

Grolnick, W. S., Benjet, C., Kurowski, C. O., & Apostoleris, N. H. (1997). Predictors of parent involvement in children's schooling. *Journal of Education and Psychology, 89*, 538–548.

Grolnick, W., Frodi, A., & Bridges, L. (1984). Maternal control styles and the mastery motivation of one-year-olds. *Infant Mental Health Journal, 5*, 72–82.

Grolnick, W. S., Gurland, S. T., DeCourcey, W., & Jacob, K. (2002). Antecedents and consequences of mothers' autonomy support: An experimental investigation. *Developmental Psychology, 38*, 143–155.

Grolnick, W. S., & Ryan, R. M. (1989). Parent styles associated with children's self-regulation and competence in school. *Journal of Education and Psychology, 81*, 143–154.

Hart, C. H., Nelson, D. A., Robinson, C. C., Olsen, S. F., & McNeilly-Choque, M. K. (1998). Overt and relational aggression in Russian nursery-school-age children: Parenting style and marital linkages. *Developmental Psychology, 34*, 687–697.

Hodgins, H. S., Brown, A. B., & Carver, B. (2007). Autonomy and control motivation and self-esteem. *Self and Identity, 6*, 189–208.

Hodgins, H. S., Koestner, R., & Duncan, N. (1996). On the compatibility of autonomy and relatedness. *Personality and Social Psychology Bulletin, 22*, 227–237.

Houlfort, N., Koestner, R., Joussemet, M., Nantel-Vivier, A., & Lekes, N. (2002). The impact of performance-contingent rewards on perceived autonomy and competence. *Motivation and Emotion, 26*, 279–295.

Iyengar, S. S., & DeVoe, S. E. (2003). Rethinking the value of choice: Considering cultural mediators of intrinsic motivation. In V. Murphy-Berman & J. J. Berman (Eds.), *Nebraska symposium on motivation: Cross-cultural differences in perspectives on self* (Vol. 49, pp. 129–174). Lincoln, NE: University of Nebraska Press.

Iyengar, S. S., & Lepper, M. R. (2000). When choice is demotivating: Can one desire too much of a good thing? *Journal of Personality and Social Psychology, 79*, 995–1006.

Jang, H., Reeve, J., & Deci, E. L. (2010). Engaging students in learning activities: It is not autonomy support or structure but autonomy support and structure. *Journal of Education and Psychology, 102*, 588–600.

Jordan, J. V. (1997). Do you believe that the concepts of self and autonomy are useful in understanding women? In J. V. Jordan (Ed.), *Women's growth in diversity: More writings from the Stone Center* (pp. 29–32). New York: The Guilford Press.

Joussemet, M., Vitaro, F., Barker, E. D., Côté, S., Nagin, D. S., Zoccolillo, M., et al. (2008). Controlling parenting and physical aggression during elementary school. *Child Development, 79*, 411–425.

Kanat-Maymon, M., & Assor, A. (2010). Perceived maternal control and responsiveness to distress as predictors of young adults' empathic responses. *Personality and Social Psychology Bulletin, 36*, 33–46.

Kasser, T., & Ryan, R. M. (1996). Further examining the American dream: Differential correlates of intrinsic and extrinsic goals. *Personality and Social Psychology Bulletin, 22*, 280–287.

Kauffman, S., & Clayton, P. (2006). On emergence, agency, and organization. *Biology and Philosophy, 21*, 501–521.

Kelley, H. H., & Thibaut, J. W. (1978). *Interpersonal relations: A theory of interdependence*. New York: Wiley.

Kidd, C., Piantadosi, S. T., & Aslin, R. N. (2012). The goldilocks effect: Human infants allocate attention to visual sequences that are neither too simple nor too complex. *PLoS ONE, 7*, e36399.

Koestner, R., Ryan, R. M., Bernieri, F., & Holt, K. (1984). Setting limits on children's behavior: The differential effects of controlling versus informational styles on children's intrinsic motivation and creativity. *Journal of Personality, 54*, 233–248.

La Guardia, J. G., & Patrick, H. (2008). Self-determination theory as a fundamental theory of close relationships. *Canadian Psychology, 49*, 201–209.

La Guardia, J. G., Ryan, R. M., Couchman, C. E., & Deci, E. L. (2000). Within-person variation in security of attachment: A self-determination theory perspective on attachment, need fulfillment, and well-being. *Journal of Personality and Social Psychology, 79*, 367–384.

Landry, R., Whipple, N., Mageau, G., Joussemet, M., Koestner, R., DiDio, L., et al. (2008). Trust in organismic development, autonomy support, and adaptation among mothers and their children. *Motivation and Emotion, 32*, 173–188.

Levy-Warren, M. H. (1999). I am, you are, and so are we: A current perspective on adolescent separation-individuation theory. In A. Esham, L. T. Flaherty, & H. A. Horowitz (Eds.), *Adolescent psychiatry: Vol. 24. Developmental and clinical studies* (pp. 3–24). Hillsdale, NJ: Analytic Press.

Loevinger, J. (1976). *Ego development*. San Francisco: Jossey-Bass.

Lopez, F. G., Campbell, V. L., & Watkins, C. E. (1988). Family structure, psychological separation, and college adjustment: A canonical analysis and cross-validation. *Journal of Counseling Psychology, 35*, 402–409.

Luyckx, K., Soenens, B., Vansteenkiste, M., Goossens, L., & Berzonsky, M. D. (2007). Parental psychological control and dimensions of identity formation in emerging adulthood. *Journal of Family Psychology, 21*, 546–550.

Markus, H. R., & Kitayama, S. (1991). Culture and the self: Implications for cognition, emotion, and motivation. *Psychological Review, 92*, 224–253.

Markus, H. R., & Kitayama, S. K. (2003). Models of agency: Sociocultural diversity in the construction of action. In V. Murphy-Berman & J. J. Berman (Eds.), *Nebraska symposium on motivation: Cross-cultural differences in perspectives on self* (Vol. 49, pp. 1–57). Lincoln, NE: University of Nebraska Press.

Maslow, A. H. (1968). *Toward a psychology of being*. New York: Van Nostrand.

Murray, S. L., Holmes, J. G., Aloni, M., Pinkus, R. T., Derrick, J. L., & Leder, S. (2009). Commitment insurance: Compensating for the autonomy costs of interdependence in close relationships. *Journal of Personality and Social Psychology, 97*, 256–278.

Niemiec, C. P., & Deci, E. L. (2012). *The effects of provision and deprivation of autonomy on interaction quality between strangers*. Unpublished manuscript, University of Rochester, Rochester, NY.

Niemiec, C. P., Lynch, M. F., Vansteenkiste, M., Bernstein, J., Deci, E. L., & Ryan, R. M. (2006). The antecedents and consequences of autonomous self-regulation for college: A self-determination theory perspective on socialization. *Journal of Adolescence, 29*, 761–775.

Niemiec, C. P., & Ryan, R. M. (2009). Autonomy, competence, and relatedness in the classroom: Applying self-determination theory to educational practice. *Theory and Research in Education, 7*, 133–144.

Niemiec, C. P., & Ryan, R. M. (2013). What makes for a life well lived? Autonomy and its relation to full functioning and organismic wellness. In S. A. David, I. Boniwell, & A. C. Ayers (Eds.), *The oxford handbook of happiness* (pp. 214–226). Oxford, UK: Oxford University Press.

Niemiec, C. P., Ryan, R. M., & Deci, E. L. (2009). The path taken: Consequences of attaining intrinsic and extrinsic aspirations in post-college life. *Journal of Research in Personality, 43*, 291–306.

Niemiec, C. P., Ryan, R. M., & Deci, E. L. (2010). Self-determination theory and the relation of autonomy to self-regulatory processes and personality development. In R. H. Hoyle (Ed.), *Handbook of personality and self-regulation* (pp. 169–191). Malden, MA: Blackwell Publishing.

Niemiec, C. P., Ryan, R. M., Deci, E. L., & Williams, G. C. (2009). Aspiring to physical health: The role of aspirations for physical health in facilitating long-term tobacco abstinence. *Patient Education and Counseling, 74*, 250–257.

Niemiec, C. P., Ryan, R. M., Patrick, H., Deci, E. L., & Williams, G. C. (2010). The energization of health-behavior change: Examining the associations among autonomous self-regulation, subjective vitality, depressive symptoms, and tobacco abstinence. *The Journal of Positive Psychology, 5*, 122–138.

Patall, E. A., Cooper, H., & Robinson, C. (2008). The effects of choice on intrinsic motivation and related outcomes: A meta-analysis of research findings. *Psychological Bulletin, 134*, 270–300.

Patrick, H., Knee, C. R., Canevello, A., & Lonsbary, C. (2007). The role of need fulfillment in relationship functioning and well-being: A self-determination theory perspective. *Journal of Personality and Social Psychology, 92*, 434–457.

Peterson, A. C., & Taylor, B. (1980). The biological approach to adolescence: Biological change and psychological adaptation. In J. Adelson (Ed.), *Handbook of adolescent psychology* (pp. 117–155). New York: Wiley.

Piaget, J. (1971). *Biology and knowledge*. Chicago: University of Chicago Press.

Plant, R. W., & Ryan, R. M. (1985). Intrinsic motivation and the effects of self-consciousness, self-awareness, and ego-involvement: An investigation of internally controlling styles. *Journal of Personality, 53*, 435–449.

Reeve, J. (2002). Self-determination theory applied to educational settings. In E. L. Deci & R. M. Ryan (Eds.), *Handbook of self-determination research* (pp. 183–203). Rochester, NY: University of Rochester Press.

Rogers, C. R. (1957). The necessary and sufficient conditions of therapeutic personality change. *Journal of Consulting Psychology, 21*, 95–103.

Rogers, C. R. (1963). The actualizing tendency in relation to "motives" and to consciousness. In M. R. Jones (Ed.), *Nebraska symposium on motivation* (Vol. 11, pp. 1–24). Lincoln, NE: University of Nebraska Press.

Roth, G., Assor, A., Niemiec, C. P., Ryan, R. M., & Deci, E. L. (2009). The emotional and academic consequences of parental conditional regard: Comparing conditional positive regard, conditional negative regard, and autonomy support as parenting practices. *Developmental Psychology, 45*, 1119–1142.

Ryan, R. M. (1982). Control and information in the intrapersonal sphere: An extension of cognitive evaluation theory. *Journal of Personality and Social Psychology, 43*, 450–461.

Ryan, R. M. (1991). The nature of the self in autonomy and relatedness. In J. Strauss & G. R. Goethals (Eds.), *The self: Interdisciplinary approaches* (pp. 208–238). New York: Springer.

Ryan, R. M. (1995). Psychological needs and the facilitation of integrative processes. *Journal of Personality, 63*, 397–427.

Ryan, R. M., Chirkov, V. I., Little, T. D., Sheldon, K. M., Timoshina, E., & Deci, E. L. (1999). The American dream in Russia: Extrinsic aspirations and well-being in two cultures. *Personality and Social Psychology Bulletin, 25*, 1509–1524.

Ryan, R. M., & Deci, E. L. (2000). Self-determination theory and the facilitation of intrinsic motivation, social development, and well-being. *American Psychologist, 55*, 68–78.

Ryan, R. M., & Deci, E. L. (2001). On happiness and human potentials: A review of research on hedonic and eudaimonic well-being. In S. T. Fiske, D. L. Schacter, & C. Zahn-Waxler (Eds.), *Annual review of psychology* (Vol. 52, pp. 141–166). Palo Alto, CA: Annual Reviews, Inc.

Ryan, R. M., & Deci, E. L. (2002). Overview of self-determination theory: An organismic dialectical perspective. In E. L. Deci & R. M. Ryan (Eds.), *Handbook of self-determination research* (pp. 3–33). Rochester, NY: University of Rochester Press.

Ryan, R. M., & Deci, E. L. (2006). Self-regulation and the problem of human autonomy: Does psychology need choice, self-determination, and will? *Journal of Personality, 74*, 1557–1585.

Ryan, R. M., Huta, V., & Deci, E. L. (2008). Living well: A self-determination theory perspective on eudaimonia. *Journal of Happiness Studies, 9*, 139–170.

Ryan, R. M., La Guardia, J. G., Solky-Butzel, J., Chirkov, V., & Kim, Y. (2005). On the interpersonal regulation of emotions: Emotional reliance across gender, relationships, and cultures. *Personal Relationships, 12*, 145–163.

Ryan, R. M., & Lynch, J. H. (1989). Emotional autonomy versus detachment: Revisiting the vicissitudes of adolescence and young adulthood. *Child Development, 60*, 340–356.

Ryan, R. M., Mims, V., & Koestner, R. (1983). Relation of reward contingency and interpersonal context to intrinsic motivation: A review and test using cognitive evaluation theory. *Journal of Personality and Social Psychology, 45*, 736–750.

Ryan, R. M., & Powelson, C. L. (1991). Autonomy and relatedness as fundamental to motivation and education. *The Journal of Experimental Education, 60*, 49–66.
Ryan, R. M., Stiller, J., & Lynch, J. H. (1994). Representations of relationships to teachers, parents, and friends as predictors of academic motivation and self-esteem. *Journal of Early Adolescence, 14*, 226–249.
Schwartz, B. (2000). Self-determination: The tyranny of freedom. *American Psychologist, 55*, 79–88.
Shapira, Z. (1976). Expectancy determinants of intrinsically motivated behavior. *Journal of Personality and Social Psychology, 34*, 1235–1244.
Sheldon, K. M., & Niemiec, C. P. (2006). It's not just the amount that counts: Balanced need satisfaction also affects well-being. *Journal of Personality and Social Psychology, 91*, 331–341.
Sierens, E., Vansteenkiste, M., Goossens, L., Soenens, B., & Dochy, F. (2009). The synergistic relationship of perceived autonomy support and structure in the prediction of self-regulated learning. *British Journal of Educational Psychology, 79*, 57–68.
Soenens, B., Neyrinck, B., Vansteenkiste, M., Dezutter, J., Hutsebaut, D., & Duriez, B. (2012). How do perceptions of God as autonomy supportive or controlling relate to individuals' social-cognitive processing of religious contents? The role of motives for religious behavior. *The International Journal for the Psychology of Religion, 22*, 10–30.
Soenens, B., & Vansteenkiste, M. (2010). A theoretical upgrade on the concept of parental psychological control: Proposing new insights on the basis of self-determination theory. *Developmental Review, 30*, 74–99.
Soenens, B., Vansteenkiste, M., Goossens, L., Duriez, B., & Niemiec, C. P. (2008). The intervening role of relational aggression between psychological control and friendship quality. *Social Development, 17*, 661–681.
Soenens, B., Vansteenkiste, M., Lens, W., Luyckx, K., Goossens, L., Beyers, W., et al. (2007). Conceptualizing parental autonomy support: Adolescent perceptions of promotion of independence versus promotion of volitional functioning. *Developmental Psychology, 43*, 633–646.
Soenens, B., Vansteenkiste, M., Luyten, P., Duriez, B., & Goossens, L. (2005). Maladaptive perfectionistic self-representations: The mediational link between psychological control and adjustment. *Personality and Individual Differences, 38*, 487–498.
Soenens, B., Vansteenkiste, M., & Niemiec, C. P. (2009). Should parental prohibition of adolescents' peer relationships be prohibited? *Personal Relationships, 16*, 507–530.
Soenens, B., Vansteenkiste, M., & Sierens, E. (2009). How are parental psychological control and autonomy-support related? A cluster-analytic approach. *Journal of Marriage and Family, 71*, 187–202.
Soenens, B., Vansteenkiste, M., Vandereycken, W., Luyten, P., Sierens, E., & Goossens, L. (2008). Perceived parental psychological control and eating-disordered symptoms: Maladaptive perfectionism as a possible intervening variable. *Journal of Nervous and Mental Disease, 196*, 144–152.
Stephens, N. M., Markus, H. R., & Townsend, S. S. M. (2007). Choice as an act of meaning: The case of social class. *Journal of Personality and Social Psychology, 93*, 814–830.
Taylor, I. M., & Ntoumanis, N. (2007). Teacher motivational strategies and student self-determination in physical education. *Journal of Education and Psychology, 99*, 747–760.
Thøgersen-Ntoumani, C., Ntoumanis, N., & Nikitaras, N. (2010). Unhealthy weight control behaviours in adolescent girls: A process model based on self-determination theory. *Psychology and Health, 25*, 535–550.
Vallerand, R. J., & Reid, G. (1984). On the causal effects of perceived competence on intrinsic motivation: A test of cognitive evaluation theory. *Journal of Sport Psychology, 6*, 94–102.
Van den Broeck, A., Vansteenkiste, M., De Witte, H., Soenens, B., & Lens, W. (2010). Capturing autonomy, competence, and relatedness at work: Construction and initial validation of the Work-related Basic Need Satisfaction scale. *Journal of Occupational and Organizational Psychology, 83*, 981–1002.
van IJzendoorn, M. (1995). Adult attachment representations, parental responsiveness, and infant attachment: A meta-analysis on the predictive validity of the Adult Attachment Interview. *Psychological Bulletin, 117*, 387–403.

Vansteenkiste, M., Lens, W., Soenens, B., & Luyckx, K. (2006). Autonomy and relatedness among Chinese sojourners and applicants: Conflictual or independent predictors of well-being and adjustment? *Motivation and Emotion, 30*, 273–282.

Vansteenkiste, M., Neyrinck, B., Niemiec, C. P., Soenens, B., de Witte, H., & Van den Broeck, A. (2007). On the relations among work value orientations, psychological need satisfaction and job outcomes: A self-determination theory approach. *Journal of Occupational and Organizational Psychology, 80*, 251–277.

Vansteenkiste, M., Niemiec, C. P., & Soenens, B. (2010). The development of the five mini-theories of self-determination theory: An historical overview, emerging trends, and future directions. In T. C. Urdan & S. A. Karabenick (Eds.), *Advances in motivation and achievement, v. 16A—The decade ahead: Theoretical perspectives on motivation and achievement* (pp. 105–165). London: Emerald Group Publishing Limited.

Vansteenkiste, M., Simons, J., Lens, W., Sheldon, K. M., & Deci, E. L. (2004). Motivating learning, performance, and persistence: The synergistic effects of intrinsic goal contents and autonomy-supportive contexts. *Journal of Personality and Social Psychology, 87*, 246–260.

Vohs, K. D., Mead, N. L., & Goode, M. R. (2006). The psychological consequences of money. *Science, 314*, 1154–1156.

Weinstein, N., Hodgins, H. S., & Ryan, R. M. (2010). Autonomy and control in dyads: Effects on interaction quality and joint creative performance. *Personality and Social Psychology Bulletin, 36*, 1603–1617.

White, R. W. (1959). Motivation reconsidered: The concept of competence. *Psychological Review, 66*, 297–333.

Williams, G. C., Niemiec, C. P., Patrick, H., Ryan, R. M., & Deci, E. L. (2009). The importance of supporting autonomy and perceived competence in facilitating long-term tobacco abstinence. *Annals of Behavioral Medicine, 37*, 315–324.

Wong, M. M. (2008). Perceptions of parental involvement and autonomy support: Their relations with self-regulation, substance use and resilience among adolescents. *North American Journal of Psychology, 10*, 497–518.

Zuckerman, M., Porac, J. F., Lathin, D., Smith, R., & Deci, E. L. (1978). On the importance of self-determination for intrinsically motivated behavior. *Personality and Social Psychology Bulletin, 4*, 443–446.

Chapter 5
On the Flexibility of the Automatic Us-Them Divide

Jen-Ho Chang, Holley S. Hodgins, Yi-Cheng Lin, and Chin-Lan Huang

Henri Tajfel (1982; Tajfel & Turner, 1979) proposed that humans readily divide the social world into "us" and "them", and quickly associate 'us' with 'good' and 'them' with 'bad'. This constructed psychological distance between self and others often is referred to as the "us-them divide". There is much evidence that humans do indeed divide the social world into "us" and "them". For example, individuals use categorization rules to make distinctions between self and others, individuals and groups, and 'us' and 'them' (Brewer, 1991; Tajfel, 1982; Turner, Oakes, Haslam, & McGarty, 1994).

Tajfel predicted that us-them divide processes would lead to prejudice (Tajfel & Turner, 1979, p. 41); Dharmakirti, a seventh century sage, predicted even more broadly that the separation between self and others causes "all possible faults" (Karr, 2007, p. 6). Research confirms these unfavorable predictions. For example, the us-them divide relates to intergroup hostility in minimal group paradigm studies (e.g., Staub, 1988), especially among highly ethnocentric individuals and high in-group identifiers (Perreault & Bourhis, 1999). The us-them divide has been used systematically to justify intergroup violence by political leaders including Osama bin Laden, G.W. Bush, and Tony Blair (Leudar, Marsland, & Nekvapil, 2004). Other research indicates that, together with emotions, stereotypes shape behavior toward

J.-H. Chang (✉)
Department of Educational Psychology and Counseling,
National Taiwan Normal University, Taipei, Taiwan
e-mail: jenhoc@gmail.com

H.S. Hodgins
Department of Psychology, Skidmore College, NY, USA

Y.-C. Lin
Department of Psychology, National Taiwan University, Taipei, Taiwan

C.-L. Huang
Department of Humanities and Social Sciences,
National Taiwan University of Science and Technology, Taipei, Taiwan

N. Weinstein (ed.), *Human Motivation and Interpersonal Relationships: Theory, Research, and Applications*, DOI 10.1007/978-94-017-8542-6_5,

outgroup members (Fiske, 1993; Fiske, Cuddy, & Glick, 2007; Fiske & Neuberg, 1990). Recently, social neuroscience research has shown that basic neural mechanisms correlate with making self-other distinctions and are important in understanding social cognition and affect (Heatherton, 2011; Lieberman, 2007).

Consistent with Tajfel's (1982) statement, many researchers assume that the us-them divide is based in natural tendencies and that social cognitive processes that underlie the us-them divide are fairly automatic, unconscious, and inevitable. However, research shows that the tendency to divide the social world into 'us' and 'them' is potentially variable, and depends at least in part on situational factors. For example, in-group bias was not evident in a minimal group experiment that used three groups instead of two (Hartstone & Augoustinos, 1995). In another study, voluntary contributions to collective interests were a function of the salience of social categorizations (Wit & Kerr, 2002). In studies using yet different paradigms, automatic behavioral contrast that distances the self from an out-group occurred only when intergroup comparisons were salient (Spears, Gordijn, Dijksterhuis, & Stapel, 2004), and social discrimination occurred only when the comparison dimension closely fit group categorizations (Reynolds, Turner, & Haslam, 2000). Also supporting the flexibility of the us-them divide, there is evidence that intergroup bias is reduced when conceptual representations of groups are altered (Gaertner, Mann, Murrell, & Dovidio, 1989), for example, when cooperation is induced (Gaertner, Mann, Dovidio, Murrell, & Pomare, 1990), and that intergroup discrimination depends on mood (Forgas & Fiedler, 1996). Hence, use of a pronounced us-them divide is not fixed, stable, or inevitable.

The Two-Stage Process of the Us-Them Divide

In addition to the situational factors that modify the us-them divide in the research above, we propose that other motivational factors can attenuate the magnitude of the us-them divide. The purpose of this chapter is to propose a model outlining a two-stage process that underlies the us-them divide. We suggest that us-them divide processes, although common and well-documented, are not automatic or inevitable, and thus, there is flexibility in how individuals engage them. Specifically, the us-them divide occurs in two stages: The first stage involves a social cognitive distinction between ingroup and outgroup, and the second stage includes, in addition, defensive evaluation that is motivated by anxiety (see Fig. 5.1).

Tajfel's (1982) theory has generated a large and important literature on intergroup relations and prejudice. However, he clearly specified that the us-them divide is an important part of individual self-construal. That is, in-group identification serves the purpose of establishing individual identity and self-worth: Group membership is internalized as social identity so that individuals treat in-groups as extensions of the individual self (Tajfel & Turner, 1979). Thus, although much past research documents intergroup us-them processes, the us-them divide also should manifest at the level of individual cognitive functioning, and should be measurable within individuals. Our review is concerned largely with cognitive processes that are experienced and measured at the individual level, although clearly related to intergroup perception and processes.

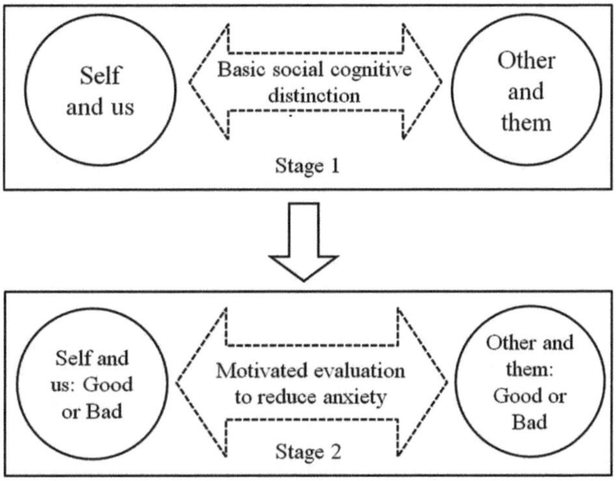

Fig. 5.1 The two-stage process of the us-them divide: a social cognitive and motivational model

Stage 1: A Natural Social Cognitive Process Underlying the Us-Them Divide

As noted above, the us-them divide often is viewed as a natural human cognitive tendency. Evidence for very basic distinction making between self and other is seen even in infants, who demonstrate the social cognitive ability to distinguish themselves from others (Stern, 1985). Moreover, individuals easily use physical features to categorize and group external stimuli, including into self and other, and us and them (Fiske, 1993; Tajfel, 1982; Tajfel, Billig, Bundy, & Flament, 1971). Psychological attributes also are applied to physical features (Tversky, 1977), as shown by the systematic work of Fiske and her colleagues (Cuddy, Fiske, & Glick, 2008; Fiske et al., 2007; Fiske, Cuddy, Glick, & Xu, 2002). Applying social perception attributes to investigate the interactive relationship between self and others, they found that individuals use two basic social perception dimensions, warmth and competence, to perceive and categorize individuals into response quadrants. Self and other perceptions, categorizations, and identification processes are cross-cultural (Cuddy et al., 2008), are seen in basic judgment processes of human perceptions of facial expressions (Oosterhof & Todorov, 2008), and thus, appear to be quite basic, possibly arising from innate tendencies.

Hence, what we refer to as the first stage of the us-them divide is based on a basic human tendency to cognitively differentiate individuals according to categories. The division is a fairly inevitable and automatic part of normal cognition, and corresponds to the associative processes discussed by Gawronski and Bodenhausen in their associative–propositional evaluation (APE) model (see 2011). The central assumption of the APE model is that humans use two qualitatively different mental processes: Associative processes lead to implicit behaviors, whereas propositional processes lead to explicit behaviors.

Consistent with the APE model, we argue that the automatic cognitive differentiation of self or in-group from others does not inevitably lead to defensive judgments or evaluation. Rather, individuals differ in how quickly they experience threat and engage in self-protective responses in stage two, and the differences in defense are related to situational and individual differences.

Stage 2: Motivated Evaluative Us-Them Divide Processes

Many theorists assume that individuals go beyond a simple cognitive distinction to the evaluation of "us" and "them," typically by devaluing others and praising themselves. This occurs because individuals seek to maintain positive self-feelings and evaluations or as an ongoing and universal preference for self-enhancement (e.g., Sedikides & Gregg, 2008). Self-protection and self-enhancement also are seen at the group level, in the form of in-group favoritism and out-group derogation (Tajfel, 1982; Turner et al., 1994). Research shows that self-enhancement bias occurs cross-culturally, in both individualistic and collectivist countries (Gaertner, Sedikides, & Chang, 2008; Sedikides, Gaertner, & Toguchi, 2003), and even with close others, such as best friends and in-group members (Yamaguchi et al., 2007). Self-enhancement sometimes is viewed as an evolution-based process that benefits well-being, both physically and psychologically (McKay & Dennett, 2009; Taylor & Brown, 1988). In other words, cognitive categorization together with motivated self-enhancement yielded such adaptive benefit that humans developed an innate social cognitive tendency to engage in both processes.

In considering whether both stages are automatic, it is important to explore the precise psychological mechanism leading to self-enhancement and other-derogation. Although many theories address this, we consider two well-known and interesting theories that explain self-enhancement according to self-worth motives (cf. Leary, 2007). The first is terror management theory (TMT; Greenberg, Solomon, & Pyszczynski, 1997; Solomon, Greenberg, & Pyszczynski, 1991), which views the pursuit of self-esteem as a way to counter existential anxiety due to fear of mortality. According to this perspective, individuals self-enhance and endorse core cultural values in order to buffer anxiety and give themselves symbolic immortality (Greenberg et al., 1992).

Consistent with TMT, much research shows that priming with mortality salience (e.g., writing about one's own death) can cause increased self-esteem (e.g., Harmon-Jones et al., 1997) and devaluation of out-group members who do not share the worldview. For instance, under manipulated mortality salience, individuals decrease positive evaluations and increase negative stereotypic evaluations of out-group members (Greenberg et al., 1990; Rosenblatt, Greenberg, Solomon, Pyszczynski, & Lyon, 1989). Moreover, when mortality salience is made accessible, individuals attack or punish out-group members who threaten their worldview (McGregor et al., 1998). These findings and others (e.g., Burke, Martens, & Faucher, 2010; Pyszczynski, Solomon, Greenberg, Arndt, & Schimel, 2004) indicate that mortality salience causes individuals to go beyond a simple cognitive division into 'us' and 'them', to derogate and aggress toward 'them'. From a TMT perspective then, individuals engage in both stages of the us-them divide, with self-enhancement and other-disparagement specifically aimed at countering existential anxiety from the underlying and inevitable fear of mortality.

Fig. 5.2 Motivated anxiety-reduction in stage two of the us-them divide process

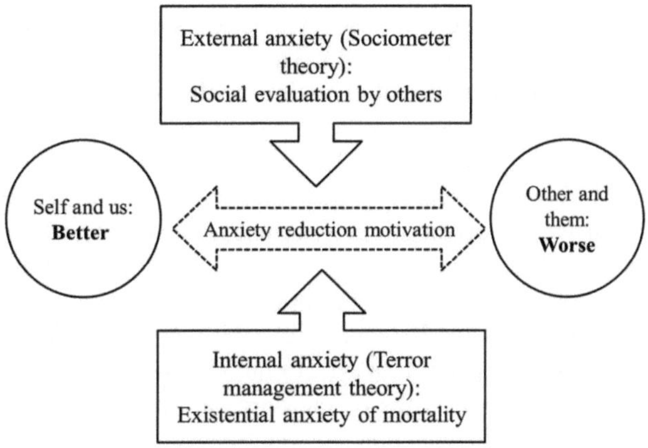

Another explanation of self-enhancement motivation is provided by the sociometer theory of self-esteem, which proposes a central human need to belong (Baumeister & Leary, 1995; Leary, 2007; Leary & Baumeister, 2000). The need for social approval – to be valued and accepted by others – leads individuals to self-enhance and present themselves in a positive manner. Much research supports this view also. For instance, Fein and Spencer (1997) conducted a series of studies showing that participants' whose self-images were threatened responded with out-group derogation and increased self-esteem. Specifically, the authors showed that degree of negative other-evaluation correlated with increased self-esteem. In a similar vein, Allen and Sherman (2011) presented a self-image threat and measured participants' implicit associations toward out-group members using the implicit association test. Results showed that, compared to a control group, threatened self-images activated negative out-group evaluations, which the authors interpreted as self-regard maintenance. Thus, consistent with the sociometer theory, research supports that devaluing others can maintain self-regard and gain social approval, giving evidence that motivated self-protection occurs in what we describe as the second stage us-them divide.

Thus, self-threats are salient in both TMT and the sociometer theory, and the theories share a core feature of motivated reduction of anxiety that arises from uncertainty. The two theories differ in terms of the source of anxiety and uncertainty, however. The sociometer theory emphasizes self-protection from the threat of negative evaluation and impaired social well-being, which is an external or interpersonal threat. In contrast, TMT posits that self-protection motivation arises from the internal, existential fear of mortality. However, the theories both predict that humans engage in motivated evaluation to avoid or reduce anxiety through the us-them divide processes that we refer to as stage two (see Fig. 5.2).

Clearly, there is much evidence that self-protection is important and frequently highly habitual in human behavior. In our view, however, the in-group/out-group distinction does not necessarily and automatically lead to defensive self-protective in-group favoritism and out-group derogation. Rather, it is possible for humans to acknowledge and integrate challenging feelings, such as anxiety, instead of responding with defensive maneuvers. Furthermore, research that documents the advantages of defensiveness might fail to consider the accompanying costs. For example, defensively accrued higher self-esteem buffers the effect of mortality salience, however, it also relates to suppression of death-related information (Harmon-Jones et al., 1997). Thus, individuals with high self-reported self-esteem who counter death-related anxiety with conscious effort and high ego-involvement should be vulnerable to the many documented costs of suppression (Butler et al., 2003; Cioffi & Holloway, 1993; Wegner, 2011).

Moreover, research shows that some so-called 'self-esteem' is insecure and defensive, involving higher explicit (i.e., self-reported) self-esteem than implicitly measured self-esteem. There is empirical evidence showing that explicit self-esteem does not correlate well with implicit self-esteem as assessed by indirect, unconscious measures (Bosson, Brown, Zeigler-Hill, & Swann, 2003; Jordan, Spencer, & Zanna, 2003; Jordan, Spencer, Zanna, Hoshino-Browne, & Correll, 2003) and that discrepancies between the two types of measures are associated with trait narcissism, ingroup bias, dissonance reduction (Jordan, Spencer, Zanna, et al., 2003), ethnic discrimination (Jordan, Spencer, & Zanna, 2005) and compensatory self-enhancement (Bosson et al., 2003). Related to the current review, research and theory that cite benefits of other-derogation and self-enhancement often rely on self-reported 'self-esteem' that reflects constructed defenses rather than genuine or securely felt self-regard.

We take the perspective that it is possible for humans to respond to challenging feelings, such as anxiety from threat, by experiencing such feelings openly and integrating them, rather than merely defending against them. Moreover, to the extent that, over time, individuals experience and integrate challenging feelings, they can respond with relatively less defense and avoidance across many situations (Hodgins, 2008; Hodgins & Knee, 2002). Lower defensiveness is a valuable interpersonal quality in itself, but also has advantages for task performance (e.g., Hodgins et al., 2010) and interpersonal functioning (e.g., Weinstein, Hodgins, & Ryan, 2010). Granted, the emotional integration that fosters nondefensiveness is established slowly and gradually, and perhaps only in part (Ryan, 1991; Ryan, Deci, & Grolnick, 1995). Thus, the differences between more and less defensive individuals are relative, rather than absolute differences. In other words, we do not suggest that some individuals defend and some do not, but that emotional integration is negatively associated with defense.

Another way of stating this is that the well-documented and familiar defensive processes represented in the second stage of the us-them divide can be attenuated by emotional integration. Basic stage one differentiation of individuals into groups based on social cognitive processes occurs naturally; however, the second stage of the us-them divide, involving self-enhancement and other-derogation, is potentially flexible. Essentially, our view allows for threat and anxiety to be experienced and integrated so that when individuals encounter 'others', there is less need and less motivation to view them negatively.

Potential Flexibility in the Us-Them Divide

We review three approaches that can account for flexibility in us-them divide processes: Self-determination theory (Deci & Ryan, 2000; Ryan & Deci, 2000), a theory of interpersonal goals (Crocker, 2008), and a Buddhist perspective on self

(Brown, Ryan, & Crewell, 2007; Hwang & Chang, 2009). The three approaches describe different mechanisms that potentially can attenuate the us-them divide, but are not mutually exclusive. Indeed, the accounts overlap and have been connected empirically (e.g., Brown & Ryan, 2003). However, each approach also can stand alone as an explanation for flexibility in the defensive stage two us-them divide processes.

Self-Determination Theory and the Us-Them Divide

One way to conceptualize attenuated defensiveness is through motivational processes described by self-determination theory (SDT; Deci & Ryan, 2000; Ryan & Deci, 2000). SDT holds that there are general motivational orientations, referred to as autonomy and control orientations, that predict behavior and thought across diverse domains. Autonomy orientation involves a sense of agency and choicefulness about behavior, and is associated with intrinsic motivation. In contrast, controlled motivation orientation is associated with feeling coerced and pressured to respond in particular ways (i.e., I "ought" or "should") and is associated with extrinsic motivation (Deci & Ryan).

Hodgins and Knee (2002) proposed that autonomy and control motivation orientations are related to readiness to experience threat, such that autonomy leads to relatively lower defensiveness compared to controlled motivation (also see Hodgins, 2008). This has been described in terms of thresholds for threat (see Hodgins, Liebeskind, & Schwartz, 1996; Hodgins et al., 2010), with autonomy orientation causing a higher threshold. This means that to the extent that individuals are autonomy-oriented, they are less quick to perceive and respond to threat, compared to controlled-oriented individuals. Relating this prediction to the Fig. 5.1 model, it can be said that autonomous motivation orientation should relate to less use of the stage 2 us-them divide processes, which essentially are defensive (e.g., other-derogation).

Evidence That Autonomy and Intrinsic Motivation Relate to Lower Defense

Much empirical support is consistent with Hodgins and Knee's (2002) predictions that autonomy is associated with lower defensiveness. For example, research measuring individual differences has shown that, relative to dispositional control orientation, autonomy relates to greater interpersonal openness in naturally-occurring interactions (Hodgins, Koestner, & Duncan, 1996; Knee, Lonsbary, Canevello, & Patrick, 2005), more effective written emotional expression (Weinstein & Hodgins, 2009), and taking responsibility openly and honestly after harming others (Hodgins & Liebeskind, 2003; Hodgins, Liebeskind, et al., 1996). In a consistent way, in intimate relationships, autonomous orientation predicts greater use of positive communication strategies (e.g., positive reinterpretation) and fewer defensive behaviors (e.g., denial) while discussing relationship conflict, whereas controlled orientation predicts the reverse (Knee et al., 2005; Knee, Patrick, Vietor, Nanayakkara, & Neighbors, 2002).

In other defense-related behavior, autonomous orientation predicts less use of self-serving attributions (Knee & Zuckerman, 1996), self-handicapping and defensive coping strategies (Knee & Zuckerman, 1998), less driving aggression (Neighbors, Vietor, & Knee, 2002) and a less easily threatened identity (Soenens, Berzonsky, Vansteenkiste, Beyers, & Goossens, 2005). In the same direction, a social comparison study showed that autonomy orientation moderated comparison consequences such that less autonomous individuals experienced increased negative affect and decreased self-esteem when paired with a better performing other (Neighbors & Knee, 2003).

In the domain of prosocial engagement, autonomous orientation positively predicts helping behavior (e.g., volunteer work; Gagne, 2003), and benefit in well-being for both the helper and receiver (Weinstein & Ryan, 2010). Interestingly, in the latter study, the benefit to well-being for both helper and recipient was mediated by gratitude, such that autonomous motivation for helping increased both the helper's and recipient's gratitude (Weinstein, DeHaan, & Ryan, 2010). Evidence for the *opposite* of prosocial behavior comes from a resource dilemma study: Groups with more extrinsic value oriented members harvested more on average than groups with more intrinsic motivation value members, and extrinsic value orientation positively correlated with resource acquisition strategies (Sheldon & McGregor, 2000). Thus, extrinsic values predicted acting in self-interest and against the interest of others.

More recently, experimental studies have provided causal evidence that addresses the direction of the relation between motivation and defense. In these studies, motivation orientations were primed, which is analogous to situationally manipulated motivation. Taken together, they show that, relative to a controlled orientation, autonomous orientation leads to lower defense. For example, primed autonomy orientation causes less desire to escape, less self-serving bias, and among collegiate rowers, less self-handicapping for athletic performance and better performance (Hodgins, Yacko, & Gottlieb, 2006). It is possible that performance effects are related to underlying self-esteem: in two studies, Hodgins, Brown, and Carver (2007) showed that, compared to controlled orientation, primed autonomy causes higher implicit self-esteem and lower defensive self-esteem. Extending the inquiry to dyadic experience, Weinstein, Hodgins, & Ryan (2010) primed unacquainted dyads with motivation and examined interaction quality and joint performance on two creative tasks. Results showed that autonomy-primed dyads were more attuned and encouraging to one another and performed better on the creative joint tasks, showing again, that autonomy, in the SDT sense of choicefulness, improves interpersonal experience. The advantage of autonomy for interpersonal relating also is seen in a set of studies on the enjoyment of hostile humor, which is a type of interpersonal aggression (Weinstein, Hodgins, & Ostvik-White, 2011). Specifically, relative to primed autonomy, primed control motivation increased the appreciation of hostile (compared with nonhostile) humor, as measured by nonverbal behavior and self-report. It is likely that the higher aggression demonstrated under control orientation is related to greater threat responsiveness, as was demonstrated by Hodgins et al. (2010). In that study, participants who were primed with autonomy and control motivations were physiologically monitored and videotaped during a stressful one-on-one interview. Results showed consistently lower threat response in autonomy-primed relative to controlled-primed participants across very diverse behavioral measures. Specifically, autonomy-primed participants had lower defensiveness on measures of verbal, paralinguistic, smiling, vocal fundamental frequency, and cardiovascular responses. Moreover, autonomy-primed participants also performed better on a subsequent speech task, and their better performance was mediated by interview defensiveness. In other words, nondefensiveness during the stressful interview allowed autonomy-primed participants to give better speeches subsequently.

Hence, taken together, the experimental research shows that, relative to controlled motivation orientation, autonomous orientation *causes* less behavioral defensiveness across diverse domains. As mentioned above, the lower defense under autonomous motivation has been described as reflecting a higher threshold for threat (Hodgins, Liebeskind, et al., 1996; Hodgins et al., 2010), which means that autonomously behaving individuals are slower to perceive and react defensively to potential threat. We believe that the cognitive processes underlying a lower threshold for threat involve differently constructed concepts of 'self' or 'us' and 'other'. Specifically, a higher threshold for threat is associated with less distance between 'us' and 'them', or a lower us-them divide. A lower magnitude us-them divide would still involve a stage one cognitive differentiation between 'us' and 'them', however, there would be less defensively motivated self-protection or stage two process.

We suggested above that stage two defenses represent an attempt to reduce anxiety. Related to this, SDT suggests that extrinsic values are adopted to compensate for the lack of fulfillment of innate psychological needs (Deci & Ryan, 2000). Not surprisingly, given that extrinsic motivation is compensatory following need thwarting, extrinsic motivation also predicts anxiety. Specifically, anxiety, depression, and ill-being are positively correlated with extrinsic central life aspirations (e.g., financial wealth, appearance, status), and negatively correlated with intrinsic aspirations (e.g., personal growth, relatedness, community; Kasser & Ryan, 1993, 1996). Hence, just as defensive responses are motivated by anxiety-reduction in TMT and the sociometer theory, in SDT, defensiveness associated with extrinsic and controlled motivation are related to anxiety and threat susceptibility. Table 5.1 summarizes the relation of autonomous and controlled motivation orientations to positive and negative social experience, as reviewed above.

Direct Evidence That Autonomy Relates to Less Stage Two Us-Them Divide

We believe that us-them divide processes are based largely on unconscious, rather than consciously reportable cognitions. After all, threat and defense are not primarily rooted in conscious intellectual experience, but in affective experience that is at

Table 5.1 Autonomous and controlled motivation orientations and positive and negative social experience

Categories and reference	Autonomous or intrinsic	Controlled or extrinsic
Positive and nondefensive social experience		
Prosocial behavior (Gagne, 2003)	High	Low
Implicit self-esteem (Hodgins et al., 2007)	High	Low
Helping behaviors (Weinstein & Ryan, 2010)	High	Low
Gratitude to others (Weinstein, DeHaan et al., 2010)	High	Low
Interaction quality (Hodgins, Koestner, et al., 1996; Weinstein, Hodgins, et al., 2010)	High	Low
Taking responsibility for harm (Hodgins & Liebeskind, 2003; Hodgins, Liebeskind, et al., 1996)	High	Low
Joint creative performance (Weinstein, Hodgins, et al., 2010)	High	Low
Romantic relationships (Knee et al., 2002, 2005)	High	Low
Negative and defensive social experience		
Self-serving bias (Knee & Zuckerman, 1996)	Low	High
Self-protection (Hodgins et al., 2010; Knee & Zuckerman, 1998)	Low	High
Social evaluative pressures and anxiety (Neighbors & Knee, 2003)	Low	High
Defensive self-esteem (Hodgins et al., 2007)	Low	High
Hostile/aggressive humor (Weinstein et al., 2011)	Low	High
Self-centered resource use (Sheldon & McGregor, 2000)	Low	High

least partly unaware. Accordingly, the best way to empirically investigate automaticity versus flexibility in us-them processes is with indirect measures of cognition.

Recently, Hodgins (2010) used such a measure to perform preliminary tests to examine directly the relations between motivation and automatic us-them divide cognition. Specifically, she used a lexical decision test paradigm to measure individual differences in the automatic association of "us" with "good" and "them" with "bad". Participants categorized letter strings according to whether they were words (positive and negative trait adjectives such as energetic, irritable) or non-words (e.g., crantick, walon). Each letter string was preceded by a subliminal pronoun related to us or them; reaction times (RTs) were measured. The logic of lexical decision task is that subliminal primes speed the processing (i.e., RTs) of consistent target items and slow down the processing of inconsistent targets. Thus, the pattern of RTs indicate the extent to which individuals unconsciously associate "us" with "good" and "them" with "bad", or in other words, have an automatic us-them divide. Previous use of a similar measure revealed the presence of an unconscious us-them divide (Perdue, Dovidio, Gurtman, & Tyler, 1990, Exp. 2); however, the authors did not examine correlates of individual differences.

Replicating Perdue et al. (1990), Hodgins (2010) found clear evidence for an automatic, or unconscious, us-them divide. Moreover, motivation orientation moderated the divide, with autonomy predicting a smaller us-them divide compared to controlled orientation. A second study replicated the presence of the us-them divide, and the same relation to motivation orientations. Furthermore, Study 2 showed that controlled orientation and the lexical decision task us-them divide both predicted the interpretation of ambiguous visual images as threatening. Finally, there was evidence for partial mediation of the effects: The effect of motivation orientation on threat perception occurred at least in part because individuals with higher controlled orientation had a larger magnitude automatic cognitive us-them divide.

The results provide preliminary evidence that the lower defensiveness under autonomous, relative to controlled orientation, as shown in much past research, is associated with differing unconscious cognition. Specifically, relative to control orientation, autonomy predicted less automatic association between 'us' and 'good' and 'them' and 'bad'. Thus, the higher threshold for threat under autonomy orientation relates to less automatic cognitive us-them divide. Relating this to Fig. 5.1, autonomy motivation orientation allows individuals to engage the us-them more flexibly so that stage two defenses are less automatic.

Egosystem and Ecosystem Interpersonal Goals and the Us-Them Divide

A second perspective that allows for flexibility in stage two of us-them divide processes is a theory of interpersonal goals by Crocker and her colleagues (Crocker, 2008; Crocker & Canevello, 2008). The researchers proposed that broad and differing motivations, referred to as egosystem and ecosystem, underlie human relationships. Egosystem motivation focuses on pursuing self-esteem, which is similar to self-enhancement motivation, and can include self-image goals. In contrast, those with ecosystem motivation tend to pursue compassionate goals and focus on caring for others. Their more global scope considers a larger human interaction system, and allows transcending self-interest to pay attention to group interests.

Crocker's (2008) motivated interpersonal goals can be connected to us-them divide processes in that stage two motivated self-enhancement should be more likely under egosystem than ecosystem motivation. Ecosystem motivation is not self-sacrificing or self-effacing, but allows for integrating the interests of self and other (Crocker, Olivier, & Nuer, 2009) and feeling compassion that can lead to growth. That is, in addition to concern for others, compassionate feelings can entail self-elevating moral emotion that benefits individuals themselves (Haidt, 2003; Haidt & Morris, 2009).

Accordingly, ecosystem and egosystem motivations should involve different us-them processes. Specifically, the compassionate goals and other-concern of ecosystem motivation are incompatible with self-enhancement and devaluing others, whereas the self-image goals of egosystem motivation are consistent with those responses. Research by Crocker and her colleagues has systematically investigated interpersonal correlates of the two motivations and supports this prediction. For example, roommate dyads were recruited for weekly evaluation of the dynamics of their self-images and compassionate goals. Results showed that those with self-image egosystem goals were more likely to feel anxious and depressed (Crocker, Canevello, Breines, & Flynn, 2010) and have lower self-esteem (Canevello &

Table 5.2 Egosystem and ecosystems and positive and negative social experience

Categories and reference	Egosystem motivation: self-image goals	Ecosystem motivation: compassionate goals
Positive social experience		
Perceived social support (Crocker & Canevello, 2008)	Low	High
Received social support (Crocker & Canevello, 2008)	Low	High
Perceived responsiveness (Canevello & Crocker, 2010, 2011)	Low	High
Received responsiveness (Canevello & Crocker, 2010, 2011)	Low	High
Negative social experience		
Zero sum beliefs (Crocker & Canevello, 2008)	High	Low
Hostile toward others (Moeller et al., 2009)	High	Low
Psychological entitlement (Moeller et al., 2009)	High	Low

Crocker, 2011). They also were more hostile to roommates, had higher self-entitlement (Moeller, Crocker, & Bushman, 2009), and perceived and received less social support (Canevello & Crocker, 2010; Crocker & Canevello, 2008). Moreover, egosystem motivated individuals were more likely to endorse zero sum beliefs and to perceive lower inclusion with others (Crocker & Canevello). The findings show that egosystem goals predict engaging in the us-them divide cognitively and motivationally, that is, both differentiating from and then devaluing other people.

In contrast, those with compassionate goals were less anxious and depressed (Crocker et al., 2010), had higher self-esteem (Canevello & Crocker, 2011), were less hostile to roommates, showed lower self-entitlement (Moeller et al., 2009), reported receiving more social support (Canevello & Crocker, 2010; Crocker & Canevello, 2008), lower endorsement of zero sum beliefs, and higher inclusion with others (Crocker & Canevello). These findings suggest that, although those with compassionate goals make the natural cognitive differentiation between self and other, they are less likely to engage in the stage two motivated devaluation of others.

In sum, past research is consistent with the prediction that the lower intrapersonal and interpersonal adjustment among individuals with egosystem motivation is associated with greater us-them divide. In contrast, the better social relations among ecosystem individuals should be associated with an attenuated us-them divide.

It is interesting to consider that us-them divide processes under egosystem motivation might be similar to the mechanisms underlying TMT and sociometer theory explanations, in that self-image goals might serve the purpose of anxiety reduction. Pursuing self-image goals leads to a negative cycle that provokes more anxiety and social evaluative pressure (Crocker & Park, 2004; Crocker & Wolfe, 2001), which in turn may cause greater us-them divide. Thus, the egosystem approach to anxiety could be a self-perpetuating cycle, creating an endless negative feedback loop that increases anxiety (Table 5.2) (Canevello & Crocker, 2010, 2011).

Buddhist Perspective of Self and the Us-Them Divide

A third and final way to envision flexibility in us-them divide processes is from a Buddhist perspective of self. This approach to 'self' seems paradoxical because the Buddhist view is that there *is no* independent and separate self (Hwang, 2009; Hwang & Chang, 2009), and that the most optimal self-functioning occurs when there is non-attachment to mental representations of self (Sahdra, Shaver, & Brown, 2010). Nonattachment refers to living in the present, fully mindful that existence occurs moment by moment, and does not depend on constructed ideas about the self, past or future (Brown & Ryan, 2003; Brown et al., 2007). Importantly and interestingly, then, the Buddhist perspective of self is as a totally dynamic process that cannot be captured in stable conceptualized representations, but that is fully experiential (Williams, 2010). Stated differently, in Buddhism, "self" is a constructed delusion. The delusion causes anxiety and suffering because vigilant self-protection becomes necessary to preserve the construction. To the extent that individuals gain insight into the constructed nature of self, and are nonattached to the constructed self-representations, they become free of anxiety and suffering. Thus, happiness and well-being are a result of freedom from attachment to constructed self-representations.

A common question that arises is whether the Buddhist nonattached self is similar to an avoidant attachment style. However, nonself or non-attachment and insecure attachment differ both conceptually and empirically. A recent measure of non-attachment shows that it is negatively correlated with both avoidant attachment (Sahdra et al., 2010) and dissociation (Baer, Smith, Hopkins, Krietemeyer, & Toney, 2006).

The Buddhist perspective of self also can be considered in terms of "mindfulness", a state of present moment awareness without judgment of experience (Bishop et al., 2004). Interestingly, mindful individuals are more aware of environmental information in the present moment. In some Buddhist practices and training methods, such as meditation, participants are instructed to simply observe thoughts, without evaluating or engaging in analytic processing (Williams, 2010). Meditation instruction also can include awareness of internal and external stimuli, either internally and or in the environment (Lutz, Slagter, Dunne, & Davidson, 2008). Consequently, with intensive and long-term training (possibly exceeding 40,000 h), meditators can distinguish stimuli from internal thoughts and the external world more accurately (Brefczynski-Lewis, Lutz, Schaefer, Levinson, & Davidson, 2007; Hodgins & Adair, 2010; Slagter et al., 2007), and are less disturbed by distraction and interference, including the flanker effect (Tang et al., 2007) and the Stroop effect (Moore & Malinowski, 2009). This mindful cognitive flexibility also can influence self-related and social perceptions. For instance, people who are highly mindful are sensitive to detecting themselves and others (Baer et al., 2006), suggesting that meditators easily make the self-other distinction in the first stage of the us-them divide. However, the second stage, of motivated self-enhancement and other-derogation, should be attenuated in highly mindful individuals.

Recent evidence supports this. For example, in a neuroimaging study, Creswell, Way, Eisenberger, and Lieberman (2007) measured trait mindfulness and then asked participants to match facial expressions to appropriate affect words (e.g., angry, sad, or sacred). Results showed that trait mindfulness was negatively correlated with amygdala activation. This implies that negative facial expressions did not arouse negative affect in more mindful individuals, and that mindfulness is associated with less evaluation of others. In line with this, compared to a control group, individuals who engaged in mindfulness practice had less biased attitudes about both positive and negative information (Kiken & Shook, 2011).

On the interpersonal level, Heppner et al. (2008) showed that trait mindfulness correlates negatively with aggressive behavior and hostile attribution bias in ambiguous interpersonal contexts. Furthermore, participants who engaged in mindfulness practice and then received social rejection feedback showed less aggressive behavior compared to rejected participants without mindfulness practice. Extending this to intimate relationships, Barnes, Brown, Krusemark, Campbell, and Rogge (2007) measured dispositional mindfulness and asked couples to discuss relationship conflict. Results revealed that trait mindfulness negatively predicted anxiety and anger-hostility both pre- and post-conflict discussion. Interestingly, pre-conflict discussion anxiety and anger-hostility mediated the relationship between trait mindfulness and post-conflict discussion anxiety and anger-hostility. The result indicates that those high in trait mindfulness have lower perceived anxiety and anger-hostility toward their partners. In terms of the us-them divide, it suggests that trait mindfulness might decrease the ego-involved motivation of stage two us-them divide processes, because more mindful individuals experience less anxiety.

In the same direction, at the more global level of group interactions, Niemiec et al. (2010) showed that trait mindfulness can decrease us-them divide processes under mortality salience. Specifically, they conducted a series of studies indicating that trait mindfulness was negatively correlated with self-esteem enhancing and worldview defense for participants primed with mortality salience. Furthermore, acceptance of death thoughts was the mechanism that mediated between trait mindfulness and less defensive responding. Highly mindful individuals were willing to spend more time writing about their own deaths and were less likely to suppress death-related thoughts, as measured by a word fragment test. Thus, results suggest that the non-judgmental component of mindfulness, which involves an open attitude toward the self and others, decreases defense.

Several studies have connected mindfulness and intrinsic motivation; for example, in an experience sampling study, Brown and Ryan (2003) found that trait mindfulness correlated positively with state autonomy. Using the same paradigm, Levesque and Brown (2007) revealed that those who were highly mindful reported more explicit autonomous behaviors day-to-day, regardless of their dispositional implicit orientation toward autonomy or heteronomy. This means that trait mindfulness can moderate the relationship between implicit and explicit levels of autonomy. People high in mindfulness could also be autonomous in daily behaviors, even if their implicit autonomy was low.

Interestingly, some studies have linked the Buddhist perspective of self with compassion motivation, which is similar to ecosystem motivation, using a paradigm from Buddhist training practices called loving-kindness meditation. Loving-kindness meditation is similar to traditional mindfulness meditation in that both involve training attention toward the here and now. However, while mindfulness meditation focuses on a nonjudgmental attitude toward self and other involvement, loving-kindness involves directing positive other-oriented emotions, such as warmth and caring, in an open-hearted way. Individuals are asked to focus on a person for whom they feel great warmth and caring (e.g., parents, a lover), and asked to extend these feelings first to themselves and then to others (e.g., siblings, friends, strangers). In one study, working adults were randomly assigned to loving-kindness meditation or a control group (Fredrickson, Cohn, Coffey, Pek, & Finkel, 2008). Results showed that individuals who engaged in loving-kindness meditation reported increased daily experiences of positive emotions over time. The degree of increased positive emotion in turn predicted beneficial psychological outcomes, including trait mindfulness and well-being. In addition, over time, individuals who engaged in loving-kindness meditation provided more support to others and felt more gratitude and love from them. Similarly, in a single shot priming study, participants were randomly assigned to loving-kindness meditation or a simple imagery condition (Hutcherson, Seppala, & Gross, 2008). Results showed that loving-kindness meditation enhanced social connections and positive other-evaluation in explicit and implicit measures, even for targets who were strangers.

Recently, Lin, Huang, Hodgins, and Chang (2011) directly investigated the relationship between mindfulness and the us-them divide using measures of trait mindfulness and Hodgins' (2010) us-them lexical decision task. Results showed that mindful individuals had faster reaction times on *us/positive* than *us/negative* trials, but the same reaction times on *them/positive* and *them/negative* trials. This means that more mindful individuals maintained positive self-feelings without derogating others, a pattern similar to that in Perdue et al. (1990). In contrast, the pattern among more mindless individuals was faster RTs on *us/positive* than *them/positive* trials, but slower RTs on *us/negative* than *them/negative* trials. Thus, mindless individuals showed both self-enhancement and other-derogation. Together results show that mindfulness is associated with less automatic cognitive other-derogation.

To summarize, research shows that meditation practice and mindfulness predict lower negative affect and less aggression and hostility across several contexts, including in partner relationships and following social rejection. Mindfulness also predicts attenuated defense following mortality salience and less other-derogation at the level of automatic cognitive processes.

It might seem paradoxical that "non-attached" individuals have better quality interpersonal experience. In a Buddhist context, however, "nonattachment" is in relation to one's own concepts, rather than to people. Nonattachment allows freedom from the compulsion to maintain and protect and rigid self-representations because those representations are realized to be constructed, ever-changing, and insubstantial. Thus the freedom of nonattachment reduces anxiety, allowing better interpersonal relations.

A concept seemingly similar to nonattachment is seen in work by Leary, Adam, and Tate (2006, 2010), in their term, hypo-egoic self-regulation. Those who are hypo-egoic paradoxically regulate *better* than those who consciously and intentionally self-regulate, referred to as hyper-egoic self-regulation (Leary et al., 2006). Under hyper-egoic self-regulation, high ego-involvement causes affective loading that limits and drains cognitive and social resources. In contrast, hypo-egoic self-regulation is anxiety-free, allowing individuals to engage in tasks mindfully and fully, with less distraction. Hypo-egoic self-regulation is reminiscent of Masicampo and Baumeister's (2007) proposal that mindfulness allows self-regulation that is characterized by peace of mind, and occurs among individuals who free themselves from unwanted worries. Indeed, without the burden of anxiety, individuals perform better on self-regulatory tasks and other performance tasks (e.g., Hodgins et al., 2010). Thus, several perspectives converge on the conclusion that to the extent the self recedes into the background, is nonattached or hypo-egoic, the defensive, second stage us-them divide processes become less necessary, and self-enhancement and other-derogation decrease.

Conclusion: Flexibility in the Us-Them Divide

Tajfel's (1982; Tajfel & Turner, 1979) original statement about the human proclivity for dividing the social world into ingroups and outgroups has stimulated a tremendous amount of research, much of which confirms the predicted negative outcomes of the us-them divide. We have suggested that the process of dividing the social world into 'us' and 'them' can be thought of as occurring in two stages. Stage one is the basic cognitive differentiation into categories of 'us' and 'them', which occurs quite automatically due to basic human cognitive capacities. The second stage goes beyond categorization and involves judging 'us' as better than 'them,' an evaluation motivated by the need to reduce anxiety. Stage two us-them divide processes are self-serving, self-protective, and defensive.

However, in our view, stage two us-them divide processes are characterized by considerable flexibility. That is, whether and to what extent individuals engage in defensive maneuvers of the stage two us-them divide varies with self and motivation-related factors. We reviewed three theoretical approaches that can account for attenuation of the defensive processes of the second stage – Self-determination theory (Deci & Ryan, 2000; Ryan & Deci, 2000), a theory of interpersonal goals (Crocker, 2008), and a Buddhist perspective on self (Brown et al., 2007; Hwang & Chang, 2009). These three are not mutually exclusive, nor are they the only possible explanations of the effects.

Nonetheless, all three approaches propose that motivation and self-related factors allow less defensive other-evaluation. That is, each proposes that defensive anxiety reduction responses, such as self-enhancement and other-derogation, which often are conceived of as normal or pervasive, are modifiable and not inevitable. Those defensive responses probably are in large part unaware, or unconscious, and thus are best investigated with indirect measures that assess unaware cognitive processes. Accordingly, we describe unpublished data collected in our laboratories that used a lexical decision task measure of unconscious cognitive associations related to the us-them divide. The results from these preliminary studies support the predictions that individual differences in mindfulness (Lin et al., 2011) and in autonomy and controlled motivation orientations (Hodgins, 2010) correlate with the magnitude of us-them divide. Furthermore, there is evidence that the lower us-them divide mediates the effect of motivation orientation on threat perception in the predicted direction (Hodgins, 2010).

Finding even preliminary evidence for flexibility in stage two us-them processes is exceedingly good news. The widespread human tendencies for self-enhancement and other-derogation have tremendous ill consequences, both for the actors and targets of such behaviors. The list of consequences includes impaired performance, increased psychological and physiological stress, disrupted interpersonal functioning, aggression, hostility, loneliness and much more. Defensive responses have paradoxical effects – individuals avoid threat to gain immediate protection of so-called "self-esteem." However, sources of threat, for example, in social exchanges and in mortality itself, are inevitable; they lurk and re-appear without warning. Thus, habitual defensive responding offers a momentary warding off of threat-related experience, but it requires continual vigilance, draining emotional and cognitive resources, and interfering with the quality of life. Fortunately, it does not have to be that way.

References

Allen, T. J., & Sherman, J. W. (2011). Ego threat and intergroup bias: A test of motivated-activation versus self-regulatory accounts. *Psychological Science, 22*, 331–333.

Baer, R. A., Smith, G. T., Hopkins, J., Krietemeyer, J., & Toney, L. (2006). Using self-report assessment methods to explore facets of mindfulness. *Assessment, 13*, 27–45.

Barnes, S., Brown, K. W., Krusemark, E., Campbell, W. K., & Rogge, R. D. (2007). The role of mindfulness in romantic relationship satisfaction and responses to relationship stress. *Journal of Marital and Family Therapy, 33*, 482–500.

Baumeister, R. F., & Leary, M. R. (1995). The need to belong: Desire for interpersonal attachment as a fundamental human motive. *Psychological Bulletin, 117*, 497–529.

Bishop, S. R., Lau, M., Shapiro, S., Carlson, L., Anderson, N. D., Carmody, J., et al. (2004). Mindfulness: A proposed operational definition. *Clinical Psychology-Science and Practice, 11*, 230–241.

Bosson, J. K., Brown, R. P., Zeigler-Hill, V., & Swann, W. B., Jr. (2003). Self-enhancement tendencies among people with high explicit self-esteem: The moderating role of implicit self-esteem. *Self and Identity, 2*, 169–187.

Brefczynski-Lewis, J. A., Lutz, A., Schaefer, H. S., Levinson, D. B., & Davidson, R. J. (2007). Neural correlates of attentional expertise in long-term meditation practitioners. *Proceedings of the National Academy of Sciences of the United States of America, 104*, 11483–11488.

Brewer, M. B. (1991). The social self – On being the same and different at the same time. *Personality and Social Psychology Bulletin, 17*, 475–482.

Brown, K. W., & Ryan, R. M. (2003). The benefits of being present: Mindfulness and its role in psychological well-being. *Journal of Personality and Social Psychology, 84*, 822–848.
Brown, K. W., Ryan, R. A., & Creswell, J. D. (2007). Mindfulness: Theoretical foundations and evidence for its salutary effects. *Psychological Inquiry, 18*, 211–237.
Burke, B. L., Martens, A., & Faucher, E. H. (2010). Two decades of terror management theory: A meta-analysis of mortality salience research. *Personality and Social Psychology Review, 14*, 155–195.
Butler, E., Egloff, B., Wlhelm, F. H., Smith, N. C., Erickson, E. A., & Gross, J. J. (2003). The social consequences of expressive suppression. *Emotion, 3*, 48–67.
Canevello, A., & Crocker, J. (2010). Creating good relationships: Responsiveness, relationship quality, and interpersonal goals. *Journal of Personality and Social Psychology, 99*, 78–106.
Canevello, A., & Crocker, J. (2011). Interpersonal goals, others' regard for the self, and self-esteem: The paradoxical consequences of self-image and compassionate goals. *European Journal of Social Psychology, 41*, 422–434.
Cioffi, D., & Holloway, J. (1993). Delayed costs of suppressed pain. *Journal of Personality and Social Psychology, 64*, 274–282.
Creswell, J. D., Way, B. M., Eisenberger, N. I., & Lieberman, M. D. (2007). Neural correlates of dispositional mindfulness during affect labeling. *Psychosomatic Medicine, 69*, 560–565.
Crocker, J. (2008). From egosystem to ecosystem: Implications for learning, relationships, and wellbeing. In H. Wayment & J. Brauer (Eds.), *Transcending self-interest: Psychological explorations of the quiet ego* (pp. 63–72). Washington, DC: American Psychological Association.
Crocker, J., & Canevello, A. (2008). Creating and undermining social support in communal relationships: The role of compassionate and self-image goals. *Journal of Personality and Social Psychology, 95*, 555–575.
Crocker, J., Canevello, A., Breines, J. G., & Flynn, H. (2010). Interpersonal goals and change in anxiety and dysphoria in first-semester college students. *Journal of Personality and Social Psychology, 98*, 1009–1024.
Crocker, J., Olivier, M.-A., & Nuer, N. (2009). Self-image goals and compassionate goals: Costs and benefits. *Self and Identity, 8*, 251–269.
Crocker, J., & Park, L. E. (2004). The costly pursuit of self-esteem. *Psychological Bulletin, 130*(3), 392–414.
Crocker, J., & Wolfe, C. T. (2001). Contingencies of self-worth. *Psychological Review, 108*, 593–623.
Cuddy, A. J. C., Fiske, S. T., & Glick, P. (2008). Warmth and competence as universal dimensions of social perception: The stereotype content model and the bias map. In M. P. Zanna (Ed.), *Advances in experimental social psychology* (Vol. 40, pp. 61–149). New York: Academic.
Deci, E. L., & Ryan, R. M. (2000). The "what" and "why" of goal pursuits: Human needs and the self-determination of behavior. *Psychological Inquiry, 11*, 227–268.
Fein, S., & Spencer, S. J. (1997). Prejudice as self-image maintenance: Affirming the self through derogating others. *Journal of Personality and Social Psychology, 73*, 31–44.
Fiske, S. T. (1993). Social cognition and social-perception. *Annual Review of Psychology, 44*, 155–194.
Fiske, S. T., Cuddy, A. J. C., & Glick, P. (2007). Universal dimensions of social cognition: Warmth and competence. *TRENDS in Cognitive Sciences, 11*, 77–83.
Fiske, S. T., Cuddy, A. J. C., Glick, P., & Xu, J. (2002). A model of (often mixed) stereotype content: Competence and warmth respectively follow from perceived status and competition. *Journal of Personality and Social Psychology, 82*, 878–902.
Fiske, S. T., & Neuberg, S. L. (1990). A continuum of impression-formation, from category-based to individuating processes – Influences of information and motivation on attention and interpretation. In M. P. Zanna (Ed.), *Advances in experimental social psychology* (Vol. 23, pp. 1–74). San Diego, CA: Academic.
Forgas, J. P., & Fiedler, K. (1996). Us and them: Mood effects on intergroup discrimination. *Journal of Personality and Social Psychology, 70*, 28–40.

Fredrickson, B. L., Cohn, M. A., Coffey, K. A., Pek, J., & Finkel, S. M. (2008). Open hearts build lives: Positive emotions, induced through Loving-kindness meditation, build consequential personal resources. *Journal of Personality and Social Psychology, 95*, 1045–1062.

Gaertner, S. L., Mann, J. A., Dovidio, J. F., Murrell, A. J., & Pomare, M. (1990). How does cooperation reduce intergroup bias? *Journal of Personality and Social Psychology, 59*, 692–704.

Gaertner, S. L., Mann, J. A., Murrell, A., & Dovidio, J. F. (1989). Reducing intergroup bias: The benefits of recategorization. *Journal of Personality and Social Psychology, 57*, 239–249.

Gaertner, S. L., Sedikides, C., & Chang, K. (2008). On pancultural self-enhancement – Well-adjusted Taiwanese self-enhance on personally valued traits. *Journal of Cross-Cultural Psychology, 39*, 463–477.

Gagne, M. (2003). The role of autonomy support and autonomy orientation in prosocial behavior engagement. *Motivation and Emotion, 27*, 199–223.

Gawronski, B., & Bodenhausen, G. V. (2011). The associative-propositional evaluation model: Theory, evidence, and open questions. In J. M. Olson & M. P. Zanna (Eds.), *Advances in experimental social psychology* (Vol. 44, pp. 59–127). San Diego, CA: Academic.

Greenberg, J., Pyszczynski, T., Burling, J., Simon, L., Solomon, S., Rosenblatt, A., et al. (1992). Why do people need self-esteem – Converging evidence that self-esteem serves an anxiety-buffering function. *Journal of Personality and Social Psychology, 63*, 913–922.

Greenberg, J., Solomon, S., & Pyszczynski, T. (1997). Terror management theory of self-esteem and cultural worldviews: Empirical assessments and conceptual refinements. In M. P. Zanna (Ed.), *Advances in experimental social psychology* (Vol. 29, pp. 61–139). San Diego, CA: Academic.

Greenberg, J., Solomon, S., Veeder, M., Lyon, D., Pyszczynski, T., Rosenblatt, A., et al. (1990). Evidence for terror management theory II: The effects of mortality salience on reactions to those who threaten or bolster the cultural worldview. *Journal of Personality and Social Psychology, 58*, 308–318.

Haidt, J. (2003). The moral emotions. In R. J. Davidson, K. R. Scherer, & H. H. Goldsmith (Eds.), *Handbook of affective sciences* (pp. 852–870). Oxford, NY: Oxford University Press.

Haidt, J., & Morris, J. P. (2009). Finding the self in self-transcendent emotions. *Proceedings of the National Academy of Sciences of the United States of America, 106*, 7687–7688.

Harmon-Jones, E., Simon, L., Greenberg, J., Pyszczynski, T., Solomon, S., & McGregor, H. (1997). Terror management theory and self-esteem: Evidence that increased self-esteem reduces mortality salience effects. *Journal of Personality and Social Psychology, 72*, 24–36.

Hartstone, M., & Augoustinos, M. (1995). The minimal group paradigm: Categorization into two versus three groups. *European Journal of Social Psychology, 25*, 179–193.

Heatherton, T. F. (2011). Neuroscience of self and self-regulation. *Annual Review of Psychology, 62*, 363–390.

Heppner, W. L., Kernis, M. H., Lakey, C. E., Campbell, W. K., Goldman, B. M., Davis, P. J., et al. (2008). Mindfulness as a means of reducing aggressive behavior: Dispositional and situational evidence. *Aggressive Behavior, 34*, 486–496.

Hodgins, H. S. (2008). Motivation, threshold for threat, and quieting the ego. In H. A. Wayment & J. J. Bauer (Eds.), *Transcending self-interest: Psychological explorations of the quiet ego* (pp. 117–124). Washington, DC: American Psychological Association.

Hodgins, H. S. (2010). *Dividing the social world into 'Us' and 'Them'*. Paper presented at the 4th International Self-determination theory Conference, Ghent, Belgium.

Hodgins, H. S., & Adair, K. C. (2010). Attentional processes and meditation. *Consciousness and Cognition, 19*, 872–878.

Hodgins, H. S., Brown, A. B., & Carver, B. (2007). Autonomy and control motivation and self-esteem. *Self and Identity, 6*, 189–208.

Hodgins, H. S., & Knee, C. R. (2002). The integrating self and conscious experience. In E. L. Deci & R. M. Ryan (Eds.), *Handbook of self-determination research* (pp. 87–100). Rochester, NY: University of Rochester Press.

Hodgins, H. S., Koestner, R., & Duncan, N. (1996). On the compatibility of autonomy and relatedness. *Personality and Social Psychology Bulletin, 22*, 227–237.

Hodgins, H. S., & Liebeskind, E. (2003). Apology versus defense: Antecedents and consequences. *Journal of Experimental Social Psychology, 39*, 297–316.
Hodgins, H. S., Liebeskind, E., & Schwartz, W. (1996). Getting out of hot water: Facework in social predicaments. *Journal of Personality and Social Psychology, 71*, 300–314.
Hodgins, H. S., Weibust, K. S., Weinstein, N., Shiffman, S., Miller, A., Coombs, G., et al. (2010). The cost of self-protection: Threat response and performance as a function of autonomous and controlled motivations. *Personality and Social Psychology Bulletin, 36*, 1101–1114.
Hodgins, H. S., Yacko, H., & Gottlieb, E. (2006). Autonomy and nondefensiveness. *Motivation and Emotion, 30*, 283–293.
Hutcherson, C. A., Seppala, E. M., & Gross, J. J. (2008). Loving-kindness meditation increases social connectedness. *Emotion, 8*, 720–724.
Hwang, K. K. (2009). The development of indigenous counseling in contemporary Confucian communities. *Counseling Psychologist, 37*, 930–943.
Hwang, K. K., & Chang, J. (2009). Self-cultivation culturally sensitive psychotherapies in Confucian societies. *Counseling Psychologist, 37*, 1010–1032.
Jordan, C. H., Spencer, S. J., & Zanna, M. P. (2003). 'I love me…I love me not:' Implicit self-esteem, explicit self-esteem, and defensiveness. In S. J. Spencer, S. Fein, M. P. Zanna, & J. M. Olson (Eds.), *Motivated social perception: The Ontario symposium* (Vol. 9, pp. 117–145). Mahwah, NJ: Lawrence Erlbaum Associates.
Jordan, C. H., Spencer, S. J., & Zanna, M. P. (2005). Types of high self-esteem and prejudice: How implicit self-esteem relates to ethnic discrimination among high explicit self-esteem individuals. *Personality and Social Psychology Bulletin, 31*, 693–702.
Jordan, C. H., Spencer, S. J., Zanna, M. P., Hoshino-Browne, E., & Correll, J. (2003). Secure and defensive high self-esteem. *Journal of Personality and Social Psychology, 85*, 969–978.
Karr, A. (2007). *Contemplating reality: A practitioner's guide to the view in Indo-Tibetan Buddhism*. Boston: Shambhala.
Kasser, T., & Ryan, R. M. (1993). A dark side of the American dream: Correlates of financial success as a central life aspiration. *Journal of Personality and Social Psychology, 65*, 410–422.
Kasser, T., & Ryan, R. M. (1996). Further examining the American dream: Differential correlates of intrinsic and extrinsic goals. *Personality and Social Psychology Bulletin, 22*, 280–287.
Kiken, L. G., & Shook, N. J. (2011). Looking up: Mindfulness increases positive judgments and reduces negativity bias. *Social Psychological and Personality Science, 2*, 425–431.
Knee, C. R., Lonsbary, C., Canevello, A., & Patrick, H. (2005). Self-determination and conflict in romantic relationships. *Journal of Personality and Social Psychology, 89*, 997–1009.
Knee, C. R., Patrick, H., Vietor, N. A., Nanayakkara, A., & Neighbors, C. (2002). Self-determination as growth motivation in romantic relationships. *Personality and Social Psychology Bulletin, 28*, 609–619.
Knee, C. R., & Zuckerman, M. (1996). Causality orientations and the disappearance of the self-serving bias. *Journal of Research in Personality, 30*, 76–87.
Knee, C. R., & Zuckerman, M. (1998). A nondefensive personality: Autonomy and control as moderators of defensive coping and self-handicapping. *Journal of Research in Personality, 32*, 115–130.
Leary, M. R. (2007). Motivational and emotional aspects of the self. *Annual Review of Psychology, 58*, 317–344.
Leary, M. R., Adams, C. E., & Tate, E. B. (2006). Hypo-egoic self-regulation: Exercising self-control by diminishing the influence of the self. *Journal of Personality, 74*, 1803–1832.
Leary, M. R., Adams, C. E., & Tate, E. B. (2010). Hypo-egoic self-regulation. In R. H. Hoyle (Ed.), *Handbook of personality and self-regulation* (pp. 474–497). New York: Guilford.
Leary, M. R., & Baumeister, R. F. (2000). The nature and function of self-esteem: Sociometer theory. In M. P. Zanna (Ed.), *Advances in experimental social psychology* (Vol. 32, pp. 1–62). San Diego, CA: Academic.
Leudar, I., Marsland, V., & Nekvapil, J. (2004). On membership categorization: 'Us', 'them' and 'doing violence' in political discourse. *Discourse and Society, 15*, 2–3.

Levesque, C., & Brown, K. W. (2007). Mindfulness as a moderator of the effect of implicit motivational self-concept on day-to-day behavioral motivation. *Motivation and Emotion, 31*, 284–299.
Lieberman, M. D. (2007). Social cognitive neuroscience: A review of core processes. *Annual Review of Psychology, 58*, 259–289.
Lin, Y. C., Huang, C. L., Hodgins, H. S., & Chang, J. (2011). *Mindfulness and the us-them divide process*. Manuscript in preparation.
Lutz, A., Slagter, H. A., Dunne, J. D., & Davidson, R. J. (2008). Attention regulation and monitoring in meditation. *TRENDS in Cognitive Sciences, 12*, 163–169.
Masicampo, E. J., & Baumeister, R. R. (2007). Relating mindfulness and self-regulatory processes. *Psychological Inquiry, 18*, 255–258.
McGregor, H. A., Lieberman, J. D., Greenberg, J., Solomon, S., Arndt, J., Simon, L., et al. (1998). Terror management and aggression: Evidence that mortality salience motivates aggression against worldview-threatening others. *Journal of Personality and Social Psychology, 74*, 590–605.
McKay, R. T., & Dennett, D. C. (2009). The evolution of misbelief. *Behavioral and Brain Sciences, 32*, 493–561.
Moeller, S. J., Crocker, J., & Bushman, B. J. (2009). Creating hostility and conflict: Effects of entitlement and self-image goals. *Journal of Experimental Social Psychology, 45*, 448–452.
Moore, A., & Malinowski, P. (2009). Meditation, mindfulness and cognitive flexibility. *Consciousness and Cognition, 18*, 176–186.
Neighbors, C., & Knee, C. R. (2003). Self-determination and the consequences of social comparison. *Journal of Research in Personality, 37*, 529–546.
Neighbors, C., Vietor, N. A., & Knee, C. R. (2002). A motivational model of driving anger and aggression. *Personality and Social Psychology Bulletin, 28*, 324–335.
Niemiec, C. P., Brown, K. W., Kashdan, T. B., Cozzolino, P. J., Breen, W. E., Levesque-Bristol, C., et al. (2010). Being present in the face of existential threat: The role of trait mindfulness in reducing defensive responses to mortality salience. *Journal of Personality and Social Psychology, 99*, 344–365.
Oosterhof, N. N., & Todorov, A. (2008). The functional basis of face evaluation. *Proceedings of the National Academy of Sciences of the United States of America, 105*, 11087–11092.
Perdue, C. W., Dovidio, J. F., Gurtman, M. B., & Tyler, R. B. (1990). Us and them: Social categorization and the process of intergroup bias. *Journal of Personality and Social Psychology, 59*, 475–486.
Perreault, S., & Bourhis, R. Y. (1999). Ethnocentrism, social identification, and discrimination. *Journal of Personality and Social Psychology, 25*, 92–103.
Pyszczynski, T., Solomon, S., Greenberg, J., Arndt, J., & Schimel, J. (2004). Why do people need self-esteem? A theoretical and empirical review. *Psychological Bulletin, 130*, 435–468.
Reynolds, K. J., Turner, J. C., & Haslam, S. A. (2000). When are we better than them and they worse than us? A closer look at social discrimination in positive and negative domains. *Journal of Personality and Social Psychology, 78*, 64–80.
Rosenblatt, A., Greenberg, J., Solomon, S., Pyszczynski, T., & Lyon, D. (1989). Evidence for terror management theory.1. The effects of mortality salience on reactions to those who violate or uphold cultural-values. *Journal of Personality and Social Psychology, 57*, 681–690.
Ryan, R. M. (1991). The nature of the self in autonomy and relatedness. In J. Strauss & G. R. Goethals (Eds.), *Multidisciplinary perspectives on the self* (pp. 208–238). New York: Springer.
Ryan, R. M., & Deci, E. L. (2000). Self-determination theory and the facilitation of intrinsic motivation, social development, and well-being. *American Psychologist, 55*(1), 68–78.
Ryan, R. M., Deci, E. L., & Grolnick, W. S. (1995). Autonomy, relatedness, and the self: Their relation to development and psychopathology. In D. Cicchetti & D. J. Cohen (Eds.), *Developmental psychopathology: Vol. 1. Theory and methods* (pp. 618–655). New York: Wiley.

Sahdra, B. K., Shaver, P. R., & Brown, K. W. (2010). A scale to measure nonattachment: A Buddhist complement to western research on attachment and adaptive functioning. *Journal of Personality Assessment, 92*, 116–127.
Sedikides, C., Gaertner, L., & Toguchi, Y. (2003). Pancultural self-enhancement. *Journal of Personality and Social Psychology, 84*, 60–79.
Sedikides, C., & Gregg, A. P. (2008). Self-enhancement: food for thought. *Perspectives on Psychological Science, 3*, 102–116.
Sheldon, K. M., & McGregor, H. A. (2000). Extrinsic value orientation and "The tragedy of the commons". *Journal of Personality, 68*, 383–411.
Slagter, H. A., Lutz, A., Greischar, L. L., Francis, A. D., Nieuwenhuis, S., Davis, J. M., et al. (2007). Mental training affects distribution of limited brain resources. *Plos Biology, 5*, 1228–1235.
Soenens, B., Berzonsky, M. K., Vansteenkiste, M., Beyers, W., & Goossens, L. (2005). Identity styles and causality orientations: In search of the motivational underpinnings of the identity exploration process. *European Journal of Personality, 19*, 427–442.
Solomon, S., Greenberg, J., & Pyszczynski, T. (1991). A terror management theory of social-behavior – The psychological functions of self-esteem and cultural worldviews. In M. P. Zanna (Ed.), *Advances in experimental social psychology* (Vol. 24, pp. 93–159). San Diego, CA: Academic.
Spears, R., Gordijn, E., Dijksterhuis, A., & Stapel, D. A. (2004). Reaction in action: Intergroup contrast in automatic behavior. *Personality and Social Psychology Bulletin, 30*, 605–616.
Staub, E. (1988). The evolution of caring and nonaggressive persons and societies. *Journal of Social Issues, 44*, 81–100.
Stern, D. N. (1985). *The interpersonal world of the infant*. New York: Basic Books.
Tajfel, H. (1982). Social-psychology of inter-group relations. *Annual Review of Psychology, 33*, 1–39.
Tajfel, H., Billig, M. G., Bundy, R. P., & Flament, C. (1971). Social categorization and intergroup behaviour. *European Journal of Social Psychology, 1*, 149–178.
Tajfel, H., & Turner, J. C. (1979). An integrative theory of intergroup conflict. In W. G. Austin & S. Worchel (Eds.), *The social psychology of intergroup relations* (pp. 33–47). Monterey, CA: Brooks/Cole.
Tang, Y. Y., Ma, Y. H., Wang, J., Fan, Y. X., Feng, S. G., Lu, Q. L., et al. (2007). Short-term meditation training improves attention and self-regulation. *Proceedings of the National Academy of Sciences of the United States of America, 104*, 17152–17156.
Taylor, S. E., & Brown, J. D. (1988). Illusion and well-being – A social psychological perspective on mental-health. *Psychological Bulletin, 103*, 193–210.
Turner, J. C., Oakes, P. J., Haslam, S. A., & McGarty, C. (1994). Self and collective – Cognition and social-context. *Personality and Social Psychology Bulletin, 20*, 454–463.
Tversky, A. (1977). Features of similarity. *Psychological Review, 84*, 327–352.
Wegner, D. M. (2011). Setting free the bears: Escape from thought suppression. *American Psychologist, 66*, 671–680.
Weinstein, N., DeHaan, C. R., & Ryan, R. M. (2010). Attributing autonomous versus introjected motivation to helpers and the recipient experience: Effects on gratitude, attitudes, and well-being. *Motivation and Emotion, 34*, 418–431.
Weinstein, N., & Hodgins, H. S. (2009). The moderating role of autonomy and control on the benefits of written emotion expression. *Personality and Social Psychology Bulletin, 35*, 351–364.
Weinstein, N., Hodgins, H. S., & Ostvik-White, E. (2011). Humor as aggression: Effects of motivation on hostility expressed in humor appreciation. *Journal of Personality and Social Psychology, 100*, 1043–1055.
Weinstein, N., Hodgins, H. S., & Ryan, R. M. (2010). Autonomy and control in dyads: Effects on interaction quality and joint creative performance. *Personality and Social Psychology Bulletin, 36*, 1603–1617.

Weinstein, N., & Ryan, R. M. (2010). When helping helps: Autonomous motivation for prosocial behavior and its influence on well-being for the helper and recipient. *Journal of Personality and Social Psychology, 98*, 222–244.

Williams, J. (2010). Mindfulness and psychological process. *Emotion, 10*, 1–7.

Wit, A. P., & Kerr, N. L. (2002). "Me versus just us versus us all" categorization and cooperation in nested social dilemmas. *Journal of Personality and Social Psychology, 83*, 616–637.

Yamaguchi, S., Greenwald, A. G., Banaji, M. R., Murakami, F., Chen, D., Shiomura, K., et al. (2007). Apparent universality of positive implicit self-esteem. *Psychological Science, 18*, 498–500.

Chapter 6
The Self-Concept in Relationships

Martin F. Lynch

How people think about themselves, or their *self-concept*, is deeply rooted in the nature of their interpersonal relationships, and, further, has consequences for well-being. James (1890/1950), for example, suggested that "a man has as many social selves as there are individuals who recognize him and carry an image of him in their mind" (p. 294). Mead (1934) argued similarly that an "individual possesses a self only in relation to the selves of the other members of his social group" (p. 164). In a very real sense, it is the relationship that gives rise to the sense of self, as psychodynamic theorists long have argued (Winnicott, 1965). But what does it mean to 'be oneself,' what are the implications for well-being, and how are relationships involved? The link between self-concept and well-being is complex, and has been treated differently within different traditions. This chapter explores three perspectives on the link between self-concept and well-being: one which argues that well-being depends upon consistency in self-concept, a second which suggests that it is authenticity in self-concept that matters, and a third according to which convergence between one's actual view of self and one's ideal view of self leads to well-being. In each of these perspectives, there are consequences for well-being that suggest the existence of what some have called a 'coherence motive' (Habermas & Paha, 2001; King & Hicks, 2006; McAdams, 1985, 2001, 2006, 2008; McLean, 2005; McLean, Pasaputhi, & Pals, 2007; Pals, 2006; Swann & Bosson, 2008). That is, depending on one's theoretical starting point people strive variously to maintain consistency, to be authentic, or to approach their ideal view of self, and failing to do so has consequences for well-being. This chapter will explore each of these three traditions and will suggest how the construct of *autonomy support* may provide an integrative perspective for thinking about the self-concept and a motive toward coherence in the context of interpersonal relationships. I begin however with a review of some basic notions about the self-concept and its origins.

M.F. Lynch (✉)
Warner School of Education, University of Rochester, Rochester, NY, USA
e-mail: mlynch@warner.rochester.edu

N. Weinstein (ed.), *Human Motivation and Interpersonal Relationships: Theory, Research, and Applications*, DOI 10.1007/978-94-017-8542-6_6,

Historical Views of the Self-Concept

As noted by Harter (2006), early thinking about the self-concept was deeply influenced by the work of William James (1890/1950, 1910) and the symbolic interactionists Cooley (1902), Baldwin (1895), and Mead (1934). James made the important distinction between the *I-self*, or the self as knower, subject, agent, and the *Me-self*, or the self as known or object. The categorical representation of the Me-self is what contemporary psychologists generally refer to as the self-concept. Importantly for the present chapter, James acknowledged that a person could have different Me-selves depending on the social context, suggesting, as previously noted, that "a man has as many social selves as there are individuals who recognize him and carry an image of him in their mind" (James, 1890/1950, p. 294). In addition, he believed that self-concept played a critical role in the experience of self-esteem, based on the ratio of one's perceived successes to one's 'pretensions.' Implicit in this formulation is an understanding that self-esteem is linked to a perceived convergence between one's current or actual state and some preferred or ideal view of self toward which one strives. Further, the fact that life presents one with alternative pathways and versions of oneself requires the engagement of choice: "the seeker of his truest, strongest, deepest self must review the list [of options] carefully, and pick out the one on which to stake his salvation" (James, 1890, p. 14). James is here underscoring the fact that the I-self ultimately has a role in shaping the definition of the Me-self, and that some 'selves' may be more central to one's core, more 'true,' than others.

Despite his recognition of multiple social selves, James did not particularly emphasize the role of relationships in the development of the self. That topic was of course of great interest to later psychodynamic (Kernberg, 1975; Kohut, 1977; Winnicott, 1965), attachment theory (Ainsworth, 1979; Bowlbv, 1980), and humanistic (Rogers, 1961) thinkers, but early attention to the social construction of the self was given by the symbolic interactionists. For Cooley (1902), Baldwin (1895), and Mead (1934), the self was crafted through symbolic interactions in the form of linguistic exchanges with others, beginning in early childhood. This perspective is captured powerfully in Cooley's notion of the 'looking glass self,' according to which "significant others constituted a social mirror into which the individual gazes to detect their opinions toward the self," opinions which "in turn are incorporated into one's sense of self" (Harter, 2006, p. 511). Implied is a developmental process of internalization of others' opinions of oneself, but this process is not affectively neutral. To some extent one becomes the self one sees in the other's eyes, and this appraisal in turn has an impact on one's feelings about oneself, whether positive or negative. Within contemporary developmental approaches a corollary of the social construction viewpoint holds that, especially during adolescence, people develop "multiple selves" (Harter, 1999) such that "an individual comes to develop a self with each parent, a best friend, a romantic other, and classmates of each gender – selves that often are defined by very different self descriptors" and may be accompanied by "the pressure to be a particular self in each relational context" (Harter,

2006, p. 509). In other words, whereas James emphasized the role of the I-self in choosing one's truest self-definition, here we see an acknowledgment that relational forces 'outside' the self may conspire to impose a role-specific definition on the self.

From these early theories emerged an understanding that people can have multiple views of themselves, views which to an important degree are shaped by their interactions with others. From James as well we can draw the notion that this potential for multiplicity is linked to well-being in the form of self-esteem, that it serves a motivational role to the extent that people strive to realize their 'pretensions,' and that the I-self, or the self as agent, plays a role in choosing from among the possibilities available for self-definition. From this brief overview of early views on the self-concept I wish to turn now to a presentation of three different contemporary perspectives on the issue of self-definition which will suggest different ways in which the relationship between self-concept and well-being may be understood, whether in terms of consistency, authenticity, or ideal/actual convergence. I then turn to a discussion of how the construct of autonomy support may shed light on the optimizing role that relationships may play in this process.

The Self-Concept and Its Relation to Well-Being

As noted, the way that people think about themselves has implications for well-being. There is disagreement however on the mechanism by which self-concept influences well-being, with some suggesting that well-being is a matter of consistency, others that it is authenticity that counts, and still others that well-being is enhanced when people's self-view approaches their personal ideal. The following sections review these three perspectives.

Self-Concept Consistency

As previously noted, some have postulated that people have a motive to form and maintain a coherent self-concept (Habermas & Paha, 2001; King & Hicks, 2006; McAdams, 1985, 2001, 2006, 2008; McLean, 2005; McLean et al., 2007; Pals, 2006; Swann & Bosson, 2008). 'Being oneself,' here, means being consistent in how one views, experiences, and expresses oneself. Within Western psychology, theorists have long argued that consistency in one's identity is a hallmark of mental health, whereas inconsistency is evidence of conflict and defense. Lecky (1945), for example, argued that inconsistency among self-concepts is at the root of such unpleasant experiences as tension, anxiety, and confusion. Others have viewed inconsistency as a sign of fragmentation of the personality. Block (1961) for example referred to this as being a social 'chameleon,' and he and others (e.g., Horney, 1950; Winnicott, 1965) have seen inconsistency as indicative of a lack of a 'true self' or 'core self.' More recently, Donahue, Robbins, Roberts, and John (1993) argued that self-inconsistency is largely a defensive process that reflects an underlying fragmentation of the personality and bodes badly for well-being.

An alternative position, however, is that variability or inconsistency in self-presentation may not represent fragmentation or defense as much as it reflects social adaptation and flexibility. Along these lines, Mead (1934) argued that an "individual possesses a self only in relation to the selves of the other members of his social group" (p. 164). More recently in social constructivist accounts of the self, fluidity, flexibility, and complexity have been seen as adaptive within a postmodern world (Gergen, 1991). The more refined and 'specialized' one's sense of self under varying circumstances, the more one may be able to respond to the demands of changing and varied social circumstances (see also Linville, 1987).

These diverging takes on the meaning of variability and its relations with well-being have spawned a number of research studies (for reviews, see Campbell, Assanand, & Di Paula, 2003; Rafaeli-Mor & Steinberg, 2002). In two seminal studies, Donahue, Roberts and colleagues (Donahue, Robbins, Roberts, & John, 1993; Roberts & Donahue, 1994) employed an index they called *self-concept differentiation* (SCD) to tap the degree to which one's self-concept varied across important life roles. They found that higher SCD was associated with lower conscientiousness, agreeableness, and self-esteem, and with higher depression and neuroticism. Donahue and colleagues thus characterized SCD as *fragmentation*, a view supported by its negative association with well-being outcomes. Subsequently, Sheldon, Ryan, Rawsthorne, and Ilardi (1997) examined variability across life roles in the 'Big Five' traits, which traditionally are considered to be relatively stable and enduring over time and contexts (McCrae & Costa, 1999). They found substantial within-person variability in Big Five traits (see also McCrae, 2001) and, as Roberts and Donahue had predicted, greater within-person variability was negatively associated with well-being.

This literature, which suggests a negative relation between inconsistency and well-being, would seem to support the existence of a coherence motive which views coherence in terms of consistency; research on autobiographical memory, another tradition that has considered the issue of self-consistency, would seem to make the same point (Bluck, Alea, Habermas, & Rubin, 2005; Conway, Singer, & Tagini, 2004; Sutin & Robins, 2005, 2008).

With regard to the debate about consistency versus inconsistency, recent empirical work on personality expression has established that people do in fact display considerable variability or *inconsistency* in their self-views across situations (Baird, Le, & Lucas, 2006; Fleeson, 2001, 2004; Shoda et al., 1994). Fleeson (2001, 2004) for example, in his research on *density distributions* of personality traits, has shown that people routinely display almost every level of a given personality trait. (I make the argument that such research on personality is relevant to thinking about the self-concept to the extent that these studies make use of self-report measures of personality.) Perhaps more importantly, individuals differ significantly in the amount of situational variability in personality that they express (Baird et al., 2006; Biesanz & West, 2000; Biesanz, West, & Graziano, 1998; Fleeson, 2001, 2004; Larsen, 1989; Nesselroade, 1988; Paunonen & Jackson, 1985; Snyder, 1974), with some people departing further from their own mean levels than others do. This 'fact' of inconsistency however does not address the larger issue of *how*, or indeed *whether*, such inconsistency is related to well-being.

Baird et al. (2006) reported results of three studies they conducted that seem to have definitively answered the question. They first provided evidence that existing measures of self-concept consistency typically conflate mean-level information with variability in trait expression. Included among such studies are those that have used the 'SCD' index developed by Donahue et al. (1993). Then, Baird and colleagues demonstrated that once mean levels are removed, self-concept consistency is no longer related to well-being.

Some however have suggested that the relation of self-consistency to well-being depends upon cultural values. Clearly, cultures play a crucial role in shaping how people think (Vygotsky, 1977), and thus cultural orientations carry 'plausible consequences' for self-concept (Oyserman, Coon, & Kemmelmeier, 2002; see also Sedikides & Brewer, 2001). In terms of self-consistency, there may, for example, be different consequences for varying or failing to vary across interpersonal contexts for persons from individualist versus collectivist societies. *Idiocentrists* – those whose *self-construals* (Singelis, 1994) are primarily individualistic – have been argued to be on average less likely to modify their self-concepts to adapt to social circumstances and group demands. In contrast, *allocentrists* (people with primarily collectivistic self-construals) might more readily make accommodations in self-attributes from context to context. As Baumeister and Twenge (2003) observed, "members of independent societies see themselves and others in terms of relatively constant personality traits, whereas members of interdependent societies see personality and behavior as more dependent on the situation" (p. 344). This has suggested to some that whereas self-concept inconsistency might well represent fragmentation in individualistic cultures (and thus relate negatively to well-being), it may represent flexibility and contextual sensitivity (and thus relate positively to well-being) in collectivist cultures.

A study by Suh (2002) found support for the general negative effects of self-concept inconsistency on well-being, as well as evidence for cultural moderation of that effect. He found that inconsistency, rather than being adaptive in a collectivist context as some have argued, was negatively related to well-being in both an Asian (South Korean) and a western (U.S.) setting. However, culture did matter. This negative relation was less strong in the South Korean context. Although Suh did not directly assess participants' cultural self-construals, his findings point to the importance of considering cultural contexts as a potential moderator of variability effects.

Cross, Gore, and Morris (2003) assessed whether differences in relational self-construals within a U.S. sample would impact upon the self-consistency/well-being relation. They specifically explored whether participants whose relational self-construals were more interdependent might show less negative impact from self-concept inconsistency. They found that, although there was not a strong relation between one's self-construal style and self-concept consistency, there was a moderation effect such that self-concept consistency was less strongly related to well-being for those whose relational self-construal was highly interdependent. Although this lends support to the position that self-construals may influence the consistency-to-well-being relation, Cross et al. did not in this study assess non-Western cultural groups.

The existing research investigating the role of culture in the debate about consistency and well-being is limited in scope, and may be subject to the same methodological critique that Baird and colleagues (2006) made of the consistency literature, in general. To overcome these limitations, in addition to controlling for mean levels it would be necessary to test explicitly whether country membership or independent versus interdependent self-construals moderate the consistency-to-well-being relation. In addition, concerns raised by Baird et al. about how consistency has typically been computed can be addressed by using an experience sampling methodology. This is because experience sampling allows the researcher to track "real-time changes in self-reported personality across roles and situations" and "random moments over time while assessing the specific nature of the situation in which participants find themselves" (Baird et al., p. 515), as several researchers have already demonstrated (e.g., Bolger, Davis, & Rafaeli, 2003; Fleeson, 2001). Experience sampling would similarly allow tracking of fluctuations in self-concept across relationship contexts.

Authenticity in Self-Concept

The second approach to 'being oneself' has a long tradition in philosophy, going back at least to Kierkegaard, and emphasizes the importance of authenticity. In fact, existential and humanistic psychology (e.g., Rogers, 1961) have always seen authenticity as being important to mental health. Authenticity, genuineness, congruence are all related constructs in these traditions. 'Being oneself' is about being 'true' to oneself in the sense of being genuine and congruent. It is not so much whether one changes or adapts oneself across social contexts that is important, as whether one experiences either change or stability as reflecting one's true values and beliefs. Along similar lines, within the dynamic tradition the concept of authenticity relates to Winnicott's (1965) distinction between 'true self' and 'false self', in that, when acting from the true self, people feel real and 'in touch' with their core needs and emotions. In contrast, when acting from false self, people display 'as-if' personalities to gain approval in non-accepting social contexts. Horney (1950) similarly distinguished between one's real self and 'as-if' self-presentations.

Several researchers have provided more recent empirical evidence for the importance of authenticity in mental health. Kernis (2003), for example, showed that greater authenticity related to increased self-esteem and greater well-being in different social contexts (see also Kernis & Paradise, 2002; Ryan, La Guardia, & Rawsthorne, 2003). Sheldon and colleagues (1997), investigating both the authenticity and consistency perspectives, found that the experience of authenticity related to well-being in U.S. samples. In their study, they found that authenticity and inconsistency were negatively related to each other: the more authentic people felt themselves to be, the less inconsistent they were in their self-presentations across a number of life-roles.

It is important however to acknowledge that the relevance of authenticity to members of non-Western societies has been questioned, particularly by cross-cultural researchers (e.g., Markus, Kitayama, & Heiman, 1996), who consider authenticity to be a Western construct that may have minimal relevance in other cultural contexts. Although some have suggested that authenticity may in fact be valued in Eastern societies (Doi, 1986), to date limited empirical research has addressed the issue. In one study, Lynch and Ryan (2004) found that in three countries, China, Russia, and the United States, both authenticity and consistency were related to well-being and these associations were largely unmoderated by either independent or interdependent self-construals. When allowed to compete for variance in well-being, however, only authenticity was significant in each of the three countries. This study however did not take into account the concerns raised in the later paper by Baird and colleagues (2006) about measures of inconsistency and the need to control for mean levels in self expression, so its results need to be replicated and confirmed.

Convergence Between Ideal and Actual Self-Concept

A third perspective suggests that the coherence motive may be about convergence or movement toward an ideal view of self. James (1910) early on noted that people can discriminate between who they are and who they would like to be. 'Being oneself' means being one's ideal self. The idea that people can have different views of themselves as they actually are and as they would ideally like to be, and that these self-concept discrepancies have implications for well-being, has a long tradition in humanistic (Rogers & Dymond, 1954) and social-cognitive (Higgins, 1987) psychology, and indeed has been suggested by others as well (e.g., Lecky, 1945).

Rogers (1961) argued that the self-concept plays an important role in the regulation of behavior. In Rogers' view, the self-concept determines which aspects of experience we become aware of and which aspects have to be 'repressed' in order to minimize conflict, whether the conflict is interpersonal or intrapersonal in nature. Whether particular aspects of the self-concept are deemed acceptable or not is largely determined by the nature of our interactions with others. For Rogers, a particularly salient aspect of relationships in this regard is the experience of being conditionally regarded by important others, particularly by parents, because such experiences can impose 'conditions of worth' that shape how we think about ourselves. The child who grows up feeling that her worth or lovability depends on conforming to others' expectations may learn to stifle her true wishes, needs, and preferences and take on an incongruent, 'as-if' view of self that conforms to the other's expectations. In contrast, the child who grows up experiencing unconditional regard from her caregivers will likely develop a sense of self that is more congruent, one in which what is truly felt and experienced can be explored and given expression because it is met with interest and acceptance by the child's important others. In this regard, it is important to note that Rogers believed that people also have an ideal view of themselves, in addition to their current or actual self-concept. In a way that is reminiscent of James' (1890, 1910) earlier work, Rogers argued that the gap between the current or actual view of self and the ideal view of self serves as an important gauge of self-esteem: the larger the gap, the lower one's self-esteem, while the closer people are to their ideal the better they feel about themselves. He believed that when people become aware of a gap between their current and ideal view of self they experience discomfort. Indeed, he argued that this awareness plays a major role in motivating people to seek counseling and psychotherapy. In a number of innovative studies involving Q-sorts of idiographic self-statements, Rogers and his colleagues provided empirical support for a link between self-concept discrepancies and well-being (Rogers & Dymond, 1954). A reduction in ideal/actual discrepancies was such an important therapeutic outcome that Rogers considered it to be an indication of positive personality change (Rogers).

From a social-cognitive perspective Higgins (1987, 1989) similarly argued and provided empirical evidence that when people experience a discrepancy between their actual self-concept and their ideal self-concept, they are likely to experience distress in the form of depressed affect. Accordingly, people generally seek to reduce such ideal/actual self-concept discrepancies. Regarding the notion of a coherence motive, both the perspective of Rogers and that of Higgins are *motivational* in the sense that both predict that people are motivated to reduce perceived discrepancies between ideal and actual views of the self. While Higgins' theory suggests that what is motivating is the desire to reduce discomfort, Rogers' view is more 'organismic' in that it suggests an integrative, forward-moving, growth-oriented tendency.

These researchers suggest ideal/actual discrepancies in self-concept are associated with distress, and that well-being is therefore linked with greater congruence between ideal and actual self-views. In line with the focus of the present chapter, it is important to ask whether there are factors in the interpersonal environment that may help to reduce such discrepancies and to promote congruence. Higgins' (1987, 1989) initial work did not address this possibility. Rogers (1961) however argued that the therapeutic relationship could play an important role in this regard. To the extent that it was characterized by genuineness, empathy, and unconditional positive regard, the relationship between therapist and client could facilitate the reduction of ideal/actual discrepancies by creating an environment in which clients would feel safe to explore and integrate aspects of themselves that previously had been treated as off-limits or alien to the self. By exploring and integrating the various aspects of the self in the context of the therapeutic relationship, clients could experience greater freedom to pursue their personal ideal for the person they would like to be. Although his research focused on the therapeutic relationship, Rogers speculated that the same principles should apply to everyday, non-professional relationships, as well.

To test the prediction that discrepancies between ideal and actual self-concept would have implications for well-being across cultures, Lynch, La Guardia, and Ryan (2009) in a recent study administered self-report surveys to participants in China (N = 245), Russia (N = 192), and the United States (N = 205). In an initial session, participants were asked to complete a measure of ideal self-concept assessed in terms of a 30-item set of Big Five trait items (Sheldon et al., 1997). Participants were given the instruction, "Think of the attributes or characteristics you would ideally like to have – the type of person you wish, desire, or hope to be. Regardless of other people's opinions, these are the attributes that you feel are a reflection of how you would be ideally." The phrase, "regardless of other people's opinions," was included in order to increase the likelihood that participants' ideal ratings would reflect personally held values rather than socially desirable trait expressions. Then they were provided the stem, "Ideally, I would like to see myself as someone who is," followed by each of the Big Five adjectives. Ideal self-concept scores were the average of the six items for each subscale, yielding an ideal self-concept score for each of the Big Five dimensions (Extraversion, Neuroticism, Agreeableness, Openness to Experiences, and Conscientiousness).

Measures in Session 2 focused on within-person variations across six, everyday relationships: mother, father, best friend, romantic partner, roommate, and a self-selected teacher. The 'teacher' target was included so that a potentially hierarchical-subordinate relationship would be assessed along with parental and peer relationships, and so that temporary as well as more lasting relationships would be included. For each relationship, participants completed measures of perceived autonomy support (to be discussed in more detail, below), Big Five self-concept (using the same items administered at Session 1), and well-being (well-being within each relationship was computed as a composite of relationship satisfaction, subjective vitality, and positive and negative affect). In this way separate measures of actual self-concept, autonomy support, and well-being were obtained for each relationship.

Ideal/actual self-concept discrepancies were calculated for each of the Big Five as the absolute difference between a participant's ideal self-concept, measured at Session 1, and his or her actual self-concept within each particular relationship as assessed at Session 2.

A preliminary analysis using paired-sample t-tests determined that, indeed, in each of the three countries participants in general ideally preferred to see themselves as more extraverted, conscientious, agreeable, and open to experience, but as less neurotic, than they actually saw themselves.

Multilevel modeling (Fleeson, 2007; Lynch, 2012) was used in order to test the prediction that there would be a within-person process relating self-concept discrepancies to well-being. As expected, in each country, for the typical individual the larger the gap between actual self-concept and one's ideal the greater the decrement to well-being.

Lynch et al. (2009) performed the same analyses after combining data from the three countries in order to test whether country membership would moderate any of the associations. For the analysis testing the association between ideal/actual discrepancies and well-being, there were no main effects by country. There were, however, several significant interactions. The interactions indicated that, although larger discrepancies were associated with poorer well-being outcomes for the typical individual in all three countries, for extraversion, neuroticism, agreeableness, and openness these associations were stronger (more negative) for participants from the United States compared to those from China. The associations were stronger among Russian compared to Chinese participants for neuroticism and agreeableness.

Lynch et al. (2009) thus provided initial evidence for a within-person process relating ideal/actual self-concept discrepancies with decrements to well-being. Although it is notable that the findings held across three countries that likely differ in important respects, it remains important to test these associations in other countries and to test whether a measured dimension of culture, such as independent versus interdependent self-construals (Singelis, 1994), might moderate these associations. As well, because these results were obtained in a lab-based survey study, it is important to test whether they are generalizable to daily experiences in various interpersonal settings.

Building on this initial research, Przybylski, Weinstein, Murayama, Lynch, and Ryan (2012) conducted two studies to test the notion that one reason people play video games is that games allow them to "try on" ideal aspects of themselves that they might not otherwise be able to express. One study (N=144) used a within-subjects design in which participants responded to introductory questionnaires, played three different video games in the media laboratory, and completed questionnaires after each game. A second study (N=979) used a between-subjects design in which players were recruited from an online gaming community and completed a set of questionnaires. In both laboratory and observational designs, the researchers found that convergence between people's experience of themselves during play and their concept of their ideal selves (both measured in terms of the Big Five personality dimensions) was related to enjoyment of play and positive shifts in affect after play. Among other things, these studies provide evidence from another domain of behavior that a gap between ideal and actual self-concept has implications for important outcomes related to motivation and well-being.

Autonomy Support, Self-Concept, and the Relationship Context: An Integrative Framework

From the preceding sections it seems clear that how people think about themselves has implications for well-being, and that, in one way or another, their interpersonal relationships are implicated in the process. Harter (2006) for example recognized that relationships can create pressures for people to view themselves in particular ways, and others from the psychodynamic tradition understood how the early relationship between caregiver and child can create conditions that facilitate the expression of either a true self or, alternatively, a false, 'as-if' self (Horney, 1950; Winnicott, 1965). From the humanistic perspective, Rogers (1961) understood how self-views can be influenced either by unconditional positive regard or by 'conditions of worth,' with very different results for the child's integration and well-being. In this section, I wish to explore how an aspect of relationships known as autonomy support may provide a positive and integrative framework for understanding the role of relationships in promoting both the self-concept and well-being.

Within contemporary psychology, the construct of autonomy has been most clearly articulated from within the self-determination theory tradition (Deci & Ryan, 1985; Ryan & Deci, 2000). Self-determination theory (SDT) in turn derives its understanding of the construct from the phenomenological (Husserl, 1980; Pfander, 1908/1967; Ricoeur, 1966) and analytic (Dworkin, 1988; Frankfurt, 1969) traditions in philosophy and emphasizes *self-rule* in contrast to heteronomy or *rule by the other*.

Autonomy, as conceptualized by SDT, concerns the need to feel oneself able to make personally meaningful choices, to take initiative, and to pursue personally held goals and ideals. Thus, within SDT autonomy is conceptualized as a basic psychological need, the satisfaction of which conduces toward intrinsically motivated behavior, well-being, and the facilitation of inherent, organismic processes of integration. Importantly, social contexts generally and interpersonal relationships in particular can either support, fail to support, or even undermine the satisfaction of autonomy as a basic need. Relationship partners who are experienced as autonomy supportive provide opportunities for choice, initiative-taking, and personal goal-pursuit, avoid pressuring or controlling verbal or nonverbal behaviors, and generally engage in trying to understand the other person's internal frame of reference (Grolnick & Ryan, 1989; Reeve, 2002; Reeve, Bolt, & Cai, 1999; Ryan & Lynch, 2003). Importantly for the self-concept, a relationship that is experienced as supportive of the need for autonomy (in contrast to a relationship experienced as controlling or pressuring) should promote healthy self-esteem (Deci & Ryan, 1995).

In terms of the coherence motive and the three perspectives under discussion in the present chapter, in general, SDT does not make any specific predictions pertaining to consistency, *per se*, viewing it as an essentially neutral phenomenon, but the constructs of autonomy and autonomy support do lend themselves to specific predictions relative to the other two perspectives discussed herein. Specifically, in the context of the current chapter, autonomy supportive relationships provide a likely context in which to feel free to pursue the self one would ideally like to be. Thus, it would be logical to expect that there should be greater convergence between ideal and actual self-concept in autonomy supportive relationships. Similarly, autonomy is closely related to the idea of authenticity (Ryan & Deci, 2004), and SDT argues that people generally feel it easier to be authentic in relationships experienced as autonomy supportive.

There is some initial empirical evidence linking autonomy supportive relationships with both authenticity in self-concept and convergence between ideal and actual self-concept. In the cross-cultural study mentioned earlier, Lynch and Ryan (2004) found that autonomy supportive relationships conduced toward greater well-being, more 'positive' expressions of Big Five self-concept (that is, more extraversion, openness to experience, agreeableness, and conscientiousness, and less neuroticism), and authenticity, in three cultures. These relations held even when independent and interdependent self-construals were taken into account. Thus, this study provided evidence that support for autonomy is an optimizing quality in relationships, with particular implications for self-concept.

In their cross-cultural study investigating the relation between well-being and ideal/actual self-concept discrepancies, Lynch and colleagues (2009) also tested the role of autonomy supportive relationships in helping people to approach their self-endorsed ideal view of self, arguing, in line with self-determination theory, that interpersonal autonomy support should facilitate people's innate propensities toward integration and should allow people to pursue their personally held ideal. They also reasoned that this would provide a further test of Rogers' (1961) prediction that everyday relationships have the potential to facilitate integration of the self-concept and personality. Using multilevel modeling, Lynch and colleagues found that there was, indeed, a within-person process linking autonomy support with self-concept discrepancies, in line with predictions made by Rogers and self-determination theory. Specifically, people reported feeling closer to their personal ideal view of self when with partners they experienced as being autonomy supportive, and, conversely, reported being further from their personal ideal with partners experienced as controlling. This association held in all three countries – China, Russia, and the United States – and was not moderated by country membership. In addition, autonomy support partially mediated the association between ideal/actual discrepancies and well-being, suggesting not only that autonomy support plays an important role in the expression of self-concept, but that ideal/actual discrepancies in themselves carry important implications for well-being that are not wholly accounted for by satisfaction of the need for autonomy.

The empirical evidence thus far is limited, but it suggests that the experience of autonomy and its support in interpersonal relationships may indeed be an optimizing quality in the expression of the self-concept. When in relationships experienced as autonomy supportive, people see themselves as being more authentic in their self-expressions and, additionally, as being closer to their personally held ideal view of self. Further, greater authenticity and closer convergence with one's ideal seem clearly to be associated with greater well-being. These associations have been found to hold in several different cultures around the world, to date. What is not yet clear is the relation between authenticity and attaining one's ideal view of self, because it is possible that one's ideals could be either introjected or personally endorsed, that is, one's ideal view of self could in theory be more or less autonomously internalized (see, e.g., Lynch et al., 2009; Rogers & Dymond, 1954). Presumably, given the links between autonomy support and authenticity (Lynch & Ryan, 2004) and autonomy support and ideal/actual self-concept convergence (Lynch et al., 2009), one's ideal self-concept will often be one's authentic self-concept. Those associations however need to be tested, and may be moderated for example by the experience of parental conditional regard (Rogers, 1961): ideal views of self may well be less authentic and less congruent, in Rogers' sense, for the child who, while growing up, learned to value a self that conformed to the wishes, demands, and expectations of others rather than to his or her own inner needs and personal preferences. I suspect that, developmentally speaking, experiencing one's parents as conditionally regarding forces children to sacrifice the need for autonomy for the need for relatedness. This is because, in evolutionary terms, given the human child's prolonged period of dependence preserving relatedness to one's caregivers is probably more essential for survival than is autonomy. When forced to sacrifice autonomy for relatedness, however, there should be predictable consequences for the self-concept and for well-being. Specifically, in order to preserve the relationship with one's parents, ideal views of self will likely become more introjected (false, as-if) and less authentic, and there should be decrements to well-being as a result. Parents who provide unconditional regard for their children, on the other hand, allow the needs for relatedness and autonomy to be met in tandem, likely promoting the internalization of ideal self-views that are more genuine, true, and authentic. In this model, it is autonomy, specifically, that promotes the internalization of ideals that are authentic and whose realization leads to well-being, while experiences of conditional regard effectively force the child to choose relatedness over autonomy, thereby interrupting and moderating these associations. These predictions however, need to be tested.

In light of James' (1890) argument that the I-self plays an important role in self-definition, and Harter's (2006) understanding of the way in which social contexts may pressure people to adopt particular self-definitions, it is indeed exciting that this contemporary line of research underscores the important role played by autonomy and interpersonal autonomy support in the way that people think about themselves. In light of these findings, I suggest that future research further investigate the possibility that to the extent that a motive for coherence exists, what it more accurately represents is not so much a motive toward consistency, *per se*, but a motive toward realizing one's truest, most authentic and ideal self, a motive that can be fostered or undermined by one's interpersonal relationships to the degree that they are experienced as either autonomy supportive or controlling.

References

Ainsworth, M. (1979). Infant-mother attachment. *American Psychologist, 34*, 932–937.

Baird, B. M., Le, K., & Lucas, R. E. (2006). On the nature of intraindividual personality variability: Reliability, validity, and associations with well-being. *Journal of Personality and Social Psychology, 90*, 512–527.

Baldwin, J. M. (1895). *Social and ethical interpretations in mental development: A study in social psychology*. New York: Macmillan.

Baumeister, R. F., & Twenge, J. M. (2003). The social self. In M. J. Lerner (Ed.), *Handbook of psychology: Personality and social psychology* (Vol. 5, pp. 327–352). New York: Wiley.

Biesanz, J. C., & West, S. G. (2000). Personality coherence: Moderating self-other profile agreement and profile consensus. *Journal of Personality and Social Psychology, 79*, 425–437.

Biesanz, J. C., West, S. G., & Graziano, W. G. (1998). Moderators of self-other agreement: Reconsidering temporal stability in personality. *Journal of Personality and Social Psychology, 75*, 467–477.

Block, J. (1961). Ego-identity, role variability, and adjustment. *Journal of Consulting and Clinical Psychology, 59*, 392–397.

Bluck, S., Alea, N., Habermas, T., & Rubin, D. R. (2005). A TALE of three functions: The self-reported uses of autobiographical memory. *Social Cognition, 23*, 91–117.
Bolger, N., Davis, A., & Rafaeli, E. (2003). Diary methods: Capturing life as it is lived. *Annual Review of Psychology, 54*, 579–616.
Bowlbv, J. (1980). *Attachment and loss: Vol. 3. Loss, sadness, and depression*. New York: Basic Books.
Campbell, J. D., Assanand, S., & Di Paula, A. (2003). The structure of the self-concept and its relation to psychological adjustment. *Journal of Personality, 71*, 115–140.
Conway, M. A., Singer, J. A., & Tagini, A. (2004). The self and autobiographical memory: Correspondence and coherence. *Social Cognition, 22*, 491–529.
Cooley, C. H. (1902). *Human nature and the social order*. New York: Charles Scribner & Sons.
Cross, S. E., Gore, J. S., & Morris, M. L. (2003). The relational-interdependent self-construal, self-concept consistency, and well-being. *Journal of Personality and Social Psychology, 85*, 933–944.
Deci, E. L., & Ryan, R. M. (1985). *Intrinsic motivation and self-determination in human behavior*. New York: Plenum.
Deci, E. L., & Ryan, R. M. (1995). Human autonomy: The basis for true self-esteem. In M. Kernis (Ed.), *Efficacy, agency, and self-esteem* (pp. 31–49). New York: Plenum Publishing Co.
Doi, T. (1986). *The anatomy of the self: The individual versus society* (M. A. Harbison, Trans.). New York: Harper & Row.
Donahue, E. M., Robbins, R. W., Roberts, B. W., & John, O. P. (1993). The divided self: Concurrent and longitudinal effects of psychological adjustment and social roles on self-concept differentiation. *Journal of Personality and Social Psychology, 64*, 834–846.
Dworkin, G. (1988). *The theory and practice of autonomy*. New York: Cambridge University Press.
Fleeson, W. (2001). Toward a structure- and process-integrated view of personality: Traits as density distributions of states. *Journal of Personality and Social Psychology, 80*(6), 1011–1027.
Fleeson, W. (2004). Moving personality beyond the person-situation debate: The challenge and opportunity of within-person variability. *Current Directions in Psychological Science, 13*, 83–87.
Fleeson, W. (2007). Studying personality processes: Explaining change in between-persons longitudinal and within-person multilevel models. In R. W. Robins, R. C. Fraley, & R. F. Krueger (Eds.), *Handbook of research methods in personality psychology* (pp. 523–542). New York: Guilford.
Frankfurt, H. G. (1969). Alternate possibilities and moral responsibility. *The Journal of Philosophy, 66*, 829–839.
Gergen, K. J. (1991). *The saturated self: Dilemmas of identity in contemporary life*. New York: Basic Books.
Grolnick, W. S., & Ryan, R. M. (1989). Parent styles associated with children's self-regulation and competence in school. *Journal of Educational Psychology, 81*, 143–154.
Habermas, T., & Paha, C. (2001). The development of coherence in adolescents' life narratives. *Narrative Inquiry, 11*, 35–54.
Harter, S. (1999). *The construction of the self*. New York: Guilford Press.
Harter, S. (2006). The self. In N. Eisenberg, W. Damon, & R. M. Lerner (Eds.), *Handbook of child psychology: Vol. 3. Social, emotional, and personality development* (pp. 505–570). Hoboken, NJ: Wiley.
Higgins, E. T. (1987). Self-discrepancy: A theory relating self and affect. *Psychological Review, 94*, 319–340.
Higgins, E. T. (1989). Self-discrepancy theory: What patterns of self-beliefs cause people to suffer? *Advances in Experimental Social Psychology, 22*, 93–136.
Horney, K. (1950). *Neurosis and human growth: The struggle toward self-realization*. New York: W.W. Norton & Company.
Husserl, E. (1980). *Ideas pertaining to a pure phenomenology and to a phenomenological philosophy—Third book: Phenomenology and the foundations of the sciences* (T. E. Klein & W. E. Pohl, Trans.). Dordrecht: Kluwer.

James, W. (1890/1950). *The principles of psychology*. Cambridge, MA: Harvard University Press.
James, W. (1910). *Psychology: The briefer course*. New York: Holt.
Kernberg, O. F. (1975). *Borderline conditions and pathological narcissism*. New York: Aronson.
Kernis, M. H. (2003). Toward a conceptualization of optimal self-esteem. *Psychological Inquiry, 14*, 1–26.
Kernis, M. H., & Paradise, A. W. (2002). Distinguishing between secure and fragile forms of high self-esteem. In E. L. Deci & R. M. Ryan (Eds.), *Handbook of self-determination research* (pp. 339–360). Rochester, NY: University of Rochester Press.
King, L. A., & Hicks, J. A. (2006). Narrating the self in the past and the future: Implications for maturity. *Journal of Research in Human Development, 3*, 121–138.
Kohut, H. (1977). *The restoration of the self*. New York: International Universities Press.
Larsen, R. J. (1989). A process approach to personality: Utilizing time as a facet of data. In D. Buss & N. Cantor (Eds.), *Personality psychology: Recent trends and emerging directions* (pp. 177–193). New York: Springer.
Lecky, P. (1945). *Self-consistency: A theory of personality*. New York: Island.
Linville, P. W. (1987). Self-complexity as a cognitive buffer against stress-related illness and depression. *Journal of Personality and Social Psychology, 52*, 663–676.
Lynch, M. F. (2012). Using multilevel modeling in counseling research. *Measurement and Evaluation in Counseling and Development, 45*, 211–224.
Lynch, M. F., La Guardia, J. G., & Ryan, R. M. (2009). On being yourself in different cultures: Ideal and actual self-concept, autonomy support, and well-being in China, Russia, and the United States. *The Journal of Positive Psychology, 4*, 290–304.
Lynch, M. F., & Ryan, R. M. (2004). On being yourself: Consistency versus authenticity of self-concept in cultural and interpersonal contexts. In H. W. Marsh, J. Baumert, G. E. Richards, & U. Trautwein (Eds.), *Self-concept, motivation and identity: Where to from here? Proceedings of the third international biennial SELF research conference, in Berlin*. Sydney, Australia: SELF Research Centre, University of Western Sydney.
Markus, H. R., Kitayama, S., & Heiman, R. J. (1996). Culture and "basic" psychological principles. In E. T. Higgins & A. W. Kruglanski (Eds.), *Social psychology: Handbook of basic principles* (pp. 857–913). New York: Guilford Press.
McAdams, D. P. (1985). *Power, intimacy, and the life story: Personological inquiries into identity*. New York: Guilford Press.
McAdams, D. P. (2001). *The person: An integrated introduction to personality psychology* (3rd ed.). Fort Worth, TX: Harcourt.
McAdams, D. P. (2006). The problem of narrative coherence. *Journal of Constructivist Psychology, 19*, 109–125.
McAdams, D. P. (2008). Personal narratives and the life story. In O. John, R. Robins, & L. Pervin (Eds.), *Handbook of personality: Theory and research* (3rd ed., pp. 241–261). New York: Guilford Press.
McCrae, R. R. (2001). Facts and interpretations of personality trait stability: A reply to Quackenbush. *Theory & Psychology, 11*, 837–844.
McCrae, R. R., & Costa, P. T. (1999). A five-factor theory of personality. In L. A. Pervin & O. P. John (Eds.), *Handbook of personality: Theory and research* (2nd ed., pp. 139–153). New York: Guilford Press.
McLean, K. C. (2005). Late adolescent identity development: Narrative meaning-making and memory telling. *Developmental Psychology, 41*, 683–691.
McLean, K. C., Pasaputhi, M., & Pals, J. L. (2007). Selves creating stories creating selves: A process model of self development. *Personality and Social Psychology Review, 11*, 262–278.
Mead, G. H. (1934). *Mind, self, and society: From the standpoint of a social behaviorist*. Chicago: University of Chicago Press.
Nesselroade, J. R. (1988). Some implications of the trait-state distinction for the study of development across the life span: The case of personality research. In P. B. Baltes, D. L. Featherman, & R. M. Lerner (Eds.), *Life-span development and behavior* (Vol. 8, pp. 163–189). Hillsdale, NJ: Lawrence Erlbaum Associates.

Oyserman, D., Coon, H. M., & Kemmelmeier, M. (2002). Rethinking individualism and collectivism: Evaluation of theoretical assumptions and meta-analyses. *Psychological Bulletin, 128*, 3–72.

Pals, J. L. (2006). Authoring a second chance in life: Emotion and transformational processing within narrative identity. *Research in Human Development, 3*, 101–120.

Paunonen, S. V., & Jackson, D. N. (1985). Idiographic measurement strategies for personality and prediction: Some unredeemed promissory notes. *Psychological Review, 92*, 486–511.

Pfander, A. (1908/1967). *Phenomenology of willing and motivation* (H. Spiegelberg, Trans.). Evanston, IL: Northwestern University Press.

Przybylski, A. K., Weinstein, N., Murayama, K., Lynch, M. F., & Ryan, R. M. (2012). The ideal self at play: The appeal of videogames that let you be all you can be. *Psychological Science, 23*, 69–76.

Rafaeli-Mor, E., & Steinberg, J. (2002). Self-complexity and well-being: A review and research synthesis. *Personality and Social Psychology Review, 6*, 31–58.

Reeve, J. (2002). Self-determination theory applied to educational settings. In E. L. Deci & R. M. Ryan (Eds.), *Handbook of self-determination research* (pp. 183–203). Rochester, NY: University of Rochester Press.

Reeve, J., Bolt, E., & Cai, Y. (1999). Autonomy-supportive teachers: How they teach and motivate students. *Journal of Educational Psychology, 91*, 537–548.

Ricoeur, P. (1966). *Freedom and nature: The voluntary and the involuntary* (E. V. Kohak, Trans.). Chicago: Northwestern University Press.

Roberts, B. W., & Donahue, E. M. (1994). One personality, multiple selves: Integrating personality and social roles. *Journal of Personality, 62*, 199–218.

Rogers, C. R. (1961). *On becoming a person: A therapist's view of psychotherapy*. Boston: Houghton Mifflin.

Rogers, C. R., & Dymond, R. F. (Eds.). (1954). *Psychotherapy and personality change*. Chicago: University of Chicago Press.

Ryan, R. M., & Deci, E. L. (2000). Self-determination theory and the facilitation of intrinsic motivation, social development, and well-being. *American Psychologist, 55*, 68–78.

Ryan, R. M., & Deci, E. L. (2004). Autonomy is no illusion: Self-determination theory and the empirical study of authenticity, awareness, and will. In J. Greenberg, S. L. Koole, & T. Pyszczynski (Eds.), *Handbook of experimental existential psychology* (pp. 449–479). New York: Guilford Press.

Ryan, R. M., La Guardia, J. G., & Rawsthorne, L. J. (2003). *Self-complexity and the authenticity of self-aspects: Effects on well being and resilience to stressful events*. Unpublished manuscript, University of Rochester.

Ryan, R. M., & Lynch, M. F. (2003). Motivation and classroom management. In R. Curren (Ed.), *A companion to the philosophy of education* (pp. 260–271). Oxford, UK: Blackwell.

Sedikides, C., & Brewer, M. B. (Eds.). (2001). *Individual self, relational self, collective self.* Philadelphia: Psychology Press.

Sheldon, K. M., Ryan, R. M., Rawsthorne, L. J., & Ilardi, B. (1997). Trait self and true self: Cross-role variation in the Big-Five personality traits and its relations with psychological authenticity and subjective well-being. *Journal of Personality and Social Psychology, 73*, 1380–1393.

Shoda, Y., Mischel, W., & Wright, J. C. (1994). Intraindividual stability in the organization of patterning behavior: Incorporating psychological situations into the idiographic analysis of personality. *Journal of Personality and Social Psychology, 67*, 674–687.

Singelis, T. M. (1994). The measurement of independent and interdependent self-construals. *Personality and Social Psychology Bulletin, 20*, 580–591.

Snyder, M. (1974). Self-monitoring of expressive behavior. *Journal of Personality and Social Psychology, 30*, 526–537.

Suh, E. M. (2002). Culture, identity consistency, and subjective well-being. *Journal of Personality and Social Psychology, 83*, 1378–1391.

Sutin, A. R., & Robins, R. W. (2005). Continuity and correlates of emotions and motives in self-defining memories. *Journal of Personality, 73*, 793–824.

Sutin, A. R., & Robins, R. W. (2008). When the "I" looks at the "me": Autobiographical memory, visual perspective, and the self. *Consciousness and Cognition, 17*, 1386–1397.
Swann, W. B., Jr., & Bosson, J. (2008). Identity negotiation: A theory of self and social interaction. In O. John, R. Robins, & L. Pervin (Eds.), *Handbook of personality psychology: Theory and research*. New York: Guilford.
Vygotsky, L. (1977). The development of higher psychological functions. *Soviet Psychology, 15*, 60–73.
Winnicott, D. W. (1965). *The maturational processes and the facilitating environment*. New York: International Universities Press.

Chapter 7
Self-Determination and Regulation of Conflict in Romantic Relationships

C. Raymond Knee, Ben Porter, and Lindsey M. Rodriguez

Self-Determination and Regulation of Conflict in Romantic Relationships

Even the most established, stable romantic relationships have their moments of friction. Sometimes these moments devolve into far longer patterns of ups and downs (or mostly just downs). Other times, a little bit of friction stimulates a deeper understanding and negotiation of partners' needs and improved mutual need fulfillment. Much of the essential negotiation between partners in romantic relationships requires that partners be aware of their own needs, and are able to communicate these effectively to each other, without lying, defending, accusing or blaming. Indeed, a cycle of negative reciprocity in which partners respond to each other's negative communication with equally negative responses, is one characteristic of distressed relationships that strongly predicts later relationship dissolution (Gottman & Notarius, 2000).

According to self-determination theory (Deci & Ryan, 1985b, 2000), being self-determined means that one's actions are autonomous, freely chosen, and fully endorsed by the self rather than coerced or pressured by external forces or internal expectations. This definition emphasizes authenticity of choices and behaviors that are congruent with one's needs, a mindful, reflective awareness of those needs, and the capacity of one's social environment to support them. Within romantic relationships, self-determination also refers to fully endorsing one's own involvement in the relationship, rather than feeling coerced, guilty, or not knowing why one is involved in the relationship (Knee, Lonsbary, Canevello, & Patrick, 2005). Additionally, autonomy in romantic relationships has been characterized as growth motivation, or the tendency to approach relationship conflicts nondefensively, seeing them as

DRAFT ONLY: For the edited volume *Integrating Human Motivation and Interpersonal Relationships: Theory, Research, and Applications.*

C.R. Knee (✉) • B. Porter • L.M. Rodriguez
Department of Psychology, University of Houston, Houston, TX, USA
e-mail: knee@uh.edu

N. Weinstein (ed.), *Human Motivation and Interpersonal Relationships: Theory, Research, and Applications*, DOI 10.1007/978-94-017-8542-6_7,

opportunities for understanding, acceptance, and improvement of the relationship rather than indications of threat or signs of a bad investment (Knee, Patrick, Vietor, Nanayakkara, & Neighbors, 2002). In this way, personally endorsing and feeling authentically invested in one's relationship allow individuals to be more understanding and less defensive in the presence of conflict (Hodgins & Knee, 2002).

Imagine that Clive and Hillary have been dating for 9 months. They met on a vacation in Cabo San Lucas through mutual friends. Clive and Hillary hit it off on that trip and decided to pursue a committed relationship. Imagine that, in the relationship realm, Hillary is relatively low in self-determination, and that her relationship behavior emerges not from awareness of her authentic needs, but from internalized expectations, avoidance of conflict, and fear of abandonment. Though unaware of this, she is also relatively low in relationship autonomy and is in the relationship for the wrong reasons. The beginning of their relationship was defined by extremes – periods of extreme highs and extreme lows. When Clive went out of his way to do something nice for Hillary, she would express jubilance beyond what would normally be expected. However, when small disappointments occurred, even for reasons beyond Clive's control, she would become upset, anxious, angry, and withdrawn. Further, she pines for her former partner, who left her a year ago, suddenly and with no explanation. Instead of admitting this to Clive, she instead begins lying about her recent contact with her former partner. Seemingly innocent inquiries by Clive lead Hillary to react defensively and even aggressively, often causing heated arguments. The frequency and intensity of these arguments leave both Hillary and Clive questioning the future potential of their relationship at times. Eventually, Hillary tells Clive that she is no longer interested in him, citing their recent disagreements, though she is still not fully aware of the true source of her dissatisfaction. She breaks up with Clive precipitously, and having to justify her sudden change, claims that she was never really "into him" and that she had simply been telling him what she thought he wanted to hear since they met. This example illustrates the main content of this chapter – that a self-determined awareness of one's basic psychological needs within a relationship, along with being in a relationship for self-determined reasons, facilitates openness rather than defensiveness, honest communication rather than deception, and promotes positive mutual regulation of conflict rather than avoidance or exacerbation of it.

We discuss different operationalizations of self-determination in relationships, emphasizing the ways in which self-determination is associated with more open, authentic interaction with less response to threat and less ego-defensiveness. We then briefly review a number of current theories and perspectives on close relationships with regard to how a self-determination theory perspective both integrates and goes beyond them in important ways.

Operationalizing Self-Determination in Relationships

In this chapter, we focus on research that is particularly relevant to regulation of conflict in romantic relationships, and the measures and manipulations of self-determination employed in those studies. Self-determination and autonomy have been operationalized in several ways, depending on the particular study, the level of analysis, and the domain of research.

First, self-determination has been operationalized as causality orientations, which are relatively stable individual differences in how one orients toward the social environment (Deci & Ryan, 1985a, 2002). Causality orientations (i.e., autonomy, controlled, and impersonal) are thought to be broadly integral to the regulation of behavior, and the three orientations vary in the degree to which they reflect self-determination. Autonomy orientation involves regulating behavior according to one's interests, self-endorsed values, and growth both in oneself and in others. Controlled orientation reflects a tendency to become ego-involved in one's daily experiences, and to regulate behavior according to external and internalized controls, pressures, expectations, and demands. Impersonal orientation involves a lack of intention and feeling despondent and ineffective. General causality orientations have been studied in relation to interpersonal defensiveness, explanations for social offenses, empathy and taking another's point of view, as well as engagement in coping strategies and observed behavior during romantic relationship conflict (Hodgins & Liebeskind, 2003; Hodgins, Liebeskind, & Schwartz, 1996; Hodgins, Yacko, & Gottlieb, 2006; Knee et al., 2002). The original General Causality Orientations Scale (GCOS; Deci & Ryan, 1985a) consisted of 12 vignettes, most of which were achievement-related. The revised GCOS (Hodgins, Koestner, & Duncan, 1996; Ryan, 1989) added 5 more interpersonal scenarios for 17 total vignettes and 51 items. Each vignette is followed by an autonomous response, a controlled response, and an impersonal response. Participants rate the extent to which each item accurately represents their reaction to the vignette. Scores for each subscale are averaged over the 17 responses. Each person is thought to possess some level of each orientation to varying degrees.

Another way that self-determination has been operationalized is as trait autonomy. The Self-Determination Scale (Sheldon, Ryan, & Reis, 1996) was designed to assess individual differences in the extent to which people tend to function in a self-determined way. It consists of ten items that reflect both (a) being more aware of one's feelings and sense of self, and (b) feeling a sense of choice with respect to one's behavior. The two subscales are often combined into an overall trait self-determination score. Trait self-determination has been examined in relation to understanding versus defensive coping responses to both reported, daily experienced, and laboratory-induced conflicts in romantic relationships (Knee et al., 2005).

Self-determination has also been operationalized as having more self-determined reasons for being in the relationship (Blais, Sabourin, Boucher, & Vallerand, 1990). The Couple Motivation Questionnaire (Blais et al., 1990) assesses one's autonomy in terms of one's reasons for being in the relationship. The questionnaire begins with the stem, "Why are you in the relationship?" Each of the 18 items then provides a reason for being in the relationship that varies along a continuum from those that are less self-determined (e.g., "There is nothing motivating me to stay in my relationship with my partner"), to more self-determined (e.g., "Because I value the way my relationship with my partner allows me to improve myself as a person"). An overall index of relationship autonomy can be computed by weighting the items according to where they fall on the relative autonomy continuum. Relationship autonomy (being in the relationship for relatively more self-determined reasons) has been found to predict perceived agreement, which in turn predicts relationship satisfaction for men and women (Blais et al.), as well as more understanding and less defensive reports and observed behaviors during actual couple conflicts (Knee et al., 2005).

Finally, self-determination has been operationalized as the degree of satisfaction of basic needs for autonomy, competence and relatedness within one's relationship (La Guardia, Ryan, Couchman, & Deci, 2000). According to self-determination theory, optimal psychological health and well-being emerge from the satisfaction of these three basic psychological needs. Need for autonomy reflects the need to feel that one's behavior is personally endorsed and initiated. Need for competence reflects the need to feel effective at what one does. Need for relatedness reflects the need to feel a sense of belonging, attachment, and intimacy with others. When applied specifically to romantic relationships, the need fulfillment questionnaire begins with the stem, "When I am with______ (my partner)..." The nine items reflect subscales of autonomy (e.g., "I feel free to be who I am"), competence (e.g., "I feel very capable and effective"), and relatedness (e.g., "I feel a lot of closeness and intimacy"). Items on each subscale are typically averaged and used as three subscales, as indicators of a latent variable, or as an overall index of self-determined need satisfaction. People are more securely attached to and are more likely to emotionally rely on those who meet their needs for autonomy, competence, and relatedness (La Guardia et al., 2000; Ryan, La Guardia, Solky-Butzel, Chirkov, & Kim, 2005). Within romantic relationships, the fulfillment of each need individually predicts both individual and relationship well-being (Patrick, Knee, Canevello, & Lonsbary, 2007). Further, both partners' levels of need fulfillment uniquely predict one's own relationship functioning and well-being. Finally, those who experience greater need fulfillment within their romantic relationship show better relationship quality after disagreements, due to their tendency to have more self-determined reasons for being in the relationship (Patrick et al., 2007).

Self-Determination and Openness Versus Defensiveness

Self-determination has been shown to have benefits for romantic relationships in several ways. For example, when autonomously motivated, one is more open and receptive to events and information, regardless of whether autonomy is measured as a general motivation orientation, or whether it is experimentally induced (Hodgins, 2008; Hodgins & Knee, 2002; Hodgins et al., 2010). In contrast, when motivated by feeling controlled, one feels pressured or guilty for one's decisions and actions, and tends to behave from a defensive interpersonal stance, being less reflective and more reactive, displaying more avoidance, denial, and behavioral disengagement (Hodgins, Yacko, & Gottlieb, 2006; Knee & Zuckerman, 1998). Among couples, autonomous motivation in terms of having more intrinsic reasons for being in the relationship, predicts less defensive responses to disagreements, and in turn, more relative satisfaction following those disagreements (Knee et al., 2005). Further, in another study of couples, those muted defensive responses were observable in actual behaviors during a laboratory-induced conflict (Knee et al.).

One reason that self-determination promotes less defensive responses is because autonomy reflects an integrated sense of self and authentic, genuine self-esteem whereby one's ego is not "on the line" and one is less concerned about proving oneself or feeling pressured to think about oneself in a particular way (Deci & Ryan, 1995; Kernis, 2003; Ryan, 1995). Being less focused on proving oneself and less pressured to behave in particular ways allows one to be more aware and present in the moment, and reflect rather than react to stimuli (Hodgins et al., 2010). According to Hodgins and her colleagues (2010; Hodgins, 2008), one consequence of a lack of ego-involvement is a higher threat threshold and a shift in emotional regulation toward less avoidance, denial, and defensiveness, all of which can facilitate open, honest communication in times of disagreement and conflict. These effects have recently been observed from experimentally induced (primed) autonomous motivation, relative to experimentally induced (primed) controlled motivation. Thus, it appears that situationally induced autonomous motivation promotes more openness and less defensiveness as does a more general autonomous motivation (either measured as a trait or as reasons for engaging in behavior).

The open, authentic stance that is promoted by experiencing autonomy is not limited to romantic relationships. Autonomous motivation has also been found to predict more satisfying and honest, naturally occurring interactions with family and friends (Hodgins, Koestner, & Duncan, 1996), and fewer attempts to "save face," blame others, and aggravate the distress when awkward social events occur (Hodgins & Liebeskind, 2003; Hodgins, Liebeskind, & Schwartz, 1996). The more open and accepting orientation that autonomy promotes extends beyond interpersonal events. Being self-determined also minimizes the typical defensive attributions when one attempts to explain one's own behavior. For example, when higher on autonomy and lower on controlled orientations (as measured by the GCOS, Deci & Ryan, 1985a), one tends to make similar attributions after success and failure on a task, as opposed to the more typical acceptance of more responsibility for success, but less responsibility for failure (Knee & Zuckerman, 1996). Thus, the benefits of experiencing autonomy likely carry over to romantic relationships both in terms of having less defensive self-perceptions and attributions as well as less defensive perceptions and reactions to one's partner. When motivated autonomously, one is more able to reflect than react, and conflict or criticism is perceived and experienced as less threatening.

Another byproduct of autonomous motivation is less of a desire to present a particular self-image to others (Hodgins & Knee, 2002). Although people generally monitor and adjust their behavior to fit the demands and expectations of specific environments and social settings, this tendency is likely to be weaker when autonomously motivated. While flexibility is a hallmark of being autonomously motivated, the feeling that one must present a desirable (rather than authentic) image of oneself is likely to be less of a "prime directive." The ability to freely and mutually share oneself with close others, disclosing and responding with honest, emotionally relevant information, are major ingredients for the development of intimacy (Reis &

Patrick, 1996). From a self-determination theory perspective, we can see why Clive and Hillary's relationship never reached its true potential. Genuine intimacy is less likely to emerge if partners are merely projecting the image they think the other person wants to see. The most profound connections are likely to emerge when two authentic selves are relating and responding to each others' true needs openly and freely. That said, substantial research indicates that people generally prefer to be viewed favorably, and viewing one's partner more favorably than the partner views him or herself predicts satisfaction in both dating relationships and marriages (e.g., Murray, Holmes, & Griffin, 1996). Still, "positive illusions" about one's romantic partner are probably not necessary for high relationship quality when one is autonomously motivated to be in one's relationship.

Along these lines, Knee et al. (2002) reasoned that self-determination is related to an openness and acceptance of differences, whether those differences come in the form of the qualities one seeks in an ideal partner or one's current partner's different perceptions and expectations of the relationship. When motivated by growth, one tends to embrace rather than attack differences in others and one is less likely to judge others through one's own eyes (i.e., expecting others to be just like oneself). In contrast, when one is ego-involved, judging others through one's own eyes may be second nature. Thus, a controlled, ego-involved individual may be more likely to expect the ideal romantic partner to be exactly like him or herself. Consistent with this notion, having a controlled orientation was associated with rating an ideal partner according to how one viewed oneself, whereas this was weaker with autonomy orientation (Knee et al.). In other words, when ego-involved, what one wants in an ideal partner is based largely on how one views oneself, whether positively or negatively. In contrast, when higher in autonomy orientation, this projection of self onto one's ideals is particularly weak.

A less defensive stance also explains the association between autonomous reasons for being in one's relationship and more adaptive couple behaviors and greater satisfaction with one's relationship (Blais et al., 1990). A key part of why this occurs concerns how feeling autonomous promotes more understanding and less defensive responses and behaviors during conflicts and disagreements (Knee et al., 2002, 2005). Both those who are autonomous and, more specifically, those who are autonomously invested in a romantic relationship show less defensiveness and more understanding behavioral responses in the context of disagreements and in turn remain more satisfied with the relationship. In the earlier example, if Hillary had a less defensive reaction to Clive's inquiries, the resulting conversations likely would not have initiated arguments and fights, enabling both Hillary and Clive's perceptions of the relationship to remain positive.

Need Fulfillment in Romantic Relationships

The concept of need fulfillment is central to why self-determination theory is so relevant to understanding the dynamics of optimal close relationships (La Guardia & Patrick, 2008). As mentioned earlier, one way to study self-determination in relationships is through the satisfaction of basic psychological needs for autonomy, competence, and relatedness. Self-determination theory is an especially powerful theory because its concept of basic psychological needs explicitly defines what kinds of experiences are needed for optimal development (Deci & Ryan, 2008; La Guardia & Patrick, 2008).

Along these lines, an important series of studies by La Guardia and her colleagues (2000) examined the role of need fulfillment within attachment security. Across three studies, people tended to have different levels of attachment security in different relationships (e.g., friends, parents, romantic partners). More importantly, a significant degree of this within-person variation in attachment styles was predicted by the degree of need fulfillment within those specific relationships. People were more securely attached to those with whom they felt autonomous, competent, and related. Similarly, Ryan and his colleagues (2005) found substantial within-person variation in emotional reliance across various relationship partners (i.e., close friends and romantic partners). Importantly, the degree to which people's needs for autonomy, competence, and relatedness were met mediated the association between emotional reliance and well-being.

Another line of evidence that need fulfillment is beneficial for relationship well-being comes from studies that have assessed the degree to which romantic partners felt that their needs for autonomy, competence, and relatedness were met, and tested whether this fulfillment predicted various relationship outcomes (Patrick et al., 2007). Just as research has shown that satisfaction of the three basic needs predicts positive health and well-being outcomes, it was hypothesized that satisfaction of the three basic needs in the context of one's close relationship would predict positive relational health and well-being outcomes. Study 1 found that fulfillment of autonomy uniquely predicted stronger relationship satisfaction and commitment, less perceived conflict, and more understanding and less defensive responses to conflict, even beyond the degree to which competence and relatedness were met. Study 2 found that the need fulfillment of each member within romantic couples uniquely predicted relationship outcomes such that one's partner's fulfillment of autonomy uniquely predicts one's own relationship outcomes. Thus, one's own feelings of autonomy in a relationship are not only important for how one feels about the relationship, but also uniquely extend to how the partner feels about it as well.

Similarly, individuals whose needs are relatively fulfilled are better able to communicate truthfully with their partner. A recent set of studies found that higher need fulfillment was associated with less self-presentation (Hadden, Overup, & Knee, in press). In Study 1, participants reported how much a close friendship fulfills their basic psychological needs, their levels of self-image goals, and the extent to which they engage in self-presentation with their friend. In Study 2, participants answered the same questions about a romantic partner. Results showed that need fulfillment was associated with less desire to maintain a specific self-image, and this in turn predicted lower levels of self-presentation (Hadden et al., in press).

Overall, self-determination theory is a powerful theory of close relationships because it explicitly defines three basic psychological needs that are at the core of developing optimal psychological well-being, and the degree of satisfaction of these needs primarily occurs in interpersonal contexts such as one's close relationships with romantic partners, family, and friends. Our interactions with others can either support or thwart the satisfaction of any of these three basic needs, which in turn predicts the quality of these relationships. Whereas many relationship theories rely heavily on relatedness-type needs such as perceived responsiveness, intimacy, or felt security, self-determination theory posits that more than the satisfaction of relatedness is at stake; without significant others also supporting one's autonomy and competence, the quality of those relationships will be suboptimal. In our earlier example neither Clive nor Hillary is able to address the other's needs because the dynamic between them is not one in which open honest communication can take place. If their psychological needs were met within the relationship, Hillary would be able to engage her current partner (rather than her ex-partner) more fully and Clive would not have reservations about the relationship's eventual outcome.

Self-Determination and Self-Esteem

One reason that self-determination facilitates regulation of conflict is through the kind of self-esteem that emerges when one's basic psychological needs are met and when one is autonomously motivated. When basic psychological needs for autonomy, competence, and relatedness are fulfilled over time, an authentic, noncontingent, optimal sense of self-esteem that is based on "being who one is rather than what one does," is promoted (Hodgins, 2008). When these basic psychological needs are thwarted over time, a defensive, contingent, suboptimal sense of self-esteem evolves. Hodgins, Brown, and Carver (2007) tested whether experimentally primed autonomous and controlled orientations influence implicit self-esteem in two studies, using a reaction time measure of self-esteem that is based on subliminal stimuli. This kind of implicit self-esteem may be more likely to reflect true or genuine self-esteem because, unlike self-report measures of self-esteem, its measurement bypasses one's own conscious awareness and thus cannot be defensively bolstered. As hypothesized, the results showed that inducing a controlled orientation decreased implicit self-esteem relative to inducing an autonomous orientation.

One type of self-esteem that is especially relevant to romantic relationships – and how one responds to conflict in particular – has been termed relationship-contingent self-esteem (RCSE; Knee, Canevello, Bush, & Cook, 2008). RCSE is an unhealthy form of self-esteem that involves depending heavily on one's romantic relationship for self-validation. RCSE is thought to partly derive from a lack of autonomy and personal endorsement of one's involvement in the relationship, a lack of feeling competent in one's relationship, and a lack of feeling genuinely validated, cared for, and understood by one's partner. In contrast to the benefits of noncontingent self-esteem, when self-worth is contingent within a particular domain, success or failure in that domain, or even cues that might imply success or failure, can result in intense affect and extreme fluctuations in self-esteem that carry over to evaluations of self as "good" or "bad." In romantic relationships, this means that when higher in RCSE, one is more reactive in response to disagreements and conflicts, even small, insignificant ones, because of what those events imply about the self. Support for these notions comes from four studies conducted by Knee and his colleagues (2008) that assessed RCSE and examined daily reports of emotions and self-esteem over time, as a function of positive and negative events in the relationship. Study 1 found that those higher in RCSE were also higher in other domains of contingent self-esteem, self-consciousness, social anxiety, attachment anxiety, manic and selfless love styles, romantic beliefs, and negative affect, and tended to view situations as more controlling and hopeless. Studies 2 and 3 employed an event-contingent diary procedure to examine reports of self-esteem as a function of everyday relationship events. Results showed a stronger association between the valence of relationship events (positive versus negative) and changes in daily self-esteem, among those higher in RCSE. In other words, when one's self-esteem is highly contingent on the relationship, self-esteem fluctuates more wildly with daily positive and negative relationship experiences. When the self is contingent on one's relationship, emotions related to those events and outcomes are experienced *reflexively* instead of *reflectively*, and in turn carry over to affect one's view of self as "good" or "bad." Thus, this line of work on RCSE suggests that a relatively more self-determined orientation to romantic relationships, in which one's self-validation is less contingent on the relationship, facilitates stability of emotional reactions to disagreements and conflicts on a daily basis, and thus facilitates stable self-esteem at those times.

In our hypothetical relationship, Hillary likely has a high level of RCSE. She entered into her relationship to "get over" her previous partner, and expects the relationship to automatically fulfill her expectations of what a relationship should be. When the relationship fails to fulfill these expectations, her sense of self is threatened and she experiences dramatic fluctuations within her emotional state.

Autonomy and Interpersonal Conflict

Does being autonomously motivated pose a problem when a friend or partner wants to do something that one does not? While this has been an issue of some debate (see Ryan & Deci, 2000), the disagreement largely stems from confusion about what autonomy is; self-determination theory defines "autonomy" in a vastly different manner than it is defined in other literatures (e.g., Murray, 1938). In self-determination theory, autonomy is not defined as independence, detachment, avoidance, or rebelliousness. To the contrary, Deci and Ryan's construct of autonomy reflects a deep personal endorsement of one's actions and involvements with others, and is associated with better personal and social adjustment (Hodgins et al., 1996; Koestner & Losier, 1996). Investigators have clarified these constructs by distinguishing between reactive and reflective autonomy, with the latter capturing the self-determination theory notion (Koestner et al., 1999; Koestner & Losier, 1996). Reactive autonomy involves resisting influence, defying authority and striving for independence.

On the other hand, reflective autonomy is about making informed choices based on an awareness of one's needs, interests, and values.

As explained above, autonomy also comes with an openness to information that reduces defensiveness and promotes a full exploration and consideration of all the various features of one's situation, including the consideration of others' needs (Hodgins & Knee, 2002). It is perhaps this openness to information that most facilitates how conflicts are more successfully negotiated when autonomously motivated. Indeed, research has shown that autonomous motivation predicts more relative satisfaction after disagreements, and that this is accompanied by less defensive, more understanding perceptions and observable behaviors (Knee et al., 2005).

Self-determination is important in understanding how people approach and manage conflict in romantic relationships. Those who are autonomous and, more specifically, those who are autonomously invested in a romantic relationship, show less defensiveness and more understanding in the context of disagreements and, therefore, remain more satisfied with the relationship. The benefits of relationship autonomy for how one approaches and responds to conflict are not limited to one's own autonomy but carry over to one's partner as well. Specifically, a partner's relationship autonomy uniquely predicts an individual's own satisfaction and defensiveness, controlling for the individual's own relationship autonomy. Feeling more autonomous toward the relationship may allow one's partner to feel supported unconditionally and thus behave in a more understanding, less defensive manner when discussing and experiencing conflict. Indeed, recent literature suggests that people are more open and disclosing in times of emotional distress with those who are more autonomy supportive (Ryan et al., 2005). These benefits apply to romantic partners as well. It may be easier to respond to conflict with more understanding and less defensiveness when one's partner feels autonomous and supports one's perceptions and feelings. Again, Knee et al. (2005) found that relationship autonomy predicted observed behavioral responses during a videotaped conflict in a controlled setting. Indeed, the potential benefits of relationship autonomy go beyond self-reported responses to conflict. One's own relationship autonomy predicted more observed understanding and less observed defensiveness during actual conflict. Further, one's partner's relationship autonomy uniquely predicted more observed understanding and somewhat less observed defensiveness.

Thus, self-determination with regard to one's relationship relates both to what people say they do during relationship conflict and to what they actually do during relationship conflict in a controlled setting. Further, self-determination has simultaneous influences as an individual difference and as a dyadic process in how partners approach and respond to conflict. The fact that trait autonomy, relationship autonomy, and partner autonomy have unique associations with conflict responses and satisfaction suggests that conflict responses are based on qualities that partners bring to their relationship, as well as more emergent, dyadic properties of autonomy in the relationship. Theoretically, a person who is autonomous has more optimal capacities for interpersonal functioning and is more personally committed, volitional, and persistent in maintaining relations with others. As past research has shown, higher trait autonomy is associated with more ability to take another's perspective, more empathy, and more honesty in social interactions (Hodgins & Liebeskind, 2003; Hodgins et al., 1996). Not only does autonomy involve attributes that are associated with better interpersonal functioning, but it has also been shown to promote commitment and persistence in a variety of other domains such as school dropout and weight loss attempts (e.g., Vallerand & Bissonnette, 1992; Williams, Grow, Freedman, Ryan, & Deci, 1996).

Returning to our relationship example, Hillary displays the classic defensive reactions to perceived conflict and relationship dissatisfaction. When Clive asks innocently about her feelings and behaviors in order to better understand what is happening from her perspective, she protectively lashes out assuming that he is attempting to uncover her recent contact with her former partner. In this way, an interaction which could potentially allow Clive to acknowledge Hillary's feelings and reaffirm their affection for the other, is doomed from the beginning, devolving into major conflict and disappointment.

Autonomy Support in Close Relationships

Self-determination theory defines autonomy support in terms of one relational partner acknowledging the other's perspective, providing choice, encouraging self-initiation, and being responsive to the other (Deci, La Guardia, Moller, Scheiner, & Ryan, 2006). Perceiving autonomy support from others is likely to reduce one's feelings of pressure to behave in a controlled fashion, which reduces the threat of potential disagreements and conflicts. Within self-determination theory, receiving autonomy support is theorized to be beneficial as it provides satisfaction of the basic psychological needs. Deci and colleagues (2006) studied how perceived autonomy support within close friendships was related to need fulfillment and relationship quality variables. In Study 1, the perception of autonomy support was associated with greater need fulfillment, emotional reliance, attachment security, dyadic adjustment, and inclusion of the friend in the self. There was also evidence of mutuality within friendships such that friends perceived similar degrees of autonomy support, need fulfillment, emotional reliance, attachment security, dyadic adjustment, and inclusion of the friend in the self. After controlling for dyad-level variance, the associations between perceived autonomy support and the relationship quality variables were no longer significant, but the association between received autonomy support and need fulfillment remained. In Study 2, Deci et al. extended this line of research to examine how both friends' perceived autonomy support contributes to each friend's own relationship quality and personal well-being outcomes. Perceived autonomy support was assessed in terms of one's own perceptions of both giving and receiving autonomy support. Results showed that giving autonomy support uniquely predicted need satisfaction and relationship quality beyond that accounted for by receiving autonomy support. Regarding well-being outcomes, results indicated that giving autonomy support was more strongly related to the person's well-being than was receiving autonomy support. Collectively, the findings from these studies support the importance of both giving and receiving autonomy support in one's close relationships. It is the mutuality of this dynamic that may be particularly important in facilitating adaptive regulation of conflict in the dyadic context of romantic relationships.

Self-determination theory emphasizes the dynamic between the individual and the social context in terms of supporting or thwarting fulfillment of basic psychological needs. With regard to the dyadic context of romantic relationships, it seems likely that it is easier to support the autonomy of one's partner when one feels that the partner would do the same for oneself. When autonomously motivated, one is more mindful and able to take others' perspectives more reflectively and fully, without closing them out or reflexively defending against their points of view (Brown, Ryan, & Creswell, 2007; Hodgins & Knee, 2002). Orienting oneself toward supporting rather than controlling others seems far more likely to yield beneficial mutual outcomes when it comes to regulating potential conflicts with close others.

Other Theories of Romantic Relationship Dynamics

Several other theories in the literature on close relationships have addressed many of the issues raised here such as the dynamics of motivations and fulfilling needs in relationships in a way that effectively manages conflict. However, these theories, while containing important aspects of relationships described by self-determination theory, do not encompass all mechanisms of optimal relationship functioning.

Self-Expansion Theory

Self-expansion theory (Aron & Aron, 1996; Aron, Aron, Tudor, & Nelson, 1991) states that people are motivated to expand their resources, perspectives, and characteristics by including the other person within the self. In relation to self-determination theory, a few points are worth noting. First, self-expansion and the sense of closeness that derives from "including another within one's self" seem to be largely about self-determination theory's need for relatedness. However, self-expansion theory does not address needs for autonomy and competence. Second, self-expansion theory does not explicitly discuss different qualities of self-expansion, whereas self-determination theory explicitly acknowledges and discusses healthier, more adaptive ways to expand the self via its notion of the continuum of integration (and the continuum of extrinsic to intrinsic motivations for expanding the self). In other words, self-expansion theory suggests that people are motivated to expand their resources, perspectives, and characteristics but does not distinguish between more and less self-determined expansion. It seems likely that not all motivations for relating and expanding one's self are equal. Seeking closeness from a partner to acquire resources (e.g., fame, approval from others, monetary gains) could be a less self-determined form of motivation than seeking to learn new perspectives and grow with one's partner. Furthermore, sharing activities with one's partner is a way in which one can experience novel activities and be with one's partner. If one participates in these activities because of a fear of disappointing one's partner or feels pressured to participate, the closeness that emerges will be limited, shallow, and likely restricted to that one activity at that time. Activities that are less fully endorsed by the self are restricted in their ability to fulfill basic needs for autonomy, competence, and relatedness. Relationships in which partners have a high amount of "controlled interdependence," rather than "self-determined interdependence" likely feel more instrumentally close rather than intrinsically close.

Further, relationship-contingent self-esteem (Knee et al., 2008) is an unhealthy form of self-esteem that involves depending heavily on one's romantic relationship for self-validation. In terms of self-determination theory, relationship-contingent self-esteem reflects less integrated regulation in which one is involved in the relationship for reasons other than autonomous endorsement. In essence, relationship-contingent self-esteem might be one example of what emerges from sub-optimal self-expansion, or where self-expansion occurs for the wrong reasons or by the wrong process.

Attachment Theory

One of the most prominent and empirically validated theories on close relationships is attachment theory (Bowlby, 1969; see Rholes & Simpson, 2004 for review), which views felt security and appropriate responsiveness as important for maintaining secure attachments to close others. In this way, attachment theory spells out the processes whereby attachments to close others develop and change over time, as a function of the relational context in which they emerge. Attachment theory also allows for variation in how individuals become attached to different close others. Thus, one can have a relatively secure attachment to one's spouse, but a relatively less secure attachment to one's father, and so forth. Presumably, the different attachments people develop with close others are accounted for by different kinds of relational experiences across different contexts. While attachment theory primarily relies on felt security and feelings of relatedness in accounting for different attachments, self-determination theory suggests that variations in the fulfillment of all three needs in the relational context likely determine levels of felt security and qualities of attachment to close others.

Attachment theory's account of felt security, appropriate responsiveness, and caregiving can be conceptualized, and perhaps clarified, by a discussion of basic psychological need fulfillment. That is, to provide a secure base, one must be supportive and responsive to one's partner while simultaneously allowing one's partner to freely explore (Feeney & Thrush, 2010). Essentially, one must provide a feeling of autonomy and competence to promote free, spontaneous exploration, while also fulfilling a sense of relatedness and security. In more stressful situations, a similar conceptualization applies: One must provide a sense of connectedness and support, while also supporting the partner's competence and ability to deal with the situation. The degree to which partners fulfill the roles of "secure base" and "safe haven" should further influence the formation of secure attachment bonds. Indeed, past research has found that people are more securely attached to people who they perceive as fulfilling their basic psychological needs for autonomy, competence, and relatedness (La Guardia et al., 2000).

Risk Regulation Model

The risk regulation model (Murray, Holmes, & Collins, 2006) emphasizes the importance of confidence in one's partner's regard as a regulator of whether an individual pursues self-protective relationship decisions that limit one's dependence or relationship-promotion decisions that increase one's dependence. The model states that perceptions of a partner's regard control a cognitive, affective, and behavioral system for resolving this goal conflict. Three "if–then" contingency rules are thought to operate to track the risks of rejection and resolve conflicts between self-protection and relationship-promotion goals. One rule links situations of dependence to the goal of gauging a partner's acceptance. Another rule links perceived partner acceptance or rejection to emotional and self-esteem outcomes. A third rule of dependence regulation links perceptions of a partner's acceptance or rejection to the willingness to risk future dependence. The risk regulation model emphasizes the way partners negotiate situations of dependence, in which the partner's responsiveness to one's needs is of concern, activating the threat of rejection in romantic life. The risk of rejection in such situations is said to depend on the amount of control a partner has over one's outcomes and the degree to which the partner's preferences overlap with one's own (Murray et al., 2006). When the partner's general regard for oneself is questionable and rejection seems more likely, the model says that people should tread cautiously, reserve judgment, and limit future dependence on the partner. In contrast, when confident of a partner's general regard for oneself, people can more safely risk increased dependence in the future. They can enter into situations in which the partner has control over their immediate outcomes, forgive transgressions, attach greater value to their partner's qualities, and risk a stronger sense of commitment to the partner and relationship.

The risk regulation model emphasizes both the situational and individual dynamics of partners' tendencies to perceive dependent situations as risky and threatening and as having greater potential for rejection and hurt. These dynamics are thought to drive partners' motivation to self-protect and withdraw from the relationship, or relationship-promote and invest further in the relationship. Self-determination theory augments the proposed dynamics of the risk regulation model in that it specifies a particular set of ingredients that would lead to evaluating potential indications of a partner's lack of commitment as safe and nonthreatening versus risky and harmful. Specifically, when one feels autonomously supported, competent, and genuinely intimately understood, valued, and cared for in the relationship, one becomes less defensive, avoidant, and fearful, and more open, authentic, and understanding of potential disagreements and differences (Hodgins & Knee, 2002). Alternatively, if one is high in RCSE, small possibly inadvertent indications of relationship dissatisfaction by one's partner can be interpreted as serious indicators of future rejection (Knee et al., 2008). Like the risk regulation model, self-determination theory emphasizes the interactive dynamic between the individual and the situational context, but more in terms of the degree to which basic psychological needs for autonomy, competence, and relatedness are supported versus thwarted. When supported, the dynamic moves away from perceptions of threat, risk, and avoidance of rejection and moves toward perceptions of security, nondefensive appraisals, and growth and investment in the relationship.

Communal Versus Exchange

Communal versus exchange perspectives (Mills & Clark, 2001) distinguish between a communal orientation, which carries the expectation of immediate repayment for benefits given, and an exchange orientation, which concerns the expectation of mutual responsiveness to the others' needs more generally and with a more long-term sense of equity. The motivation implied within the communal versus exchange framework is important and relates to self-determination theory in that an exchange orientation could seem more likely to go along with extrinsic motivation, whereas a communal orientation could seem more likely to go along with intrinsic motivation. Thus, when one is expecting relatively immediate "repayment" from one's partner, one is in the mindset of behaving for those more immediate reciprocal rewards rather than out of true interest in developing the relationship and enjoying it for its own sake. Similarly, when one is motivated to be responsive to the partner's needs in a more long-term fashion, one seems more motivated by appreciation and genuine desire to relate rather than by guilt or obligation. When one's psychological needs are fulfilled, it may be easier and more natural to behave out of a communal orientation. Further, a communal orientation would seem to promote trust and a deeper sense of intimacy and relatedness. It would seem difficult to be truly responsive to a partner's needs if one felt that one was being forced to do so out of guilt, obligation, or expected repayment (lack of autonomy fulfillment); if one felt incompetent or inadequate in the relationship (lack of competence fulfillment); or if one felt disconnected from one's partner or felt as if one's partner did not understand something important about oneself (lack of relatedness fulfillment). Indeed, prior research has found that being in the relationship for more intrinsic relative to extrinsic reasons predicts more adaptive couple behaviors and more understanding and less defensive responses to conflict (Blais et al., 1990; Knee et al., 2005).

Interdependence Theory

Finally, perhaps the most significant theory on regulation of potential conflict is interdependence theory (Kelley et al., 2003; Kelley & Thibaut, 1978). Interdependence theory describes how outcomes are negotiated within the interpersonal structure of dyadic situations. According to this perspective, individuals are motivated to maximize personal and relational rewards within the context of relationship decisions and behaviors. In doing this, partners transform the decisions that they would initially make (and ways that they would initially behave) that do not consider the partner's desires into different ways of deciding and behaving that do take into account the partner's desires. Interdependence as a concept seems most fundamentally about the need for relatedness, although it could also be argued that interdependence is really about the negotiation between individual outcomes and relational outcomes. However, it is important to note that individual interests and motivations in interdependence theory are not equivalent to self-determination theory's notion of autonomy. Much of the research on interdependence and transformation of motivation in close relationships has focused on two pro-relationship behaviors: accommodation (choosing not to retaliate in the face of a partner's transgression) and willingness to sacrifice (foregoing one's own immediate interests to promote the well-being of one's partner or relationship). Pro-relationship behaviors have been associated with dyadic adjustment and with a greater probability of couple persistence (Van Lange et al., 1997), and when partners perceive pro-relationship behaviors, they come to trust each other and rely on the relationship more (Wieselquist, Rusbult, Foster, & Agnew, 1999). Interdependence theory in general, and the focus on pro-relationship behaviors in particular, do not acknowledge the possibility that not all transformations of motivation or reasons for enacting pro-relationship behaviors are equal. Self-determination theory contends that one's reasons for being in the relationship and one's reasons for engaging in pro-relationship behaviors have important implications for how beneficial these behaviors may be, both for the relationship as a whole as well as for the individuals who compose it. It may be particularly beneficial to the relationship and partner when people engage in these behaviors because they truly want to and not simply to avoid an argument or to gain the approval of one's partner. Reasons for enacting pro-relationship behaviors may also impact how these behaviors are perceived by one's partner. If one's partner perceives that one is enacting these behaviors to "make points" or to gain something from the partner, pro-relationship behaviors may not be as beneficial to the relationship, as they are perceived as being motivated by one's own interests and not by one's focus on the partner or the relationship. In addition, the self-determination theory perspective suggests that, to the extent that one's autonomy, competence, and relatedness needs are fulfilled, it would be easier and more natural to take one's partner and the relationship into account and behave more interdependently.

The Dyadic Context

At its center, self-determination theory is a theory of how individuals interact with and negotiate the social dynamics that support or thwart fulfillment of basic psychological needs and facilitate or undermine intrinsic motivation in a manner that guides or restricts optimal self-development and well-being. While we know much about the ways that individual need fulfillment promotes individual development and well-being, less is known about how these processes function relationally, interpersonally, and dynamically over time. The dyadic context of romantic relationships seems like an excellent domain for studying these motivational dynamics of mutual need fulfillment over time. Such endeavors would not only extend our understanding of relationship development, but also enhance our understanding of the interpersonal processes with regard to negotiating self-determined functioning in a truly interdependent context. We feel that one of the limitations of self-determination theory, as it is currently put forth, is its emphasis on the individual's needs and outcomes rather than the dynamic processes and well-being of interdependent units and groups. The dyadic context of romantic relationships, along with modern statistical approaches for testing complex aspects of the interdependence of two-person dyads and beyond, provides a rich domain for extending and refining self-determination theory in important ways. Recent work is certainly heading in this direction (e.g., Deci et al., 2006; Wickham & Knee, 2012). We hope it continues to progress as investigators become more familiar with theorizing and hypothesizing about interdependent processes, and employ the latest statistical models for partitioning the interpersonal dynamics of need fulfillment and mutual self-determined functioning in potentially conflicting dyadic situations and beyond.

References

Aron, A., Aron, E. N., Tudor, M., & Nelson, G. (1991). Close relationships as including other in the self. *Journal of Personality and Social Psychology, 60*, 241–253. doi:10.1037/0022-3514.60.2.241.

Aron, E. N., & Aron, A. (1996). Love and the expansion of the self: The state of the model. *Personal Relationships, 3*, 45–58. doi:10.1111/j.1475-6811.1996.tb00103.x.

Blais, M. R., Sabourin, S., Boucher, C., & Vallerand, R. J. (1990). Towards a motivational model of couple happiness. *Journal of Personality and Social Psychology, 59*, 1021–1031. doi:10.1037/0022-3514.59.5.1021.

Bowlby, J. (1969). *Attachment and loss: Vol. 1. Attachment*. New York: Basic Books.

Brown, K. W., Ryan, R. M., & Creswell, J. D. (2007). Mindfulness: Theoretical foundations and evidence for its salutary effects. *Psychological Inquiry, 18*, 211–237. doi:10.1080/10478400701598298.

Deci, E. L., La Guardia, J. G., Moller, A. C., Scheiner, M. J., & Ryan, R. M. (2006). On the benefits of giving as well as receiving autonomy support: Mutuality in close friendships. *Personality and Social Psychology Bulletin, 32*, 313–327. doi:10.1177/0146167205282148.

Deci, E. L., & Ryan, R. M. (1985a). The general causality orientations scale: Self-determination in personality. *Journal of Research in Personality, 19*, 109–134. doi:10.1016/0092-6566(85)90023-6.

Deci, E. L., & Ryan, R. M. (1985b). *Intrinsic motivation and self-determination in human behavior*. New York: Plenum.

Deci, E. L., & Ryan, R. M. (1995). Human autonomy: The basis for true self-esteem. In M. H. Kernis (Ed.), *Efficacy, agency, and self-esteem* (pp. 31–49). New York: Plenum Press.

Deci, E. L., & Ryan, R. M. (2000). The "what" and "why" of goal pursuits: Human needs and the self-determination of behavior. *Psychological Inquiry, 11*, 227–268. doi:10.1207/S15327965PLI1104_01.

Deci, E. L., & Ryan, R. M. (Eds.). (2002). *Handbook of self-determination research*. Rochester, NY: University of Rochester Press.

Deci, E. L., & Ryan, R. M. (2008). A macrotheory of human motivation, development and health. *Canadian Psychology, 49*, 182–185. doi:10.1037/a0012801.

Feeney, B. C., & Thrush, R. L. (2010). Relationship influences on exploration in adulthood: The characteristics and function of a secure base. *Journal of Personality and Social Psychology, 98*, 57–76. doi:10.1037/a0016961.

Gottman, J. M., & Notarius, C. I. (2000). Decade review: Observing marital interaction. *Journal of Marriage and the Family, 62*, 927–947. doi:10.1111/j.1741-3737.2000.00927.x.

Hadden, B. W., Overup, C. S., & Knee, C. R. (in press). Removing the ego: Need fulfillment, self-image goals, and self-presentation. *Self and Identity*. July 23, 2013. doi:10.1080/15298868.2013.815398.

Hodgins, H. S. (2008). Motivation, threshold for threat, and quieting the ego. In H. A. Wayment & J. J. Bauer (Eds.), *Transcending self-interest: Psychological explorations of the quiet ego* (pp. 117–124). Washington, DC: American Psychological Association.

Hodgins, H. S., Brown, A. B., & Carver, B. (2007). Autonomy and control motivation and self-esteem. *Self and Identity, 6*, 189–208. doi:10.1080/15298860601118769.

Hodgins, H. S., & Knee, C. R. (2002). The integrating self and conscious experience. In E. L. Deci & R. M. Ryan (Eds.), *Handbook of self-determination research* (pp. 87–100). Rochester, NY: University of Rochester Press.

Hodgins, H. S., Koestner, R., & Duncan, N. (1996). On the compatibility of autonomy and relatedness. *Personality and Social Psychology Bulletin, 22*, 227–237. doi:10.1177/0146167296223001.

Hodgins, H. S., & Liebeskind, E. (2003). Apology versus defence: Antecedents and consequences. *Journal of Experimental Social Psychology, 39*, 297–316. doi:10.1016/S0022-1031(03)00024-6.

Hodgins, H. S., Liebeskind, E., & Schwartz, W. (1996). Getting out of hot water: Facework in social predicaments. *Journal of Personality and Social Psychology, 71*, 300–314. doi:10.1037/0022-3514.71.2.300.

Hodgins, H. S., Weibust, K. S., Weinstein, N., Shiffman, S., Miller, A., Coombs, G., et al. (2010). The cost of self-protection: Threat response and performance as a function of autonomous and controlled motivations. *Personality and Social Psychology Bulletin, 36*, 1101–1114. doi:10.1177/0146167210375618.

Hodgins, H. S., Yacko, H. A., & Gottlieb, E. (2006). Autonomy and nondefensiveness. *Motivation and Emotion, 30*, 283–293. doi:10.1007/s11031-006-9036-7.

Kelley, H. H., Holmes, J. G., Kerr, N. L., Reis, H. T., Rusbult, C. E., & Van Lange, P. A. M. (2003). *An atlas of interpersonal situations*. New York: Cambridge University Press.

Kelley, H. H., & Thibaut, J. W. (1978). *Interpersonal relations: A theory of interdependence*. New York: Wiley.

Kernis, M. H. (2003). Towards a conceptualization of optimal self-esteem. *Psychological Inquiry, 14*, 1–26. doi:10.1207/S15327965PLI1401_01.

Knee, C. R., Canevello, A., Bush, A. L., & Cook, A. (2008). Relationship-contingent self-esteem and the ups and downs of romantic relationships. *Journal of Personality and Social Psychology, 95*, 608–627. doi:10.1037/0022-3514.95.3.608.

Knee, C. R., Lonsbary, C., Canevello, A., & Patrick, H. (2005). Self-determination and conflict in romantic relationships. *Journal of Personality and Social Psychology, 89*, 997–1009. doi:10.1037/0022-3514.89.6.997.

Knee, C. R., Patrick, H., Vietor, N. A., Nanayakkara, A., & Neighbors, C. (2002). Self determination as growth motivation in romantic relationships. *Personality and Social Psychology Bulletin, 28*, 609–619. doi:10.1177/0146167202288005.

Knee, C. R., & Zuckerman, M. (1996). Causality orientations and the disappearance of the self-serving bias. *Journal of Research in Personality, 30*, 76–87. doi:10.1006/jrpe.1996.0005.

Knee, C. R., & Zuckerman, M. (1998). A nondefensive personality: Autonomy and control as moderators of defensive coping and self-handicapping. *Journal of Research in Personality, 32*, 115–130. doi:10.1006/jrpe.1997.2207.

Koestner, R., Gingras, I., Abutaa, R., Losier, G. F., DiDio, L., & Gagné, M. (1999). To follow expert advice when making a decision: An examination of reactive versus reflective autonomy. *Journal of Personality, 67*, 851–872. doi:10.1111/1467-6494.00075.

Koestner, R., & Losier, G. F. (1996). Distinguishing reactive versus reflective autonomy. *Journal of Personality, 64*, 465–494. doi:10.1111/j.1467-6494.1996.tb00518.x.

La Guardia, J. G., & Patrick, H. (2008). Self-determination theory as a fundamental theory of close relationships. *Canadian Psychology, 49*, 201–209. doi:10.1037/a0012760.

La Guardia, J. G., Ryan, R. M., Couchman, C. E., & Deci, E. L. (2000). Within-person variation in security of attachment: A self-determination theory perspective on attachment, need fulfillment, and well-being. *Journal of Personality and Social Psychology, 79*, 367–384. doi:10.1037/0022-3514.79.3.367.

Mills, J., & Clark, M. S. (2001). Viewing close romantic relationships as communal relationships: Implications for maintenance and enhancement. In J. Harvey & A. Wenzel (Eds.), *Close romantic relationships: Maintenance and enhancement* (pp. 13–25). Mahwah, NJ: Erlbaum Associated Publishers.

Murray, H. A. (1938). *Explorations in personality*. Oxford, UK: Oxford University Press.

Murray, S. L., Holmes, J. G., & Griffin, D. W. (1996). The benefits of positive illusions: Idealization and the construction of satisfaction in close relationships. *Journal of Personality and Social Psychology, 70*, 79–98.

Murray, S. L., Holmes, J. G., & Collins, N. L. (2006). Optimizing assurance: The risk regulation system in relationships. *Psychological Bulletin, 132*, 641–666. doi:10.1037/0033-2909.132.5.641.

Patrick, H., Knee, C. R., Canevello, A., & Lonsbary, C. (2007). The role of need fulfillment in relationship functioning and well-being: A self-determination theory perspective. *Journal of Personality and Social Psychology, 92*, 434–457. doi:10.1037/0022-3514.92.3.434.

Reis, H. T., & Patrick, B. C. (1996). Attachment and intimacy: Component processes. In E. T. Higgins & A. W. Kruglanski (Eds.), *Social Psychology: Handbook of Basic Principles* (pp. 523–563). New York: Guilford Press.

Rholes, W. S., & Simpson, J. A. (Eds.). (2004). *Adult attachment: Theory, research, and clinical implications*. New York: Guilford Publications.

Ryan, R. M. (1989). *The revised general causality orientation scale.* Unpublished manuscript, University of Rochester.

Ryan, R. M. (1995). Psychological needs and the facilitation of integrative processes. *Journal of Personality, 63*, 397–427. doi:10.1111/j.1467-6494.1995.tb00501.x.

Ryan, R. M., & Deci, E. L. (2000). The darker and brighter sides of human existence: Basic psychological needs as a unifying concept. *Psychological Inquiry, 11*, 319–338.

Ryan, R. M., La Guardia, J. G., Solky-Butzel, J., Chirkov, V., & Kim, Y. (2005). On the interpersonal regulation of emotions: Emotional reliance across gender, relationships, and cultures. *Personal Relationships, 12*, 145–163. doi:10.1111/j.1350-4126.2005.00106.x.

Sheldon, K. M., Ryan, R., & Reis, H. T. (1996). What makes for a good day? Competence and autonomy in the day and in the person. *Personality and Social Psychology Bulletin, 22*, 1270–1279. doi:10.1177/01461672962212007.

Vallerand, R. J., & Bissonnette, R. (1992). Intrinsic, extrinsic, and amotivational styles as predictors of behavior: A prospective study. *Journal of Personality, 60*, 599–620. doi:10.1111/j.1467-6494.1992.tb00922.x.

Van Lange, P. A. M., Rusbult, C. E., Drigotas, S. M., Arriaga, X. B., Witcher, B. S., & Cox, C. L. (1997). Willingness to sacrifice in close relationships. *Journal of Personality and Social Psychology, 72*, 1373–1395. doi:10.1037/0022-3514.72.6.1373.

Wickham, R. E., & Knee, C. R. (2012). Where theory and method converge: Interdependence theory and the actor-partner interdependence model. *Personality and Social Psychology Review, 16*, 375–393. doi:10.1177/1088868312447897.

Wieselquist, J., Rusbult, C. E., Foster, C. A., & Agnew, C. R. (1999). Commitment, pro-relationship behavior, and trust in close relationships. *Journal of Personality and Social Psychology, 77*, 942–966. doi:10.1037/0022-3514.77.5.942.

Williams, G. C., Grow, V. M., Freedman, Z. R., Ryan, R. M., & Deci, E. L. (1996). Motivational predictors of weight loss and weight-loss maintenance. *Journal of Personality and Social Psychology, 70*, 115–126. doi:10.1037/0022-3514.70.1.115.

Chapter 8
The Role of Autonomy in Intergroup Processes: Toward an Integration of Self-Determination Theory and Intergroup Approaches

Lisa Legault and Catherine E. Amiot

As the various chapters of this volume attest, motivation is vital in driving and shaping interpersonal relationships. Although self-determination research has given careful consideration to the *interpersonal* aspects of motivation, it is only in the past 5 years or so that a self-determination theory perspective of *intergroup* processes has begun to take form. In this chapter, we focus on the ways that self-determination can influence group-level phenomena. We divide our inquiry into two parts. The first is concerned with *outgroup*-directed motivation, and explores the role of self-determination in shaping perceptions and attitudes toward other social groups. It also includes discussion of the underlying mechanisms that help to explain the link between motivation and outgroup attitudes, such as prejudice, as well as the effects of autonomy support and social control on intergroup tension. In the second part of the chapter, we focus on *ingroup*-directed motivation, including the role of motivation, integration, and need satisfaction in the development of group identity.

This burgeoning and exciting area of research seeks to expand self-determination theory to a new level and domain of analysis. It also promises to increase our understanding of how intergroup relations thrive and falter. Indeed, as we probe further into the intersection of self-determination theory and intergroup relations research, we come closer to understanding how human autonomy might breed social tolerance, enhance social identity, foster healthy intergroup relationships,

---

To appear in N. Weinstein (Ed.), *Integrating Human Motivation and Interpersonal Relationships: Theory, Research and Applications*. New York: Springer.

The writing of this chapter was supported by a fellowship awarded to the first author from the Natural Sciences and Engineering Research Council of Canada, and a grant awarded to the second author from Fonds de recherche Santé Québec.

L. Legault (✉)
Department of Psychology, Clarkson University, Potsdam, NY, USA
e-mail: llegault@clarkson.edu

C.E. Amiot
Department of Psychology, Université du Québec à Montréal, Montreal, QC, Canada

N. Weinstein (ed.), *Human Motivation and Interpersonal Relationships: Theory, Research, and Applications*, DOI 10.1007/978-94-017-8542-6_8,

and promote social justice. At the same time, the work presented here alerts us to the need to address the potentially dark consequences of social control on intergroup relations.

Part One: Outgroup-Directed Motivation

We live in a social climate of growing diversity, with many of the great cities of the Western world becoming increasingly multicultural (United Nations, 2002). In keeping with continuous mass immigration, many countries now enforce diversity and multicultural policy, which is often accompanied by social and organizational standards of political correctness. Given our modern focus on social diversity and fairness, it is not surprising that most people are motivated to reduce prejudice toward other social groups – such as other ethnic or cultural groups, other religious groups, people of other sexual orientations, or those of the other gender (e.g., Crandall, Eshleman, & O'Brien, 2002; Legault, Green-Demers, Grant, & Chung, 2007). Indeed, nonprejudice can be considered a social norm (Crandall et al., 2002; Gaertner & Dovidio, 1986; Pettigrew & Meertens, 1995). Having the motivation to control prejudice is only half the battle, however. That is, because we are cognitively predisposed to categorize the social world based on group membership (e.g., "us" vs. "them"), and because we have the tendency to want to view our own groups in a positive light (e.g., Tajfel, 1978; Tajfel & Turner, 1979, 1986), it is hardly surprising that prejudice toward other social groups is abundant and resistant to modification (Monteith, Arthur, & Flynn, 2010; Monteith, Lybarger, & Woodcock, 2009). This motivational paradox (i.e., having the goal to reduce group-based prejudice, but being faced with the difficulty of actually doing so) highlights the importance of motivational quality and the benefits of effective self-regulation. Indeed, both motivation and self-regulation are crucial in the reduction of group-based bias. Below, we describe the important role of self-determination in enhancing the self-regulation of prejudice.

Motivation to Regulate Prejudice

Self-determination theory (SDT; Deci & Ryan, 1985a, 2008) has proven highly valuable in addressing the inherent challenge in the self-regulation of intergroup prejudice. Extending past work that has quantified motivation to regulate prejudice as either high or low (e.g., Dunton & Fazio, 1997) or dichotomized it as either internal or external (Plant & Devine, 1998), our early research (Legault et al., 2007) revealed that not all forms of motivation to regulate prejudice are created equal. In other words, motivation to regulate group-based prejudice varies in its level of self-determination, and these motivational differences have important and meaningful consequences for intergroup relations.

At the nethermost point of the self-determination continuum, those who are *amotivated* to regulate prejudice are not interested or efficacious in pursuing egalitarian ideals. In other words, motivation to regulate outgroup prejudice is absent because non-prejudice is not valued or because control over prejudice seems impossible or unattainable. Conversely, prejudice regulation can be motivated by controls in the social context – which is often the case in organizational and societal settings where antiprejudice policies and programs abound. Two forms of *controlled* motivation to regulate prejudice exist: external and introjected. *External* prejudice regulation represents wholly external motivation and involves attempts to suppress prejudice in order to satisfy external demands, such as social norms of political correctness, antiprejudice standards, or antidiscrimination laws and policies. In our politically correct society, the experience of external demands to be nonprejudiced is almost unavoidable. Despite the pervasiveness of pressure to think and feel in socially acceptable ways, the undermining influence of control on *attitudes* (such as prejudice) has been relatively under-researched. That is, the majority of self-determination research explores the effects of controlling environments on *behavior*. However, as we will describe later in this chapter, the consequences of social pressure to adopt a nonprejudiced attitude may be particularly harmful.

Moving from purely external regulation to the internal deflection of social pressure, an *introjected* motivation to regulate prejudice involves the attempt to suppress prejudice out of felt obligation and internal pressure (e.g., guilt). This type of prejudice regulation tends to be driven by anxiety and worry over prejudiced responding. In contrast to controlled forms of regulation, where nonprejudice feels like a requirement, motivation to regulate prejudice may also be seen as personally relevant and important. That is, the self-regulation of prejudice may be self-determined. Those with an *identified* regulation of prejudice place value on nonprejudice and egalitarianism and see these values as self-endorsed personal aspirations. Nonprejudice is seen as a virtue and diversity may be thought of as personally and socially beneficial. Similarly, when motivation to regulate prejudice is *integrated*, striving to be nonprejudiced is fused with the self-concept and core belief system (e.g., one sees oneself as a nonprejudiced person). For such individuals, behaving in a nonprejudiced manner constitutes an expression of self or a reflection of one's innermost values. Finally, at the height of self-determination, those with an *intrinsic* motivation to be nonprejudiced report that striving to be nonprejudiced is a source of pleasure and intergroup relating is both interesting and enjoyable. Such individuals glean satisfaction from intergroup interactions and relationships, and enjoy issues relating to diversity.

Importantly, these motivational distinctions have implications for how effective people are in their prejudice-reduction attempts (Legault & Green-Demers, 2012; Legault, Green-Demers, & Eadie, 2009; Legault et al., 2007; Legault, Gutsell, & Inzlicht, 2011; Plant & Devine, 1998). For instance, intrinsic, integrated, and identified motivations to regulate prejudice are negatively associated with symbolic racism toward Black Canadians, including the denial of race-based disadvantage and the belief that Black Canadians pose a threat to White Canadian values (Legault et al., 2007). These autonomous forms of motivation to regulate prejudice are also negatively related to negative outgroup-directed emotion and modern sexism (Legault et al., 2007).

Recently, we have extended this general finding to anti-Arab Muslim prejudice; White Canadians with an autonomous motivation to regulate prejudice (i.e., intrinsic, integrated, or identified) display more positive attitudes toward Arab-Muslims than do those with a non-autonomous motivation to regulate prejudice (i.e. introjected, external, or amotivated; Legault & Green-Demers, 2012). They are also less likely to demonstrate action tendencies toward racial discrimination (e.g., by saying that they would be more likely to eat dinner or share homework with an Arab-Muslim individual), and less likely to express anxiety or nervousness about intergroup interactions (Legault & Green-Demers).

Expanding the notion that autonomous motivation acts as a buffer against intergroup anxiety, we have also shown that the source of motivation to regulate prejudice moderates the effect of intergroup threat on prejudice. That is, when people experience intergroup threat (i.e., when they feel threatened by the economic or cultural infiltration of another group; Stephan & Renfro, 2002), only controlled prejudice regulators demonstrate the typical increase in prejudice toward those other groups. Autonomous prejudice regulators, on the other hand, do not translate feelings of threat into prejudice (Legault & Green-Demers, 2012). Motivation also modulates the effects of stereotype activation on prejudice. Specifically, when primed with non-threatening black race stereotypes (e.g., athletic, hip hop, poor), those with primarily autonomous reasons for regulating prejudice were less likely to describe a target as hostile (which is a known component of the African American stereotype), compared to those with primarily controlled reasons for regulating prejudice (Legault et al., 2009).

The pattern of association between motivation and prejudice holds at the implicit level as well (Legault et al., 2007, 2009, 2011, in prep). Thus, even when prejudice is difficult to control, autonomous prejudice regulators are more successful in reducing bias. For instance, compared to amotivation and controlled forms of prejudice regulation, autonomous forms of motivation to regulate prejudice are associated with less prejudice on the race-face implicit association test (IAT; Greenwald, McGhee, & Schwartz, 1998), which is a measure of automatic racial bias based on the strength of semantic association between group-based concepts on one hand (i.e., Black or White) and attributes on the other (i.e., pleasant or unpleasant). Using the more general concepts of internal versus external motivation to regulate prejudice, research from independent labs has supported this pattern of findings by showing that those with internal motivation to regulate prejudice exhibit less implicit prejudice than those with external motivation (e.g., Devine, Plant, Amodio, Harmon-Jones, & Vance, 2002; Plant & Devine, 1998).

Given this evidence, it seems clear that autonomous motivation to regulate prejudice is important in the pursuit of egalitarian ideals and positive intergroup relations. Those who regulate intergroup biases because they believe that nonprejudice is personally important and meaningful do a better job at being nonprejudiced than do those who are motivated primarily for external or social reasons. Next, we turn to the self-regulatory factors driving this motivational effect, in order to understand why, exactly, autonomous motivation to regulate prejudice is more effective than controlled motivation to regulate prejudice.

Why Is Autonomous Prejudice Regulation More Effective?

What mechanisms account for the relative success of autonomous motivation to regulate prejudice? SDT suggests that internalization (i.e., the process through which external goals and values become accepted as one's own) provides a basis for effective self-regulation. When behavior and motivation cohere with one's personal values and intrinsic aspirations, they become simpler to implement and they no longer require external enforcement or incentive. Indeed, when motivation is highly autonomous, it can even generate increased energy and vitality (Moller, Deci, & Ryan, 2006). However, because motivation to regulate prejudice is concerned with control over a negative (and often automatic) behavior (i.e., prejudice) as much as it is concerned with motivation toward a desired behavior (i.e., nonprejudice), it becomes important to focus on the processes of prejudice inhibition and the self-regulation of bias (e.g., Amodio & Devine, 2010; Plant & Devine, 2009). That is, because stereotypes and prejudice can often infiltrate consciousness automatically, even when motivation to suppress them is strong or autonomous (e.g., Legault et al., 2009), the capacity to implicitly monitor and regulate group-based prejudice (or, rather, lapses in the self-regulation of bias) is vital to the reduction of prejudice. In this section, we present two processes through which autonomy appears to enhance the self-regulation of prejudice; namely, the automatization of prejudice regulation and the brain-mediated monitoring of prejudiced responding.

The Automatization of Autonomous Prejudice Regulation

We recently hypothesized that autonomous motivation to regulate prejudice would be more likely to facilitate the automatic inhibition of prejudice, compared to controlled prejudice regulation (Legault et al., 2009). In other words, we expected autonomous motivation to be relatively more harmonious and automatized. Because of its self-originating nature, autonomous motivation is liable to be more consonant, chronic, and persistent than controlled motivation, and this makes it a good candidate for automatization. Indeed, the more a goal is rehearsed or entrenched, the more likely it is to become automatic (Bargh, 1990, 1999; Bargh & Chartrand, 1999; Hassin, Uleman, & Bargh, 2005) – partly because associative environmental cues can unconsciously activate deep-rooted motivational pursuits and go on to influence intentions and behavior. This suggests that well-rehearsed and highly self-concordant autonomous motivation – which is likely to be more chronically accessible because it stems from personal values – is apt to become preconsciously maintained, without the expenditure of much cognitive effort. In contrast, we expected controlled motivation to regulate prejudice to be effortful and taxing of self-control strength. Because controlled prejudice regulation is not internalized, but rather proceeds through pressure and restraint, it is not likely to operate implicitly or harmoniously – especially in the absence of external prompts.

We conducted two studies to investigate the proposed automaticity of autonomous prejudice regulation over controlled prejudice regulation. In the first study, autonomous prejudice regulators (i.e., those scoring in the top tercile of a global motivation to regulate prejudice index) and controlled prejudice regulators (i.e., those scoring the bottom tercile of the same index) were invited to complete two experimental tasks. In the first task, differences in stereotype *activation* (i.e., the semantic accessibility of the stereotype) were measured by having both groups of participants watch a video of either an Asian or a Caucasian confederate displaying a series of 12 word fragments on cue cards. Each word fragment was presented for 3 s – a period in which participants were required to complete the fragment as quickly as possible by writing down whatever word first came to mind (e.g., the word fragment S_ORT could be completed in either a stereotypical or nonstereotypical manner). A stereotype is considered activated when respondents make more stereotypical word completions than nonstereotypical word completions in the presence of a stereotype target. We concluded that this process was automatic (cf. "attentionless"; Bargh, 1999) in this study because respondents reported that they were unaware that the target's group membership exerted any influence on their responses.

In the second task, stereotype *application* was assessed by having participants complete a separate stereotype priming task and then make a judgment about a target. Participants were presented with 32 scrambled sentences that either contained words related to nonthreatening African American stereotypes (e.g., "jazz"; "basketball") or stereotype-unrelated words (e.g., "park"; "dive"). Each participant was required to create a grammatically correct sentence using the words provided. Then, participants were asked to complete an ostensibly unrelated task assessing "the way in which people form impressions of others". They read a non-evaluative story describing a man engaging in a series of ambiguously hostile behaviors, such as refusing to pay his rent and demanding his money back from a store clerk. Participants were then asked to rate their perceptions of this individual in terms of his hostility. Because hostility is a well-known African American stereotype (Devine, 1989), one would normally expect hostility ratings (i.e., stereotype application) to increase when African American stereotypes are activated.

In line with our expectations, our data revealed no motivational differences in stereotype activation (i.e., task 1; see Fig. 8.1). That is, both groups completed more Asian stereotypes when word fragments were presented by the Asian experimenter, compared to when word fragments were presented by the Caucasian experimenter (and, in fact, both motivation groups completed the same number of stereotyped word fragments.). This finding suggests that stereotypes are accessible for both groups, and that, if those with an autonomous motivation to regulate prejudice exhibit less prejudice, it cannot simply be attributed to an absence of cognitive bias (i.e., that they have no stereotypes or prejudice to regulate in the first place). In contrast, results of the stereotype application task (i.e., task 2) revealed that those with an autonomous motivation to regulate prejudice spontaneously suppress the application of stereotypes when making a negative judgment about a stereotyped target. In fact, autonomous prejudice regulators showed slightly less prejudice when

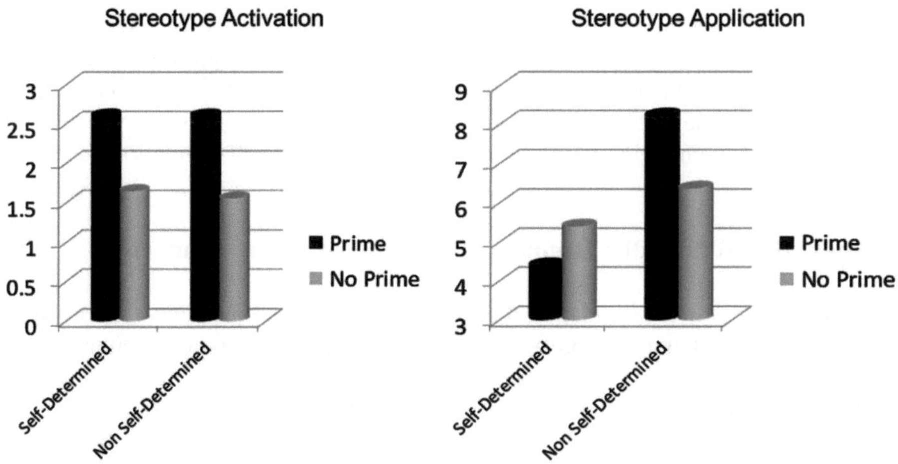

Fig. 8.1 Stereotype activation and application as a function of motivation to regulate prejudice

primed with African American stereotypes compared to when not primed. Conversely, those with a controlled motivation to regulate prejudice showed significantly more prejudice when primed with African American stereotypes compared to when not primed. Taken together, these findings support the notion that, although both autonomous and controlled prejudice regulators show a cognitive potential to be prejudiced (i.e., stereotypes are accessible in memory), only autonomous prejudice regulators implicitly inhibit negative stereotypes when making evaluations. In other words, the self-regulation of prejudice appears to be automatic for those who are autonomously motivated.

This automaticity assertion was corroborated in a second study in which autonomous and controlled prejudice regulators were depleted of self-regulatory strength (i.e., by being asked to engage in a difficult inhibition task), and then asked to respond accurately on a race-face implicit association test (the IAT). For many White participants, the IAT requires self-regulation on prejudice- or stereotype-inconsistent trials, when the ingroup category (White) shares the same response key as the negative attribute category and the outgroup category (Black) shares the same response key as the positive attribute category (e.g., Greenwald et al., 1998). Conversely, stereotype-consistent responses tend to be prepotent. In line with the strength model of self-control, we reasoned that when people are depleted of self-regulation capacity, they should perform worse on the IAT (i.e., show increased bias), to the extent that self-control on prejudice-inconsistent trials is required. In support of our hypothesis, we found that IAT scores (i.e., implicit prejudice) were higher when participants were depleted of self-regulation strength – but only when motivation to regulate prejudice was controlled. Among autonomous prejudice regulators, there were no differences in prejudice on the IAT as a function of depletion. Again, this pattern of findings lends some support to the assertion that autonomous prejudice regulation does not require self-regulatory strength, and thus operates automatically. In general, this work highlights the importance of motivation in shaping social cognition, and helps to explain why autonomous prejudice regulation is more effective and consistent in reducing prejudice; if autonomous motivation is amenable to automatization, then it should remain intact when distracted, tired, or when not actively engaging in inhibition or other forms of self-regulation.

Brain-Mediated Prejudice Regulation: The Role of Error Monitoring

Research in the self-determination theory tradition has demonstrated convincingly that behavioral regulation is improved when the motivation underlying it is autonomous rather than controlled (e.g., Teixeira et al., 2010; Williams, Grow, Freedman, Ryan, & Deci, 1996; Williams, Niemiec, Patrick, Ryan, & Deci, 2009). However, from a cognitive processes perspective, the precise mechanisms accounting for the superiority of autonomously motivated self-regulation have received little attention. Previous work has noted that autonomous motivation boosts self-regulation because it generates greater "vitality" or "energy" (e.g., Muraven, Gagné, & Rosman, 2008; Ryan & Deci, 2008). But it is not precisely or mechanistically clear what energy and vitality mean, or how they are represented. Past work on autonomy and self-regulatory processes has relied on metaphors, and less on actual information processing mechanisms – such as the monitoring and correcting of behavior in the service of optimal performance. Recently, however, research investigating how prejudice is regulated has shed light on the neurocognitive mechanisms involved in different forms of self-regulation. In particular, recent work has shown that, compared to those with an external motivation, those with an autonomous motivation to respond without prejudice demonstrate heightened neurophysiological responsiveness to lapses in prejudice regulation (e.g., Amodio, Devine, & Harmon-Jones, 2008). In other words, when motivation to regulate prejudice is autonomous, the automatic detection of discrepancy between one's ideal behavior (i.e., to respond without prejudice) and actual behavior (i.e., prejudiced responding) is enhanced, and prejudice regulation is improved.

This automatic monitoring of self-regulatory errors is a primary neurocognitive system underlying executive control. Localization research has shown that the anterior cingulate cortex (ACC) is responsible for the automatic monitoring of ongoing response tendencies and in signalling the need for enhanced regulation when conflict occurs (Botvinick, Braver, Barch, Carter, & Cohen, 2001; Bush, Luu, & Posner, 2000). Thus, the ACC plays a central role in executive function in general, and in prejudice regulation in particular. As demonstrated in various implicit measures of prejudice (e.g., Greenwald et al., 1998; Payne, 2001), self-regulation is required to override stereotype-driven biases. The ACC is crucial in signalling when such biases occur, as well as in recruiting and mobilizing self-regulation resources to reduce prejudice. In particular, the ACC gives rise to an important neurophysiological signal of this error monitoring process, namely, the error related negativity (ERN). The ERN is a negative-polarity voltage deflection observed in scalp-recorded electroencephalography (EEG) when participants make a response error on a cognitive conflict task (Dehaene, Posner, & Tucker, 1994; Falkenstein, Hohnsbein, & Hoormann, 1991; Gehring, Gross, Coles, Meyer, & Donchin, 1993). Those with larger ERN responses tend to demonstrate greater response regulation across conflict-related tasks, including the self-regulation of prejudice (Amodio et al., 2008; Gehring et al., 1993; Legault & Inzlicht, 2013). Interestingly, having an autonomous motivation to respond without prejudice, rather than a controlled motivation, is associated with increased error monitoring on prejudice inhibition tasks, as indexed by a larger ERN. In turn, this heightened ERN response is linked to greater response regulation – as demonstrated by lower implicit prejudice (Amodio et al.). Thus, because prejudice is often an ingrained consequence of categorization processes, occasional failures in responding without prejudice are inevitable – no matter how autonomously motivated one is to be nonprejudiced. ERN research suggests that, when prejudice arises, autonomous prejudice regulators are better at noticing, orienting, and reacting to race biases when they occur, so that they can learn from them and therefore minimize future instances of them.

Although not yet applied to prejudice regulation, we have recently found causal support for the effect of autonomous motivation on the ERN. Specifically, participants whose autonomy was supported via the offering of choice in a self-regulation task reported greater autonomous task motivation compared to those who were externally pressured into the task, and this increase in autonomous motivation enhanced brain-mediated error monitoring during the task, as evinced by a higher ERN (Legault & Inzlicht, 2013). From a cognitive perspective (e.g., Holroyd & Coles, 2002), this suggests that autonomous motivation amplifies the neural processes underlying the detection of self-regulation failure, which serves to improve performance. To use an affect-based explanation (e.g., Bartholow et al., 2005; Bush et al., 2000), it appears that, through increased motivational engagement, autonomous motivation enhances the neural distress signal associated with self-regulation failure. Although the link between autonomy and this distress response might at first seem counterintuitive, it is important to consider the role played by autonomy in promoting deep behavioral engagement – which indeed appears to produce a strong motivational reaction when performance is not optimal. We therefore suggest that autonomy predicts better and more accurate *awareness of negative affect and threat*, which results in improved spontaneous coping with such negative affect and threat, including dynamic adjustments to performance that can improve self-regulation. This interpretation coincides with the finding that autonomy (more than control) is related to the integrative acknowledgement of negative affect and personal flaws (Weinstein, Deci, & Ryan, 2011), and increases openness to negative feedback (Hodgins & Liebeskind, 2003; Hodgins et al., 2010). Indeed, autonomous individuals are inclined to respond to failure in a mastery-oriented fashion by accepting responsibility and focusing on self-improvement (Koestner & Zuckerman, 1994). As a result, they may be more likely to attend and react to those moments when their self-regulation efforts have failed (e.g., when responses are prejudiced). This open attending to self-regulation failure is a key adaptation to the environment that allows people to slow down, recalibrate their behavior, and ultimately improve their performance. Ongoing work in our laboratory is testing the assertion that autonomous motivation to be nonprejudiced promotes greater awareness of – and concern over – unintended biases in responding (as implemented in the brain), which in turn bolsters the automatic self-regulation of prejudice.

Influencing Prejudice Reduction: The Role of Autonomy Support and Social Control

Given the various intergroup benefits of having an autonomous motivation to regulate group-based prejudice, a natural and important question becomes: How can we promote it? That is, can the social environment encourage people to adopt self-determined reasons for behaving in nonprejudiced ways? Will this decrease prejudice? Conversely, what is the impact of using controlling anti-prejudice directives aimed at promoting external motivation to regulate prejudice? For instance, many antiprejudice and antidiscrimination programs, policies, and laws are geared toward combating or erasing prejudice, and these initiatives often stress externally prescribed outcomes based on the requirements of organizational policy or societal standards. In other words, blatant group-based prejudice is socially unacceptable in many diverse societies, and as multiculturalism rises, it is not uncommon for people to feel urged to control their biases. We were interested in assessing the impact of controlling antiprejudice tactics on prejudice reduction. At the same time, we wanted to test the hypothesis that supporting autonomous motivation would reduce prejudice.

From a SDT framework, *autonomy support* in the context of prejudice reduction involves the enhancement of perceived personal choice and volition in pursuing egalitarian ideals. It also entails the provision of information about the various benefits and virtues of nonprejudiced classrooms, workplaces, and societies. Autonomy supportive environments promote inner motivational resources by encouraging the examination of how nonprejudice and positive intergroup relations may be personally valuable, meaningful, and enjoyable. In contrast, controlling environments pressure people to comply with antiprejudice standards; use coercive language; and emphasize societal pressure and requirement to be nonprejudiced. This approach is common in organizations, where autonomy is often bypassed because individuals are forced to adhere to policy rather than encouraged to value equality on their own terms (Legault et al., 2011).

An Empirical Illustration

To examine these different environmental forces, we assessed the impact of supporting autonomous motivation to regulate prejudice and promoting controlled motivation to regulate prejudice on outgroup attitudes in two experiments (Legault et al., 2011). In the first experiment, non-Black participants were randomly assigned to read one of two prejudice intervention brochures or a neutral brochure

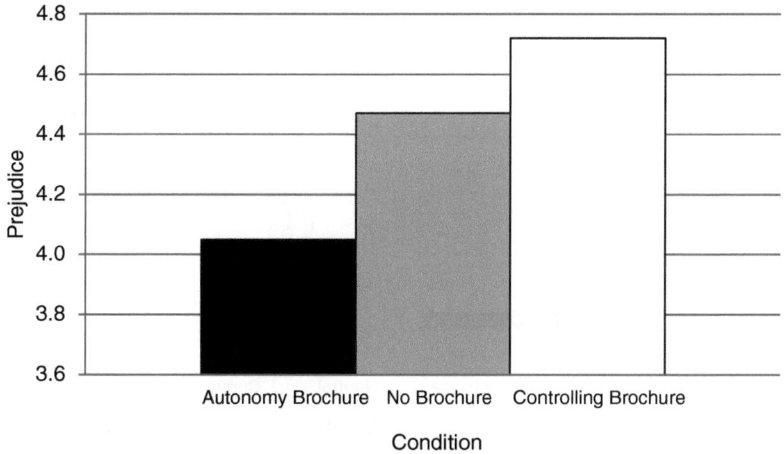

Fig. 8.2 Effect of motivational brochures on prejudice. All differences significant at $p < .05$

(i.e., an autonomy-support brochure, a controlling brochure, and a no-motivation/no-brochure condition), and then prejudice toward Black Canadians was measured using the Symbolic Racism Scale (Henry & Sears, 2002). Each motivational brochure was framed as campus initiative to reduce prejudice and, in all three conditions, participants were offered factual information about the preponderance of prejudice in society and on campus. However, the brochures differed in terms of the type of motivation they encouraged. In the autonomy-support condition, the value of nonprejudice was emphasized. Participants' inner motivational resources were targeted by encouraging volition and explaining why prejudice reduction is important and worthwhile. In the controlling-brochure condition, participants were urged to combat prejudice for external reasons and to comply with social norms of nonprejudice.

Results revealed that participants who read the autonomy-support brochure reported less prejudice than those in the neutral, no brochure condition (see Fig. 8.2). In contrast, participants assigned to read the controlling brochure actually demonstrated significantly more prejudice than those in the neutral condition – suggesting that encouraging people to control prejudice for external reasons is in fact counterproductive and produces more prejudice than doing nothing to motivate prejudice reduction.

In the second experiment, motivation to regulate prejudice was manipulated using a subtler method. Participants were induced to agree with a series of eight statements describing the need to reduce group-based prejudice. Thus, some participants were induced to agree with autonomous reasons for reducing prejudice (e.g., "being nonprejudiced is important to me"; "equality and equal rights across groups are important values") and some were induced to agree with controlled reasons for reducing prejudice (e.g., "I should avoid being racist"; "Prejudiced people are not well-liked in society"). Furthermore, participants in the autonomous motivation

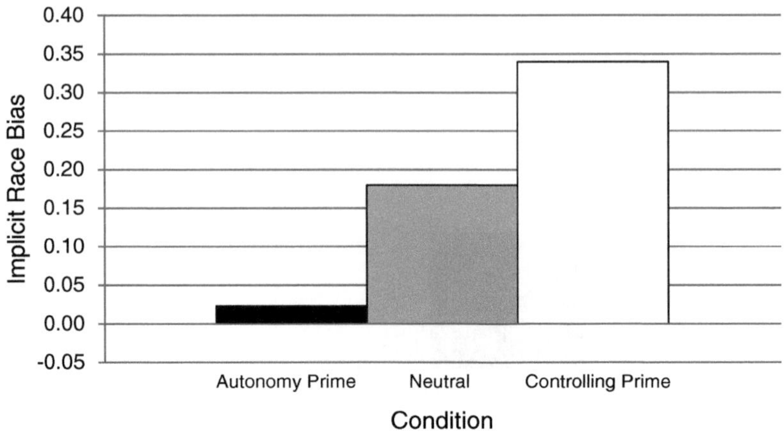

Fig. 8.3 Effect of motivational priming on implicit race bias. All differences significant at $p<.05$

condition were asked to write a few sentences describing why nonprejudice is important and enjoyable to them. In contrast, those in the controlled motivation condition were asked to describe why they felt nonprejudice is required of them by others as well as their felt obligation to be nonprejudiced. Then, prejudice was measured using both the Symbolic Racism Scale and the Race-Face Implicit Association Test. As in Experiment 1, those primed with autonomous motivation to be nonprejudiced demonstrated less explicit and implicit prejudice compared the no-manipulation group (see Fig. 8.3). Conversely, those primed with controlled motivation displayed more explicit and implicit prejudice than the other two groups. In both experiments (i.e., brochure and priming), the effect of experimental condition on prejudice was partially mediated by self-determined motivation to regulate prejudice. In other words, both the autonomy support brochure and the sentence priming manipulation reduced prejudice by increasing autonomous motivation to regulate prejudice.

Implications for Anti-prejudice Programming, Training, and Policy

The data presented in Figs. 8.2 and 8.3 demonstrate the importance of supporting and encouraging autonomous motivation to regulate prejudice. However, they also illustrate the adverse effects of pressuring people to be nonprejudiced, and show that controlling antiprejudice messages, policies, and programs can backfire to ironically increase prejudice. The ironic effect of social control found in these studies suggests that the impact of coercion on attitudes may be even more detrimental than the typical effect of external motivation on behavior. One can surely imagine a situation where increased external control and demand (e.g., the "toughening" of laws or rules) might fuel negative attitudes about the control, but nonetheless elicit behavioral compliance (e.g., you disagree with the reduced speed limit, but you obey it anyway). As such, we fear that telling people how to think and feel about other social groups actually worsens intergroup attitudes, even if these controls somehow satisfy regulations on discrimination (e.g., enacting employment equity or participating in "diversity training"). Indeed, we suggest that interventions that eliminate people's freedom to choose egalitarian goals or to value diversity and nonprejudice on their own terms may incite hostility toward the perceived source of the pressure (e.g., the stigmatized group), or a desire to rebel against the process of prejudice reduction itself. According to reactance theory (Brehm & Brehm, 1981), this "rebellion" represents a direct counterresponse (i.e., defiance) to threatened autonomy.

These findings have serious implications for the enforcement of rules and standards of nonprejudice, especially when one considers that many intervention programs and policies use controlling, antiprejudice techniques. We suggest that such antiprejudice pressure backfires—deflating personal autonomy, tapping into external and social concerns at the expense of personal ones, and ultimately increasing prejudice. Rather than relying on controlling tactics and pressuring language, it is instead important for prejudice intervention to encourage personal valuing of diversity and equality. This can be done by offering useful information regarding the virtue of egalitarianism, by discussing the importance and enjoyment of intergroup relationships, and by examining the many benefits of diverse and fair classrooms, workplaces, and communities. The notion of supplementing social policy with rationale about its merits is a humane and cost-effective (albeit highly underused) strategy that may help in shifting the locus of causality for prejudice regulation from external to internal. Thus, even if equality is externally enforced through social norms and organizational procedures, our findings indicate that such guidelines can be effectively internalized through contexts and behaviors that support autonomous motivation toward diversity and intergroup relations.

SDT and the Role of Group Norms in Shaping Intergroup Behavior

Thus far, we have suggested that the positive and prosocial norms of nonprejudice and egalitarianism can be emitted out of self-determined (as well as nonself-determined) reasons. To offer another application of SDT to the realm of intergroup relations, we have recently investigated the reasons why group members endorse not just nonprejudice and egalitarianism (i.e., parity), but also norms in favor of prejudice and discrimination (Amiot, Sansfaçon, Louis, & Yelle, 2012). Ingroup norms are potent forces that guide individual group members' behaviors and attitudes (e.g., Smith & Louis, 2008). While SDT has been mainly applied to prosocial and productive social behaviors including self-determined work motivation (e.g., Gagné & Deci, 2005), positive interpersonal relationships (LaGuardia & Patrick, 2008), persistence in sports (Pelletier, Fortier, Vallerand, & Brière, 2001), healthful behavior (Teixeira et al., 2010; Williams et al., 2009) and volunteering (Millette &

Gagné, 2008), SDT research has largely avoided the assessment of whether negative behaviors, such as prejudice and discrimination, might be emitted out of self-determined reasons. Thus, we undertook one of the first investigations of the motivations underlying harmful intergroup behaviors, such as discrimination, and the role played by group norms in shaping these motivations.

According to SDT, harmful and defensive behavior, such as discrimination, occurs when basic needs are unfulfilled (Deci & Ryan, 2000). Under these conditions, motivation for the dysfunctional behavior is not self-determined, but elicited by harmful norms and deficient environments (see also Kasser, 2002). In SDT terms, discriminatory behavior and prejudice – as forms of harmful and defensive behaviors – would hence be seen as an outcome of disturbances in need satisfaction and autonomous motivation. On the basis of this reasoning, we expected that discriminatory behavior would emanate from controlled motivations, rather than autonomous reasons.

In addition to testing whether different norms exert a significant impact on group members' behavior, we were also interested in investigating why group members behave congruently versus incongruently with different types of norms. In other words, we assessed the role of autonomous motivation in the endorsement of prosocial and harmful group norms. Although social norms are often coercive and pressuring, they can also be internalized and endorsed freely and out of choice (Amiot, Sansfaçon, & Louis, 2013; Kelman, 1961). Thus, we were interested in the conditions under which norms would be adopted (or not) for autonomous versus controlled reasons.

We investigated the effects of the relatively prosocial norm of parity/egalitarianism and the comparatively less prosocial norm of discrimination on ingroup members' own parity and discriminatory behaviors by assessing the manner in which participants distributed resources between one's ingroup and an outgroup of similar size and resource need. More specifically, after being exposed to the norms of their group, participants were asked to decide how they themselves wanted to distribute resources between the ingroup and a relevant outgroup by selecting one of two options: (1) distributing resources such that the ingroup would be advantaged (discrimination), or (2) distributing resources evenly between the ingroup and the outgroup (parity). By comparing norms of parity and discrimination, we were able to test whether the prosocial norm of parity would be more amenable to internalization than would the norm of discrimination.

In two experiments, we found that participants were more likely to discriminate when ingroup norms prescribed discrimination, and more likely to engage in parity when group norms promoted parity – a finding that replicates much research on the role of norms in shaping behavior (Smith & Louis, 2008). However, over and above this effect of norms on group members' behavior, participants were less likely to engage in discrimination than in parity behavior – suggesting that parity is a more socially valued and acceptable behavior. Moreover, as can be seen in Fig. 8.4, those who conformed to the group norm of discrimination reported lower self-determined motives for doing so (i.e., they were more likely to attribute their

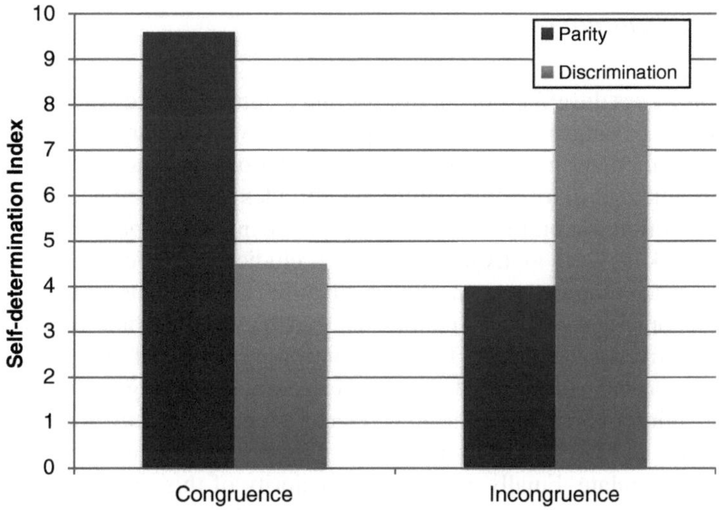

Fig. 8.4 Effects of parity and discrimination norms and participants' behavioral congruence with these norms on self-determination (Reproduced from Amiot et al., 2012)

behavior to external pressures), whereas people who conformed to the group norm of parity reported higher self-determined motivation. Interestingly, and also supporting the SDT view, participants who resisted the norm of discrimination reported high self-determination for doing so, suggesting that these participants may have been relying on deeply internalized motivation that fostered dissent against the normative tide (e.g., see: Packer, 2008). Finally, participants who resisted the parity norm, and who instead displayed discrimination, reported the lowest level of self-determination.

These findings support an SDT approach to understanding group norms, and put forth the idea that prosocial group norms are more conducive to internalization than are harmful norms, due to innate empathy and prosocial instincts. However, other interpretations of our findings exist. For instance, given that egalitarian norms are prevalent in our current democratic and diverse societies, participants may have already internalized and learned the value of egalitarian norms from their ingroups, which, in the specific experimental context, might have facilitated the learning of new egalitarian norms and inhibited the learning of discriminatory norms. This alternative explanation is more in line with a social learning/social identity explanation of intergroup behavior, which would suggest that individuals adopt the norms of their group, regardless of the norm's content (Tajfel & Turner, 1986; Turner, 1991). Future research should disentangle the effects of these alternative explanations. Indeed, given that SDT and traditional intergroup theories such as SIT have vastly divergent perspectives on human motivation, it would be advantageous for future studies to assess the relative predictive power of each theory in explaining and reducing prejudice and discrimination.

Part One: Summary

Part One discusses the effects of controlling and autonomous motivational processes on evaluations of outgroup members. In particular, we summarize the roles of both individual differences in, and situational manipulations of, autonomous motivation to be nonprejudiced in improving outgroup attitudes and reducing negative stereotyping. In addition, we outline some of the possible mediating processes that help to explain the link between motivation to be nonprejudiced and prejudice. Specifically, we suggest that, compared to controlled motivation, autonomous motivation is more likely to become automatically maintained and regulated, which accounts for its relative effectiveness, even on hard to control measures of prejudice. Moving beyond differences in automaticity, we also review evidence suggesting that autonomous motivation to be nonprejudiced is related to enhanced detection of the failure to override racial biases, as measured by increased response conflict monitoring in the anterior cingulate. Finally, whereas the majority of this section focuses on the important role of autonomy in being *non*prejudiced, we also review studies that investigated whether discrimination can be autonomously motivated. In support of SDT, we conclude that although self-determination often underlies egalitarianism, it does not underlie prejudice. Thus, even though people generally tend to adopt the prejudiced norms of their groups, they are likely to do so for controlled reasons.

Part Two: Ingroup-Directed Motivation

Until this point, we have been concerned with the role of autonomous and controlled motivation in predicting how people feel and behave toward *out*groups. We have underscored that the source of motivation guiding the perception of other groups can exert a substantive effect on attitudes and action tendencies toward those other groups. But how might motivation affect how one feels about or identifies with one's *own* group (i.e., the ingroup)?

Just as groups are prominent features of the external world, our group memberships are key features of our internal identity. In other words, our group memberships are internalized to represent who we are. When an individual thinks of him/herself in terms of "we", s/he is attaching personal significance to the group because of her/his association with it. Yet at the same time, s/he is also deriving personal meaning from the group membership itself. To varying degrees, the characteristics of the group are also characteristics of the self. Considering the focal role of the group in the self-concept, it is somewhat regrettable that self-determination theory has generally neglected the role of group processes in the organization of the self. Of course, this is not surprising given that strong traditions in social psychology have caused researchers to focus their analysis on either individual (e.g., cognition and motivation) or group level processes (e.g., social identity and intergroup relations), which has tended to prevent the study of both simultaneously. However, as we have begun to illustrate, group dynamics and human motivation are in no way mutually exclusive, and indeed the function of human autonomy and the process of internalization in group identification seems pivotal.

Bringing together motivation and intergroup approaches has several advantages. It allows us to bridge different branches of social psychology; to conduct novel and integrative research; and to compare the predictive power of these different theories in accounting for individual and intergroup consequences (Doise, 1986; see also Amiot & Hornsey, 2010). For instance, an important tenet of social identity theory – which has been one of the most important and generative approaches to intergroup relations to date – is that the feelings and values one attaches to one's own group membership play a role in shaping how one perceives other groups (Tajfel, 1982; Tajfel & Turner, 1979). Thus, whereas an abundance of research from the social identity approach examines the role of group identification in intergroup relations, SDT offers a framework for understanding how and why group members come to identify with their groups. Indeed, from a SDT perspective, it would seem that one's motivation *toward the ingroup*, and the extent to which one internalizes and integrates his or her group identity, might have implications not only for the nature of ingroup identification, but also for social wellbeing and intergroup relationships.

Motivation to Identify with the Ingroup

Building on SDT postulates of self and identity processes (Ryan & Deci, 2003), some of our recent work (Amiot & Aubin, 2013; Amiot & Sansfaçon, 2011) applies a SDT perspective to understand why group members identify with their social group. Self-determined reasons for identifying with a group include motives such as the inherent pleasure and satisfaction of being a member of the group (intrinsic motivation), the feeling that being a group member allows one to express one's deeply held values and beliefs (integrated regulation), and the feeling that group membership is important and allows one to reach valued goals (identified regulation). In contrast, nonself-determined motivations to identify with the social group include: the pressure one imposes on oneself to be a group member and the sense that one's worth is based on group identity (introjected regulation); the prestige and social recognition that group identification affords (external regulation); and the perception that identification with a social group is fruitless and will not bring about desired outcomes (amotivation).

Based on the notion that self-determined motives are generally associated with more positive consequences (Deci & Ryan, 2000), we expected that the self-determined forms of motivation to identify with one's social group would predict more positive intrapersonal (e.g., wellbeing) and intergroup outcomes (e.g., ingroup bias). This research extends a growing body of work in intergroup relations that hypothesizes that the more competitive and status-oriented forms of identification with a group predict more ingroup bias and more defensiveness, whereas identification stemming from the inherent and autonomous experience of being a group member predicts greater wellbeing and more positive attitudes toward outgroups (e.g., Hinkle & Brown, 1990; Jackson & Smith, 1999; Roccas, Klar, & Liviatan, 2006; Tyler & Blader, 2002). More generally, by applying a SDT framework to the question of why individuals identify with their groups, we sought to elucidate which specific forms of social identification are associated with detrimental versus constructive social consequences. This is an important new direction given that absolute levels of social identification (i.e., traditional measures of social identity strength, scored as high vs. low) have been associated with highly divergent outcomes, including positive outcomes such as increased wellbeing, and also negative outcomes, such as ingroup bias and intergroup competitiveness.

We have conducted several studies investigating the intergroup effects of motivation to identify with a social group – including identification as a member of one's university, identification with a specific national group (e.g., Australian), and identification as a member of one's online gaming community (Amiot & Aubin, 2013; Amiot & Hornsey, 2010; Amiot & Sansfaçon, 2011). When taken together, our findings across six studies generally confirm SDT postulates: Self-determined motivation to identify with a social group predicts more positive consequences, including patriotism, wellbeing, and more positive social identity. Conversely, nonself-determined forms of motivation tend to predict negative consequences, including nationalism, identity conflict, and ingroup bias. These effects remained even after controlling for participants' absolute degree of identification with their group (i.e., traditional measures of social identity strength). Despite this overall pattern, two findings were contrary to our expectations: intrinsic motivation to identify predicted both nationalism and ingroup bias (Amiot & Sansfaçon). These unexpected findings may be attributable to the dual nature of intrinsic motivation in certain domains. In the realm of intergroup relations and social identity, for instance, intrinsic motivation to identify with one's social group could also include an obsessive component that involves disinhibition and compulsion (Vallerand et al., 2003). It is this obsessive element that may encourage group members to engage in actions that seek to maximize a positive social identity (i.e., ingroup bias). Under such circumstances, intrinsic motivation is unlikely to be fully integrated in the self, and group membership is pursued uncontrollably or impulsively rather than thoughtfully self-endorsed. Indeed, we suggest that the integration of group identity into the self may be the critical factor in healthy group identification and positive intergroup consequences (Amiot, Sansfaçon; Legault, Weinstein, Davis, & Mitchell, in prep).

The Integration of Group Identity

Integration represents the pinnacle of authentic functioning. Accordingly, Weinstein et al. (2011) describe integration as the acknowledgment of who one is, and the experience of alignment in thoughts, actions, goals, beliefs, values, and identities. These authors echo classic theorists who note that the capacity to integrate life's many experiences into a meaningful and cohesive whole is fundamental to the development of an organized and healthy identity (e.g., Jung, 1959; Rogers, 1963). We extend their observation, and suggest that identity integration is vital not just to the individual's personal self-concept, but to *group* identity as well. In other words, we posit that the acknowledgement of the various aspects of one's group identity – regardless of whether these aspects are conflicting, inconsistent, threatening, or negative – is integrally related to the development of a healthy, integrated group identity (Legault & Upal, 2012). Given that all social groups are adorned with various divergently valenced attributes, and that, as collectives, groups experience a multitude of pleasant and unpleasant events, it is likely that the process through which people perceive and manage the content of their ingroup identity has far-reaching implications for how they perceive and interact with the social world.

Thus, applying the SDT view of integration to better understand the process of group identification and its role in intergroup relations, we suggest that the optimal development of a given group identity (e.g., ethnic identity, national identity, gender identity) rests on the incorporation and consideration of the complexity of that group's experience and the vast spectrum of group-based thoughts and feelings (Legault & Upal, 2012; Legault et al., in prep). In line with this reasoning, we refer to *group identity integration* as the process of synthesizing a coherent conceptualization of the ingroup by weaving the conflicting aspects of ingroup membership into a meaningful whole. In other words, group identity integration entails the establishment of interconnections between different, seemingly incompatible components of group identity. A more practical definition of integrated group identity, therefore, refers to the acknowledgement of both positive and negative characteristics of one's ingroup. This does not entail that group members must necessarily agree with or endorse their ingroup's negative experiences, attributes, or behavior, but rather that they acknowledge these elements as part of their overarching group identity. In contrast, defensiveness involves the rejection of certain components of identity, which leads to more guarded and fragmented functioning and diminished well-being (e.g., Weinstein et al., 2011). Under such conditions, perception becomes rigid and selective (Majstorovic, Legault, & Green-Demers, 2008). Accordingly, we refer to a *defensive group identity* as the rejection of, or defense against, certain characteristics and events (usually negative) associated with the ingroup (Legault et al., in prep).

The Motivational Antecedents of Group Identity Integration

Although not yet applied to a group processes framework, recent work suggests that motivation is crucial in the process of identity integration (Hodgins & Knee, 2002; Weinstein, et al., 2011). When people feel autonomously motivated, that is, when their actions spring from personal belief and authentic choice, they are more disposed toward integration. Because integrated people act more consistently with their needs and interests, it is not surprising that integration is robustly related to wellbeing (e.g., Deci & Ryan, 1995). In contrast, controlled motivational orientation is characterized by the internal deflection of social pressures, which constrains behavior to external contingencies – such as social approval, recognition, and reprimand. Controlled behaviour promotes defensiveness as people aim to appease external demands. As a result, openness and growth – which often involve the confrontation of undesirable behaviour and characteristics – are forestalled. Research has demonstrated that controlled motivation leads to more defensiveness in social behaviour (Hodgins, Koestner, & Duncan, 1996). Similarly, controlled individuals tend to dissociate from negative past identities, which negatively affects wellbeing (Weinstein et al., 2011).

Expanding this work to the group level, we recently assessed the link between motivational orientation and group identity integration (Legault & Upal, 2012; Legault et al., in prep). Group identity integration was assessed by asking participants to generate a range of potentially inconsistent aspects (i.e., positive and negative behaviors and qualities) of their ethnocultural ingroup, and then to indicate the extent to which they integrated these qualities into their ingroup identity (i.e., 5 items assessed the degree to which people acknowledged each quality as part of the ingroup identity). As anticipated, dispositional autonomy (as measured by the General Causality Orientations Scale; Deci & Ryan, 1985b) was positively associated with integrating both positive and negative ingroup identities to a similar degree (group identity integration). In contrast, having a controlled motivational orientation was positively related to the acceptance of positive identities, but negatively related to the integration of negative identities – suggesting that controlled individuals engage in group identity defensiveness. Interestingly, both defensive and integrated forms of group identity were comparably related to identity strength (as measured by absolute social identification). However, group identity integration was more strongly related to group esteem (i.e., feelings of positive affect and wellbeing in relation to the ingroup), compared to group identity defensiveness. And, unlike defensiveness, integration was negatively related to prejudice. Again, this finding illustrates the potential insufficiency of traditional measures of social identification in capturing important nuances in social identity processes and their implications for prejudice (see also: Croll, 2007; Goren & Plaut, 2012). This preliminary theory and data suggest that the core motivational process of integration that has proven to be vital in personality development (e.g., Deci & Ryan, 1985a, 2002; Freud, 1923; Hodgins & Knee, 2002; Jung, 1959; Rogers, 1963; Weinstein et al., 2011) is also important in group processes and intergroup relations.

The Development of New Social Identities and the Integration of Multiple Social Identities in the Self: The Role of Psychological Needs

Another line of work has looked at identity integration from a different angle, that is, by focusing on how group members integrate new and multiple group identities in their overall sense of self (Amiot, de la Sablonnière, Terry, & Smith, 2007). Given the flux of current society, our social identities are increasingly subject to change. A growing number of individuals experience organizational and career changes, migrate to new countries, change their social networks, and redefine their friendships in the process (Kammeyer-Mueller & Wanberg, 2003; United Nations, 2002; Wegmann, 1991). These life transitions lead people to join new social groups and encourage them to adopt new social, cultural, and institutional identities. Individuals also belong to multiple social groups, including their professional groups, their family, leisure groups, and social categories including one's culture(s), nation, and gender. To account for this multiplicity and change in social identities over time, we propose that multiple social identities become integrated within the self over time when they are simultaneously important to self-definition and when they are cognitively linked with one another. As a consequence, one feels coherent rather than conflicted (see also Sheldon & Kasser, 1995).

Need Satisfaction in New Group Settings

The interpersonal support and resources available within a group can directly affect a new group member's adjustment to his/her new environment, as well as the extent to which the new social identity is integrated over time. To identify the factors that facilitate the development of a new social identity and to explain the intraindividual processes involved as individuals acquire and integrate a new social identity over time, we have recently proposed the cognitive-developmental model of social identity integration (Amiot et al., 2007). One aspect of our model that is particularly relevant to the self-determination literature proposes that as individuals join their new social group, the satisfaction of their basic psychological needs in the new group context – namely, the need for autonomy, competence, and relatedness (Bettencourt & Sheldon, 2001; Sheldon & Bettencourt, 2002) – will determine which coping and adaptation strategies they will employ to adjust to the new setting. While most SDT research has focused on needs satisfied in people's lives in general (i.e., not necessarily in group contexts), it is important to note that these three fundamental psychological needs are also satisfied via our membership in social groups per se (Bettencourt & Sheldon; Sheldon & Bettencourt). When joining a new social group, we propose that the more these psychological needs are satisfied in the new group context, the more the individual will cope actively and constructively in their new environment, and the more the new social identity will develop and become an important dimension of overall self-concept.

An Empirical Illustration

We tested this proposition in two studies (Amiot, Terry, Wirawan, & Grice, 2010). Given our interest in investigating *changes* in social identification, the social identification variable in these studies was constructed so as to tap into the intraindividual changes occurring in identification over time (see also Bettencourt, Charlton, Eubanks, & Kernahan, 1999).

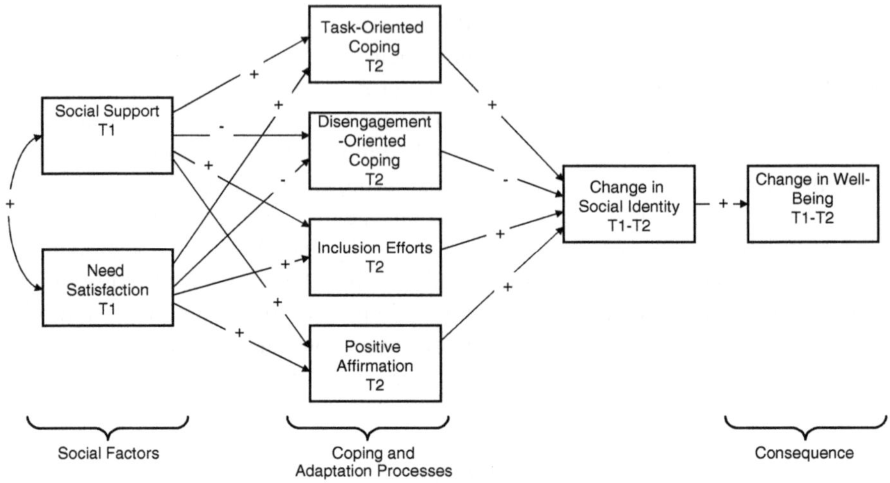

Fig. 8.5 The role of social support, need satisfaction via the new group and coping on change in social identity and well-being (Reproduced from Amiot et al., 2010)

As illustrated in Fig. 8.5, social support and need satisfaction – both conceptualized as resources that are potentially available in the new group context – were expected to predict active task-oriented coping strategies (e.g., planning, effort expenditure, problem-solving), while predicting a reduction in the use of engagement-oriented coping strategies (e.g., behavioural and mental disengagement, venting of emotions). In turn, we anticipated that these coping and adaptation strategies would lead to changes in social identification over time. In line with traditional coping research (Lazarus & Folkman, 1984), we also expected that coping and adaptation strategies would mediate the associations between the social factors (i.e., social support and need satisfaction) and changes in social identification (see also Amiot et al., 2007). Finally, and building on the increasing empirical evidence that confirms the benefits of identification with social groups (e.g., Amiot & Sansfaçon, 2011; Jetten, Haslam, & Haslam, 2011), we hypothesized that an increase in social identification would predict enhanced psychological well-being.

These associations were tested in two samples. In Study 1, we surveyed first year university students as they were experiencing an important life transition (Ruble & Seidman, 1996) and developing a new sense of identification with their university. Study 2 included members of a new online gaming community – a type of social group that is salient and important for its members (Hornsey, Grice, Jetten, Paulsen, & Callan, 2007; Reichers, Spears, & Postmes, 1995). We employed a longitudinal design in both studies and collected data at two time points. The first questionnaire took place within the first 3 months of entry into the new group and the second questionnaire was completed 3–5 months after the first questionnaire.

Findings from our path analyses supported most of the hypotheses. In Study 1, both social support and need satisfaction in the group context (at Time 1) predicted task-oriented coping (at Time 2). Social support also reduced the use of disengagement coping. Moreover, task-oriented coping predicted an increase in group identification from Time 1 to Time 2, which subsequently predicted an increase in vitality – a relevant indicator of wellbeing. Only two associations were found not to be significant, namely, the association between need satisfaction and disengagement-oriented coping and between disengagement-oriented coping and change in group identification. An alternative model that omitted the nonsignificant links (and did not significantly differ from the original model) presented satisfactory fit indices: (χ^2 (8)=11.473, p=.176, S-B χ^2=10.252, CFI=.965, adjusted CFI=.971, RMR=.059, RMSEA=.061, adjusted RMSEA=.049). Tests of mediation (Holmbeck, 1997; Shrout & Bolger, 2002) confirmed that coping strategies and changes in social identification significantly mediated the associations between the social factors (e.g., social support and need satisfaction) and wellbeing (i.e., vitality).

In Study 2, our goal was to replicate the links hypothesized in Fig. 8.5. Furthermore, in an effort to better understand the processes through which social identities change over time, we assessed two group-level coping strategies (Mummendey, Kessler, Klink, & Mielke, 1999). While individual-level strategies – which are typically assessed in the coping literature – tap into the individual's own actions to deal with the change (without reference to their social group), group-level adaptation strategies capture behaviors performed at the intragroup and intergroup levels of analysis. Thus, we assessed *inclusion efforts*, which refer to the efforts made by group members to fit in and adopt the norms of the new ingroup, and *positive affirmation*, which reflects the extent to which group members actively affirm the positive aspects of their new group relative to outgroups.

Results from the path analyses supported most of the hypothesized associations: Both social support and needs satisfied in the group context at Time 1 positively predicted each type of active coping at Time 2 (i.e., both individual task-oriented coping and group-level coping). Interestingly, only the group-level coping strategies predicted an increase in social identification from Time 1 to Time 2, suggesting the importance of group-level processes when predicting adjustment to changes that involve joining new groups and reorganizing one's social identities (Terry, Carey, & Callan, 2001). Finally, this change in identification predicted an increase in positive emotions over time. A final model that omitted the nonsignificant link (i.e., the association between task-oriented coping and change in identification) presented satisfactory fit indices (χ^2 (10)=57.564, p<.001, S-B χ^2=48.045, CFI=.938, adjusted CFI=.941, RMR=.073, RMSEA=.107, adjusted RMSEA=.096). Tests of mediation confirmed that the majority of the associations between social factors and wellbeing were mediated by coping strategies and changes in social identification.

Conclusions of These Studies

Together, these studies confirmed that the extent to which one's psychological needs are satisfied in the new group context represents an intragroup resource (i.e., a facilitator) that predicts which coping and adaptation strategies are employed by new group members to adjust to the group context. In turn, these coping and adaptation processes predict intraindividual changes in levels of identification with the new group, which in turn influences psychological wellbeing. These results suggest that providing social support to newcomers by valuing their autonomy and ability to contribute to the new group not only enhances their capacity to actively manage the transition (i.e., task-oriented coping), but also encourages them to engage in broader collective actions that will enhance their inclusion and affiliation in the group.

Over the past 5 years, we have accumulated support for the propositions of the cognitive-developmental model of social identity integration (e.g., Amiot, Terry, & Callan, 2007; Amiot, Terry, Jimmieson, & Callan, 2006; Amiot, Terry, & McKimmie, 2012; Smith, Amiot, Callan, Terry, & Smith, 2012; Smith, Amiot, Smith, Callan, & Terry, 2013; Yampolsky, Amiot, & de la Sablonnière, 2013). Building on this past work, we are currently developing novel statistical procedures and instruments to assess social identity integration (de la Sablonnière, Amiot, & Sadykova, in press; Legault et al., in prep; Yampolsky et al., 2013). Longitudinal research is also underway in the highly multicultural context of Montréal, where multiple cultural groups co-exist. This study (www.CIELmontreal.ca) investigates how the needs satisfied via a specific new social group will encourage new immigrants to develop a sense of identification with that group (Doucerain, Amiot, Mireault, & Ryder, 2012). Indeed, we expect that the advancement of research on the factors that promote the healthy integration of social identity will continue to reveal the importance of self-determination in group and intergroup processes and in the promotion of social connectedness and diversity.

Part Two: Summary

Whereas the first half of this chapter examined motivation toward other groups, Part Two investigates motivation in relation to the ingroup. In this section, we use self-determination theory to shed much-needed light on the motivation underlying social identification. That is, we show that group members vary in the extent to which their group identity is self-determined or internalized. In general, we suggest that self-determined forms of social identification are associated with positive perceptions of both the ingroup *and* the outgroup. We also suggest that self-determined motivation to identify with one's social group is an important determinant of wellbeing.

Extending our work on motivation to identify with social groups, we also delve more specifically into the process of integrating one's group identity into the self. We suggest that integration is vital not just at the level of the personal self-concept, but at the group level as well. Thus, the acknowledgement and unification of the various components of group identity, rather than its compartmentalization and defense/protection, appears to be important to group esteem, collective wellbeing, and positive attitudes toward outgroups.

Finally, we discuss the role of need satisfaction and social support in the integration of new group identities during times of social change. We show that the extent to which new groups support autonomy, competence, and relatedness is crucially related to successful coping and adjustment during life transitions (e.g., emigrating, changing schools), when people are faced with the challenge of adopting the customs and values of new groups. Taken together, our findings support the utility of integrating SDT and intergroup theories to better understand social identification processes and to specify which forms of social identification will yield which outcomes.

Concluding Remarks

The past 5 years has seen the burgeoning of a self-determination theory of group process and intergroup relations (e.g., Amiot & Aubin, 2013; Amiot & Hornsey, 2010; Amiot, Sansfaçon, et al., 2012; Legault et al., 2007, 2011, in prep; see also: Duriez, Meeus, & Vansteenkiste, 2012; Duriez, Vansteenkiste, Soenens, & De Witte, 2007). Although there is still much work to be done in this exciting and promising area of research, we have nonetheless laid some groundwork that convincingly demonstrates the role of human autonomy in strengthening group ties and in bolstering group esteem, but also in promoting the positive evaluation of other social groups. The theory and findings presented herein constitute an important extension of self-determination theory – showing that the effects of self-determination expand beyond individual and interpersonal spheres to both the group level and the intergroup dynamic. In addition to this contribution to SDT, we also highlight the extent to which intergroup relations research may benefit from the incorporation of self-determination theory; indeed, the consideration of autonomous and controlled motivations – as well as their underlying social antecedents – helps to identify various mechanisms and boundaries relevant to intergroup theory and the social identity approach. For instance, the assessment of motivation toward (and integration of) group identification adds clarity to the mixed and convoluted findings surrounding the link between group membership and intergroup bias (e.g., Brewer & Campbell, 1976; Hinkle & Brown, 1990; Reynolds & Turner, 2001). In addition, the consideration of motivational influences on intergroup processes reveals conditions under which long-standing intergroup theories no longer hold true – for instance, we have shown that the causal path between intergroup threat and prejudice, which is a fundamental intergroup process (e.g., Stephan & Renfro, 2002; Stephan & Stephan, 2000) is eliminated when motivation to be nonprejudiced is self-determined (but not when it is controlled; Legault & Green-Demers, 2012; see also: Duriez et al., 2012). More generally, we have demonstrated that intergroup attitudes and behavior can be improved when the underlying motivation is self-determined.

Although it is both fruitful and sensible to integrate SDT and intergroup research, there are also limitations. For instance, whereas SDT asserts that adequate psychological nourishment should promote prosociality and nonprejudice, the bulk of social identity theory advocates that prejudice and bias are natural, inevitable consequences of group life. We have attempted to address this discrepancy by reviewing evidence that suggests that prejudice is often a product of controlled motivation and the disruption of psychological need satisfaction. But it should be underscored that, in situations of intergroup conflict, identity integration and autonomously motivated intergroup behavior is likely to be undermined, and, from this perspective, it is not surprising that prejudice should proliferate. Similarly, many life changes are imposed upon us and can threaten our pre-existing social identities as well as our sense of personal autonomy (for instance, organizational mergers that require employees to relinquish their pre-existing organizational identity, or political changes – such as revolutions or coups – that prompt drastic sociopolitical reconfiguration). Thus, in addition to the continuation of research on the ways that need satisfaction can engender better intergroup rapport and more just and fair societies, it will also be important for future studies to assess the extent to which psychologically impoverished contexts preclude the development of autonomous social identification and self-determined motivation to be nonprejudiced. As the work we present in this chapter suggests, the thwarting of human autonomy may be a major factor in the omnipresent social problem of prejudice.

References

Amiot, C. E., & Aubin, R. M. (2013). Why and how are you attached to your social group? Investigating different forms of social identification. *British Journal of Social Psychology, 52*(3), 563–586. doi:10.1111/bjso.12004.

Amiot, C. E., de la Sablonnière, R., Terry, D. J., & Smith, J. R. (2007). Integration of social identities in the self: Toward a cognitive-developmental model. *Personality and Social Psychology Review, 11*(4), 364–388. doi:10.1177/1088868307304091.

Amiot, C. E., & Hornsey, M. J. (2010). Collective self-esteem contingency and its role in predicting intergroup bias. *Self & Identity, 9*(1), 62–86. doi:10.1080/15298860802605895.

Amiot, C. E., & Sansfaçon, S. (2011). Motivations to identify with social groups: Positive and negative consequences. *Group Dynamics, 15*(2), 105–127. doi:10.1037/a0023158.

Amiot, C. E., Sansfaçon, S., & Louis, W. R. (2013). Investigating the motivations underlying harmful social behaviors and the motivational nature of social norms. *Journal of Applied Social Psychology, 43*(10), 2146–2157. doi:10.1111/jasp.12167.

Amiot, C. E., Sansfaçon, S., Louis, W. R., & Yelle, M. (2012). Can intergroup behaviors be emitted out of self-determined reasons? Testing the role of group norms and behavioral congruence in the internalisation of discriminatory and parity behaviors. *Personality and Social Psychology Bulletin, 38*(1), 63–76.

Amiot, C. E., Terry, D. J., & Callan, V. J. (2007). Status, equity, and social identification during an intergroup merger: A longitudinal study. *British Journal of Social Psychology, 46*(3), 557–577. doi:10.1348/014466606X146015.

Amiot, C. E., Terry, D. J., Jimmieson, N. L., & Callan, V. J. (2006). A longitudinal investigation of stress and coping processes during an organizational merger: Implications for job satisfaction and organizational identification. *Journal of Management, 32*(4), 552–574. doi:10.1177/0149206306287542.

Amiot, C. E., Terry, D. J., & McKimmie, B. (2012). Social identity change and integration during an intergroup merger: The role of status, similarity, and threat. *Basic and Applied Social Psychology, 34*(5), 443–455.

Amiot, C. E., Terry, D. J., Wirawan, D., & Grice, T. (2010). Changes in social identities over time: The role of coping and adaptation processes. *British Journal of Social Psychology, 49*(4), 804–826. doi:10.1348/014466609X480624.

Amodio, D. M., & Devine, P. G. (2010). Regulating behavior in the social world: Control in the context of intergroup bias. In R. R. Hassin, K. N. Ochsner, & Y. Trope (Eds.), *Self control in society, mind and brain* (pp. 49–75). New York: Oxford University Press.

Amodio, D. M., Devine, P. G., & Harmon-Jones, E. (2008). Individual differences in the regulation of intergroup bias: The role of conflict monitoring and neural signals for control. *Journal of Personality and Social Psychology, 94*, 60–74.

Bargh, J. A. (1990). Auto-motives: Preconscious determinants of social interaction. In E. T. Higgins & R. M. Sorrentino (Eds.), *Handbook of motivation and cognition* (Vol. 2, pp. 93–132). New York: Guilford Press.

Bargh, J. A. (1999). The cognitive monster: The case against the controllability of automatic stereotype effects. In S. Chaiken & Y. Trope (Eds.), *Dual process theories in social psychology* (pp. 361–382). New York: Guilford.

Bargh, J. A., & Chartrand, T. L. (1999). The unbearable automaticity of being. *The American Psychologist, 54*, 462–479.

Bartholow, B. D., Pearson, M. A., Dickter, C. L., Fabiani, M., Gratton, G., & Sher, K. H. (2005). Strategic control and medial frontal negativity: Beyond errors and response conflict. *Psychophysiology, 42*, 33–42.

Bettencourt, B. A., Charlton, K., Eubanks, J., & Kernahan, C. (1999). Development of collective self-esteem among students: Predicting adjustment to college. *Basic and Applied Social Psychology, 21*(3), 213–222. doi:10.1207/15324839951036380.

Bettencourt, B. A., & Sheldon, K. (2001). Social roles as mechanisms for psychological need satisfaction within social groups. *Journal of Personality and Social Psychology, 81*(6), 1131–1143. doi:10.1037/0022-3514.81.6.1131.

Botvinick, M. M., Braver, T. S., Barch, D. M., Carter, C. S., & Cohen, J. D. (2001). Conflict monitoring and cognitive control. *Psychological Review, 108*, 624–652.

Brehm, S. S., & Brehm, J. W. (1981). *Psychological reactance: A theory of freedom and control.* New York: Academic.

Brewer, M., & Campbell, D. (1976). *Ethnocentrism and intergroup attitudes: East African evidence.* New York: Sage.

Bush, G., Luu, P., & Posner, M. (2000). Cognitive and emotional influences in anterior cingulate cortex. *Trends in Cognitive Sciences, 4*(6), 215–222.

Crandall, C. S., Eshleman, A., & O'Brien, L. (2002). Social norms and the expression and suppression of prejudice: The struggle for internalization. *Journal of Personality and Social Psychology, 82*, 359–378.

Croll, P. R. (2007). Modeling determinants of White racial identity: Results from a new national survey. *Social Forces, 86*, 613–642.

de la Sablonnière, R., Amiot, C. E., Cardenas, D., Sadykova, N., & Gorborukova, G. L. (under review). Identity integration: A subtractive process. *European Journal of Social Psychology.*

Deci, E. L., & Ryan, R. M. (1985a). *Intrinsic motivation and self-determination in human behavior*. New York: Plenum.

Deci, E. L., & Ryan, R. M. (1985b). The general causality orientations scale: Self-determination in personality. *Journal of Research in Personality, 19*, 109–134.

Deci, E. L., & Ryan, R. M. (1995). Human autonomy: The basis for true self-esteem. In M. H. Kernis (Ed.), *Efficacy, agency, and self-esteem* (pp. 31–49). New York: Plenum Press.

Deci, E. L., & Ryan, R. M. (2000). The "what" and "why" of goal pursuits: Human needs and the self-determination of behavior. *Psychological Inquiry, 11*(4), 227–268.

Deci, E. L., & Ryan, R. M. (2002). *Handbook of self-determination theory research.* Rochester, NY: University of Rochester Press.

Deci, E. L., & Ryan, R. M. (2008). Facilitating optimal motivation and psychological well-being across life's domains. *Canadian Psychology, 49*, 14–23.

Dehaene, S., Posner, M. I., & Tucker, D. M. (1994). Localization of a neural system for error detection and compensation. *Psychological Science, 5*, 303–305.

Devine, P. G. (1989). Stereotypes and prejudice: Their automatic and controlled components. *Journal of Personality and Social Psychology, 56*, 5–18.

Devine, P. G., Plant, E. A., Amodio, D. M., Harmon-Jones, E., & Vance, S. L. (2002). The regulation of explicit and implicit race bias: The role of motivations to respond without prejudice. *Journal of Personality and Social Psychology, 82*(5), 835–848.

Doise, W. (1986). *Levels of explanation in social psychology. European monographs in social psychology*. New York: Cambridge University Press.

Doucerain, M., Amiot, C. E., Mireault, M., & Ryder, A. G. (2012). *Acculturation et intégration des identités culturelles multiples à Montréal (Acculturation and multiple cultural identity integration in Montreal)*. Talk presented at the conference of the Société québécoise pour la recherche en psychologie, Sherbrooke, PQ, Canada.

Dunton, B. C., & Fazio, R. H. (1997). An individual difference measure of motivation to control prejudiced reactions. *Journal of Personality and Social Psychology, 23*(3), 316–326.

Duriez, B., Meeus, J., & Vansteenkiste, M. (2012). Why are some people more susceptible to ingroup threat than others? The importance of a relative extrinsic to intrinsic value orientation. *Journal of Research in Personality, 46*, 164–172.

Duriez, B., Vansteenkiste, M., Soenens, B., & De Witte, H. (2007). The social costs of extrinsic relative to intrinsic goal pursuits: Their relation with social dominance and racial and ethnic prejudice. *Journal of Personality, 75*, 757–782.

Falkenstein, M., Hohnsbein, J., & Hoormann, J. (1991). Effects of errors in choice reaction tasks on the ERP under focused and divided attention. In C. H. M. Brunia, W. K. Gailard, & A. Kok (Eds.), *Psychophysiological brain research* (Vol. 1, pp. 192–195). Tilburg, the Netherlands: Tilburg University Press.

Freud, S. (1923). *The ego and the id*. New York: Norton.

Gaertner, S. L., & Dovidio, J. F. (1986). The aversive form of racism. In J. F. Dovidio & S. L. Gaertner (Eds.), *Prejudice, discrimination, and racism* (pp. 61–89). New York: Academic.

Gagné, M., & Deci, E. L. (2005). Self-determination theory and work motivation. *Journal of Organizational Behavior, 26*, 331–362.

Gehring, W. J., Goss, B., Coles, M. G., & Meyer, D. E. (1993). A neural system for error detection and compensation. *Psychological Science, 4*, 385–390.

Goren, M. J., & Plaut, V. C. (2012). Identity form matters: White racial identity and attitudes toward diversity. *Self and Identity, 11*(2), 237–254.

Greenwald, A. G., McGhee, D. E., & Schwartz, J. L. (1998). Measuring individual differences in implicit cognition: The implicit association test. *Journal of Personality and Social Psychology, 74*(6), 1464–1480.

Hassin, R. R., Uleman, J. S., & Bargh, J. A. (2005). *The new unconscious*. New York: Oxford University Press.

Henry, P. J., & Sears, D. O. (2002). The symbolic racism 2000 scale. *Political Psychology, 23*(2), 253–283.

Hinkle, S., & Brown, R. (1990). Intergroup comparisons and social identity: Some links and lacunae. In D. Abrams & M. Hogg (Eds.), *Social identity theory: Constructive and critical advances* (pp. 48–70). New York: Springer.

Hodgins, H. S., & Knee, R. C. (2002). The integrating self and conscious experience. In E. L. Deci & R. M. Ryan (Eds.), *Handbook of self-determination research* (pp. 87–100). Rochester, NY: The University of Rochester Press.

Hodgins, H. S., Koestner, R., & Duncan, N. (1996). On the compatibility of autonomy and relatedness. *Personality and Social Psychology Bulletin, 22*, 227–237.

Hodgins, H. S., & Liebeskind, E. (2003). Apology versus defense: Antecedents and consequences. *Journal of Experimental Social Psychology, 39*, 297–316.

Hodgins, H. S., Weibust, K. S., Weinstein, N., Shiffman, S., Miller, A., & Coombs, G. (2010). The cost of self-protection: Threat response and performance as a function of autonomous and controlled motivations. *Personality and Social Psychology Bulletin, 36*(8), 1101–1114.

Holmbeck, G. N. (1997). Toward terminological, conceptual, and statistical clarity in the study of mediators and moderators. *Journal of Consulting and Clinical Psychology, 65*(4), 599–610. doi:10.1037/0022-006X.65.4.599.

Holroyd, C. B., & Coles, M. G. H. (2002). The neural basis of human error processing: Reinforcement learning, dopamine, and the error-related negativity. *Psychological Review, 109*, 679–709.

Hornsey, M. J., Grice, T. A., Jetten, J., Paulsen, N., & Callan, V. J. (2007). Group-directed criticism and recommendations for change. *Personality and Social Psychology Bulletin, 33*(7), 1036–1048. doi:10.1177/0146167207301029.

Jackson, J. W., & Smith, E. R. (1999). Conceptualizing social identity: A new framework and evidence for the impact of different dimensions. *Personality and Social Psychology Bulletin, 25*(1), 120–135. doi:10.1177/0146167299025001010.

Jetten, J., Haslam, C., & Haslam, S. A. (2011). *The social cure: Identity, health, and wellbeing*. London/New York: Psychology Press.

Jung, C. G. (1959). *Aion: Researches into the phenomenology of self* (R. F. C. Hull, Trans.). Princeton, NJ: Princeton University Press.

Kammeyer-Mueller, J. D., & Wanberg, C. R. (2003). Unwrapping the organizational entry process: Disentangling multiple antecedents and their pathways to adjustment. *Journal of Applied Psychology, 88*(5), 779–794. doi:10.1037/0021-9010.88.5.779.

Kasser, T. (2002). Sketches for a self-determination theory of values. In E. L. Deci & R. M. Ryan (Eds.), *Handbook of self-determination research* (pp. 123–140). Rochester, NY: University of Rochester Press.

Kelman, H. C. (1961). Processes of opinion change. *Public Opinion Quarterly, 25*(1), 57–78. doi:10.1086/266996.

Koestner, R., & Zuckerman, M. (1994). Causality orientations, failure, and achievement. *Journal of Personality, 62*, 321–346.

La Guardia, J. G., & Patrick, H. (2008). Self-determination theory as a fundamental theory of close relationships. *Canadian Psychology, 49*, 201–209.

Lazarus, R. S., & Folkman, S. (1984). *Stress, appraisal, and coping*. New York: Springer.

Legault, L., & Green-Demers, I. (2012). The protective role of self-determined prejudice regulation in the relationship between intergroup threat and prejudice. *Motivation and Emotion, 36*(2), 143–158. doi:10.1007/s11031-011-9242-9.

Legault, L., Green-Demers, I., & Eadie, A. L. (2009). When internalization leads to automatization: The role of self-determination in automatic stereotype suppression and implicit prejudice regulation. *Motivation and Emotion, 33*(1), 10–24.

Legault, L., Green-Demers, I., Grant, P., & Chung, J. (2007). On the self-regulation of implicit and explicit prejudice: A self-determination perspective. *Personality and Social Psychology Bulletin, 33*(5), 732–749.

Legault, L., Gutsell, J. N., & Inzlicht, M. (2011). Ironic effects of anti-prejudice messages: How motivational interventions can reduce (but also increase) prejudice. *Psychological Science, 22*(12), 1472–1477.

Legault, L., & Inzlicht, M. (2013). Self-determination, self-regulation and the brain: Autonomy improves performance by enhancing neuroaffective responsiveness to self-regulation failure. *Journal of Personality and Social Psychology, 105*(1), 123–138. doi:10.1037/a0030426.

Legault, L., & Upal, A. (2012). *Group identity integration: Its motivational antecedents and intergroup consequences.* Poster presented at the Society for Personality and Social Psychology's Group Processes and Intergroup Relations Pre-Conference, San Diego, CA.

Legault, L., Weinstein, N., Davis, C., & Mitchell, J. (in prep). The integration of positive and negative group identity: Motivational antecedents and group consequences. Manuscript in preparation.

Majstorovic, N., Legault, L., & Green-Demers, I. (2008). Measuring selfhood according to self-determination theory: Construction and validation of the Ego Functioning Questionnaire (EFQ). *Psihologija, 41*(2), 213–235.

Millette, V., & Gagné, M. (2008). Designing volunteers' tasks to maximize motivation, satisfaction and performance: The impact of job characteristics on volunteer engagement. *Motivation and Emotion, 32*, 11–22.

Moller, A. C., Deci, E. L., & Ryan, R. M. (2006). Choice and ego-depletion: The moderating role of autonomy. *Personality and Social Psychology Bulletin, 32*, 1024–1036.

Monteith, M. J., Arthur, S. A., & Flynn, S. M. (2010). Self-regulation and bias. In J. F. Dovidio, M. Hewstone, P. Glick, & V. M. Esses (Eds.), *Handbook of prejudice, stereotyping, and discrimination* (pp. 493–507). Thousand Oaks, CA: Sage.

Monteith, M. J., Lybarger, J. E., & Woodcock, A. (2009). Schooling the cognitive monster: The role of motivation in the regulation and control of prejudice. *Social and Personality Psychology Compass, 3*, 211–226.

Mummendey, A., Kessler, T., Klink, A., & Mielke, R. (1999). Strategies to cope with negative social identity: Predictions by social identity theory and relative deprivation theory. *Journal of Personality and Social Psychology, 76*(2), 229–245. doi:10.1037/0022-3514.76.2.229.

Muraven, M., Gagné, M., & Rosman, H. (2008). Helpful self-control: Autonomy support, vitality, and depletion. *Journal of Experimental Social Psychology, 44*, 573–585.

Packer, D. J. (2008). On being both with us and against us: A normative conflict model of dissent in social groups. *Personality and Social Psychology Review, 12*(1), 50–72. doi:10.1177/1088868307309606.

Payne, B. K. (2001). Prejudice and perception: The role of automatic and controlled processes in misperceiving a weapon. *Journal of Personality and Social Psychology, 81*, 181–192.

Pelletier, L. G., Fortier, M. S., Vallerand, R. J., & Brière, N. M. (2001). Associations among perceived autonomy support, forms of self-regulation, and persistence: A prospective study. *Motivation and Emotion, 25*, 279–306.

Pettigrew, T. F., & Meertens, R. W. (1995). Subtle and blatant prejudice in Western Europe. *European Journal of Social Psychology, 25*, 57–75.

Plant, E. A., & Devine, P. G. (1998). Internal and external motivation to respond without prejudice. *Journal of Personality and Social Psychology, 75*, 811–832.

Plant, E. A., & Devine, P. G. (2009). The active control of prejudice: Unpacking the intentions guiding control efforts. *Journal of Personality and Social Psychology, 96*(3), 640–652.

Reicher, S. D., Spears, R., & Postmes, T. (1995). A social identity model of deindividuation phenomena. *European Review of Social Psychology, 6*(1), 161–198. doi:10.1080/14792779443000049.

Reynolds, K., & Turner, J. (2001). Prejudice as a group process: The role of social identity. In M. Augoustinos & K. Reynolds (Eds.), *Understanding prejudice, racism, and social conflict* (pp. 159–178). London: Sage.

Roccas, S., Klar, Y., & Liviatan, I. (2006). The paradox of group-based guilt: Modes of national identification, conflict vehemence, and reactions to the in-group's moral violations. *Journal of Personality and Social Psychology, 91*(4), 698–711. doi:10.1037/0022-3514.91.4.698.

Rogers, C. R. (1963). The actualizing tendency in relation to "motives" and to consciousness. In M. R. Jones (Ed.), *Nebraska symposium on motivation* (pp. 1–24). Lincoln, NE: University of Nebraska Press.

Ruble, D. N., & Seidman, E. (1996). Social transitions: Windows into social psychological processes. In E. T. Higgins & A. W. Kruglanski (Eds.), *Social psychology: Handbook of basic principles* (pp. 830–856). New York: Guilford Press.

Ryan, R. M., & Deci, E. L. (2003). On assimilating identities to the self: A self-determination theory perspective on internalization and integrity within cultures. In M. R. Leary & J. P. Tangney (Eds.), *Handbook of self and identity* (pp. 253–272). New York: Guilford.

Ryan, R. M., & Deci, E. L. (2008). From ego-depletion to vitality: Theory and findings concerning the facilitation of energy available to the self. *Social and Personality Psychology Compass, 2*, 702–717.

Sheldon, K. M., & Bettencourt, B. A. (2002). Psychological need-satisfaction and subjective well-being within social groups. *British Journal of Social Psychology, 41*(1), 25–38. doi:10.1348/014466602165036.

Sheldon, K. M., & Kasser, T. (1995). Coherence and congruence: Two aspects of personality integration. *Journal of Personality and Social Psychology, 68*(3), 531–543. doi:10.1037/0022-3514 68.3.531.

Shrout, P. E., & Bolger, N. (2002). Mediation in experimental and nonexperimental studies: New procedures and recommendations. *Psychological Methods, 7*(4), 422–445. doi:10.1037//1082-989X.7.4.422.

Smith, L. G., Amiot, C. E., Callan, V. J., Terry, D. J., & Smith, J. R. (2012). The balancing act: The relationship between nested levels of identification and turnover intentions for newcomers at work. *British Journal of Management, 23*, 45–64.

Smith, L. G., Amiot, C. E., Smith, J. R., Callan, V. J., & Terry, D. J. (2013). The social validation and coping model of organizational identity development a longitudinal test. *Journal of Management, 39*(7). doi:10.1177/0149206313488212

Smith, J. R., & Louis, W. R. (2008). Do as we say and as we do: The interplay of descriptive and injunctive group norms in the attitude-behaviour relationship. *British Journal of Social Psychology, 47*(4), 647–666. doi:10.1348/014466607X269748.

Stephan, W. G., & Renfro, C. L. (2002). The role of threats in intergroup relations. In D. Mackie & E. R. Smith (Eds.), *Beyond prejudice: Differentiated reactions to social groups*. Mahwah, NJ: Erlbaum.

Stephan, W. G., & Stephan, C. W. (2000). An integrated threat theory of prejudice. In S. Oskamp (Ed.), *Reducing prejudice and discrimination: Claremont symposium on applied social psychology* (pp. 23–46). Hillsdale, NJ: Erlbaum.

Tajfel, H. (1978). *Differentiation between social groups: Studies in the social psychology of intergroup relations*. London: Academic.

Tajfel, H. (1982). Social psychology of intergroup relations. *Annual Review of Psychology, 33*, 1–39.

Tajfel, H., & Turner, J. (1979). An integrative theory of intergroup conflict. In W. G. Austin & S. Worchel (Eds.), *The social psychology of intergroup relations* (pp. 33–47). Monterey, CA: Brooks/Cole.

Tajfel, H., & Turner, J. C. (1986). The social identity of intergroup behaviour. In S. Worchel & W. G. Austin (Eds.), *Psychology of intergroup relations* (pp. 7–24). Chicago: Nelson Hall.

Teixeira, P. J., Silva, M. N., Coutinho, S. R., Palmeira, A. L., Mata, J., & Vieira, P. N. (2010). Mediators of weight loss and weight loss maintenance in middle-aged women. *Obesity, 18*(4), 725–735.

Terry, D. J., Carey, C. J., & Callan, V. J. (2001). Employee adjustment to an organizational merger: An intergroup perspective. *Personality and Social Psychology Bulletin, 27*(3), 267–280. doi:10.1177/0146167201273001.

Turner, J. C. (1991). *Social influence*. Belmont, CA: Thomson Brooks/Cole Publishing Co.

Tyler, T. R., & Blader, S. L. (2002). Autonomous vs. comparative status: Must we be better than others to feel good about ourselves? *Organizational Behavior and Human Decision Processes, 89*(1), 813–838. doi:10.1016/S0749-5978(02)00031-6.

United Nations. (2002). *Number of world's migrants reaches 175 million mark: Migrant population has doubled in twenty-five years*. Retrieved July 22, 2009, http://www.un.org/esa/population/publications/ittmig2002/press-release-eng.htm

Vallerand, R. J., Blanchard, C., Mageau, G. A., Koestner, R., Ratelle, C., & Léonard, M. (2003). Les passions de l'âme: On obsessive and harmonious passion. *Journal of Personality and Social Psychology, 85*(4), 756–767. doi:10.1037/0022-3514.85.4.756.

Wegmann, R. G. (1991). From job to job. *Journal of Employment Counseling, 28*(1), 8–12.

Weinstein, N., Deci, E. L., & Ryan, R. M. (2011). Motivational determinants of integrating positive and negative past identities. *Journal of Personality and Social Psychology, 100*(3), 527–544.

Williams, G. C., Grow, V. M., Freedman, Z. R., Ryan, R. M., & Deci, E. L. (1996). Motivational predictors of weight loss and weight-loss maintenance. *Journal of Personality and Social Psychology, 70*, 115–126.

Williams, G. C., Niemiec, C. P., Patrick, H., Ryan, R. M., & Deci, E. L. (2009). The importance of supporting autonomy and perceived competence in facilitating long-term tobacco abstinence. *Annals of Behavioral Medicine, 37*, 315–324.

Yampolsky, M. A., Amiot, C. E., & de la Sablonnière, R. (2013). Multicultural identity integration and well-being: A qualitative exploration of variations in narrative coherence and multicultural identification. *Frontiers in Psychology, 4*(126). doi:10.3389/fpsyg.2013.00126

Chapter 9
Autonomy Support as Acceptance for Disclosing and Developing a Healthy Lesbian, Gay, Bisexual or Transgendered Identity

Nicole Legate and William S. Ryan

Introduction

Despite recent victories in the promotion of civil rights for sexual minorities, identifying oneself as lesbian, gay, bisexual, or transgendered (LGBT) still holds a great deal of risk. 'Coming out' as LGBT can, therefore, be a difficult and sometimes dangerous task. The threat of being bullied or harassed in school or rejected by one's own family is all too real for these individuals. Among LGBT youth, 81 % reported experiencing verbal harassment, 38 % had been threatened with physical assault, and 15 % had been the victim of physical assault (D'Augelli, 2006).

It is clear that LGBT individuals have good reason to be selective in what, when, how much, and to whom they disclose. In this chapter we use a self-determination theory (SDT; Ryan & Deci, 2000) framework to understand the qualities of relationships that influence decisions about disclosure, and the psychological and relational experiences that follow. We first define coming out as a process rather than a one-time event and highlight the often difficult decisions that LGBT persons have to make around disclosure. Next, we discuss the institutional, interpersonal, and intrapersonal barriers that people face when making decisions regarding disclosing a sexual minority identity to others, as well as the potential costs and benefits of concealing versus coming out.

Throughout the chapter, we focus on how important relationship figures can impact decisions to come out or conceal. We argue that perceiving *autonomy*

Prepared for N. Weinstein (Ed.), *Integrating human motivation and interpersonal relationships: Theory, research and applications*

N. Legate (✉)
Department of Clinical & Social Sciences in Psychology,
University of Rochester, Rochester, NY, USA
e-mail: nlegate@psych.rochester.edu

W.S. Ryan
Department of Psychological & Brain Sciences,
University of California, Santa Barbara, CA, USA

N. Weinstein (ed.), *Human Motivation and Interpersonal Relationships: Theory, Research, and Applications*, DOI 10.1007/978-94-017-8542-6_9,

support, or encouragement to be oneself, from close others is an important predictor of how much people disclose their sexual minority identity. We suggest that autonomy support is important to disclosure because it leads people to feel more accepted for who they are, and safer to reveal an aspect of their identity with high potential for stigmatization. As well, we discuss how the autonomy-supportive character of relationships shapes the experiences that follow disclosure. We argue that autonomy support is also a critical element in determining the impact of disclosure on psychological well-being and physical health, such that these benefits typically occur only in autonomy-supportive environments. In contrast, coming out in controlling relationships does not have the same psychological and physical health benefits, and may in fact incur costs for the individual.

We then turn our focus to how autonomy support can impact people as they come to integrate their sexual identity with the rest of their self-concept. We review evidence illustrating the critical role of parental autonomy support in facilitating the self-acceptance and coherence of one's sexual identity. Finally, we explore some potential future directions for this burgeoning area of work, and highlight the importance of conducting research to inform interventions aimed at increasing social supports for LGBT individuals. Identifying social figures in their day-to-day lives that can facilitate beneficial coming out and integration experiences may help buffer against the deleterious effects of prejudice, discrimination, and violence that LGBT individuals too often face.

Coming Out Defined

For the purposes of this chapter we discuss coming out as gay, lesbian, bisexual, or transgender interchangeably. It is important to note, however, that the experience of coming out may vary depending on the identity being disclosed (e.g., Balsam & Mohr, 2007). In general, research on coming out has primarily sampled gay men and lesbians. Less research has addressed the bisexual experience and even fewer studies examine the experience of transgendered individuals disclosing their gender identity. Where the research reviewed implicates only specific sexual minority identities we make note accordingly. Still, we consider the potential risks and benefits of disclosure to be similar regardless of the identity disclosed. Moreover, we consider the role of important relationships in disclosure and identity integration to be equally important for all four groups. Herein we discuss the common factors and considerations of disclosing and integrating a sexual minority identity.

First, we conceptualize coming out as a continuous construct. Although the way most people talk about coming out suggests a dichotomy (i.e., one is either 'out' or 'in the closet'), such semantics obscure many aspects of what it means to come out. In fact for the vast majority of individuals, coming out is not a one-time event in which one steps 'out of the closet' and reveals his or her 'true self' to the world. Instead, both personal accounts and empirical evidence indicate that coming out is a lifelong process rather than a discrete event (e.g., Bohan, 1996; Mohr & Fassinger, 2000). Decisions about disclosure must be made throughout the lifespan as one enters new jobs, meets new people, and continues to develop relationships. Indeed, the opportunity to disclose occurs with relative frequency. A diary study by Beals, Peplau, and Gable (2009) found that lesbian and gay participants reported, on average, three disclosure opportunities over a 2-week period. Disclosure opportunities were defined as occasions in which self-identified lesbian and gay participants considered sharing their sexual orientation (whether or not they ultimately did). Such evidence highlights the regularly with which LGBT individuals are faced with the decision of whether or not to disclose their orientation to others. Moreover, most sexual minority individuals are not 'out' to all people or in all contexts. Indeed, 51 % of LGB individuals are not out to most people at work (Human Rights Campaign Report, 2010).

Even within relationships and contexts in which one has come out, one's level of *outness*, or degree of openness regarding sexual orientation, can vary (Mohr & Fassinger, 2000). For example, Jill may tell her best friend that she is a lesbian, and she may discuss aspects of her lesbian identity such as her dating life with this friend. With her mom, Jill may share that she is a lesbian, but they may never bring the topic up again. And with her coworker, Jill does not disclose her lesbian identity but she suspects that he knows. As this example implies, direct disclosure is not the only means by which one's LGBT identity can become known. This identity may also be revealed by others (i.e. 'outing') or may be deduced through various signals including clothing, style, as well as facial cues (Rule, Ambady, Adams, & Macrae, 2008) and body movement (e.g. Freeman, Johnson, Ambady, & Rule, 2010). Thus, thinking about coming out as a discrete event obscures the dynamic, ongoing nature of this process. Recognizing the complexities of coming out is integral to understanding the factors that may encourage disclosure and the consequences that follow.

Decisions Regarding Disclosure

Despite an increasingly tolerant sociopolitical climate, non-heterosexual identities are still heavily stigmatized, taking a psychological toll on those who claim them. Because LGBT individuals may be able to conceal their sexual identity from strangers, coworkers, and even close others like family members and friends, they have to make decisions around disclosure. Recent theorizing (Pachankis, 2007) and research (e.g., Legate, Ryan, & Weinstein, 2012) suggests that individuals with concealable stigmas (e.g., sexual orientation), as opposed to visible stigmas (e.g., physical disability), face additional considerations surrounding the decision, act, and aftermath of disclosing their stigmatized status to others. The challenges inherent to disclosing a concealable stigma have been documented in diverse domains including mental illness (e.g., Quinn, Kahng, & Crocker, 2004), epilepsy (Kleck, 1968), HIV, infertility, unemployment, and abortion (Major & Gramzow, 1999), among others. This decision can be very stressful, and can have important implications for psychological well-being among those with concealable stigmas. For example, results from an 11-day experience sampling study (Frable, Platt, & Hoey, 1998) showed that students with concealable stigmas reported less social confidence and self-esteem, and greater anxiety and depression than did students with a visible stigma or no stigma. Deciding whether or not to come out as LGBT may be particularly stressful because it is, in many ways, a double bind. This decision can mean choosing between two undesirable outcomes: risking discrimination or rejection from close others, or concealing an important part of oneself. These potential costs and benefits of disclosure will now be discussed in turn.

Barriers and Risks

Barriers to coming out as LGBT can arise from institutions, interpersonal relationships, and also from the LGBT individual him or herself. Together these barriers take the form of *homophobia*, or sexual prejudice, and can exist across the structural, interpersonal, and intrapersonal levels to devalue and disadvantage LGBT individuals (Herek, Gillis, & Cogan, 2009), motivating LGBT individuals to conceal their stigmatized status. People may expect or anticipate different levels of sexual prejudice from different relationships or contexts, which arguably impacts their decisions around sexual identity disclosure. Perceiving sexual prejudice from someone or from an institution conveys a message of non-acceptance, thereby inhibiting LGBT individuals from coming out. When an LGBT individual does disclose their sexual identity or it is otherwise inferred by non-accepting others, the risks can be very great and even fatal as demonstrated by the tragic hate crime committed against Matthew Shepard in 1998 and more recently against Mollie Olgin and Christine Chapa, two teenage lesbians who were shot and killed in a Texas park in June, 2012.

Structural Level: Loss of Rights and Privileges

Structural level sexual prejudice is the system of political legal, medical, and religious institutions that disadvantage sexual minorities (Herek et al., 2009). When one discloses a LGBT identity, he or she risks losing certain legal rights or services. The clearest example of this risk of disclosure is the recently repealed *Don't Ask Don't Tell* policy, under which LGB individuals were discharged from the military if their sexual orientation became known. Other examples of structural level sexual prejudice include barring legal access to marriage, refusing hospital visitation rights, as well as the standard practice of failing to provide appropriate options for non-heterosexual individuals on legal and medical forms.

When coming out means losing rights, privileges and services that one currently holds, it seems intuitive that sexual prejudice at the structural level would influence one's decision to come out. Indeed, individuals are less likely to come out in states in which anti-gay policies are upheld. For example, the number of LGB identified youth varies greatly by state with more LGB youth in states promoting LGB civil rights versus states that do not (e.g., more in Massachusetts than Minnesota; Faulkner & Cranston, 1998).

Structural level sexual prejudice not only impacts how much sexual minority individuals come out, but also their mental health. Hatzenbuehler, McLaughlin, Keyes, and Hasin (2010) found that in states with bans on same-sex marriage, LGB individuals experienced a greater prevalence of psychiatric disorders than in states without such policies. Specifically, they reported that psychiatric disorders among LGB individuals living in states that banned gay marriage increased up to 248 % between 2004 and 2005. Another study of theirs found that other state-level policies, including failure to include employment protections for sexual minorities and failure to protect against hate crimes, also had an adverse effect on the mental health and well-being of LGB individuals (Hatzenbuehler, Keyes, & Hasin, 2009). Thus, discriminatory legal policies not only discourage disclosure, but have deleterious effects on LGBT well-being.

Interpersonal Level: Discrimination and Rejection

If one does decide to come out, he or she runs the risk of facing discrimination in the workplace, jeopardizing relationships with important others, and becoming subject to verbal and/or physical harassment (e.g., D'Augelli, Hershberger, & Pilkington, 1998; Herek & Berrill, 1992). Further, one does not even need to come out as LGBT to be the target of discrimination, hostility, and unfair treatment. As the widespread accounts of school bullying have illustrated, if someone is merely perceived as sexually non-normative, he or she may become the target of discrimination or harassment. However, identifying as LGBT makes someone a clearer target for sexual prejudice, and thus represents a significant barrier to coming out.

Interpersonal discrimination and sexual prejudice can range in severity from making comments such as "that's so gay" to perpetrating violent hate crimes. Prevalence estimates of violence are difficult given variations in how crimes are categorized and how this data is reported (Herek, 2009). Still, estimates show that one in five LGB individuals reported experiencing physical and/or property violence during his or her adult life, 35 % reported threats of physical violence, and 63 % recounted verbal abuse (Herek, 2009). Derogatory comments and banter are also widespread. In the workplace, 58 % of LGB individuals reported hearing derogatory comments from their coworkers (Human Rights Campaign Report, 2010).

The numbers are particularly bleak when we look at youth, highlighting the challenges of coming out as an adolescent. D'Augelli (2006) found that rates of youth who reported victimization based on sexual orientation were high: 81 % reported verbal harassment, 38 % reported been threatened with physical assault, 15 % had been actually physically assaulted and 22 % had had objects thrown at them. Males reported being particularly at risk of physical violence. Additionally, 38 % of LGB youth feared being verbal attacked at school and 28 % feared physical assault at school (this fear was equal for men and women). It is not surprising, therefore, that those who came out at a younger age experienced more victimization, which in turn was associated with greater mental health issues and suicidal ideation (D'Augelli, 2006).

Sadly, rejection by important others is also a commonplace outcome of coming out as LGBT. One study found that 39 % of LGB youth reported losing at least one friend as a result of their sexual orientation (D'Augelli, 2006). For many, even the home does not always provide a safe haven. This same study found that only about half of mothers and one third of fathers were perceived by their LGB children to be accepting of this identity and 30 % of these youth feared verbal abuse at home. D'Augelli and colleagues (1998) found that LGB youth who had come out to their family experienced more verbal and physical abuse, and were more suicidal than those youth who had concealed their sexual orientation.

Intrapersonal Level: Self-Stigma

Internalized homophobia, or societal sexual prejudice that is incorporated into the self, is a type of self-stigma that can represent a significant barrier to coming out to others. Indeed, it is one of the most robust and consistent predictors of concealment of a lesbian, gay or bisexual identity (e.g., Balsam & Mohr, 2007; Herek, 2009; Herek, Cogan, Gillis, & Glunt, 1998; Mohr & Fassinger, 2003). This relation is not surprising, given that internalized homophobia is often experienced as feeling shame around one's identity, and that the natural behavioral reaction to shame is hiding (Kaufman & Raphael, 1996). Internalized homophobia and other forms of self-stigma also represent a significant risk factor for the development of mental health problems (e.g., Hatzenbuehler, Dovidio, Nolen-Hoeksema, & Phills, 2009; Szymanski, Chung, & Balsam, 2001; Williamson, 2000). Importantly, societal prejudice may be internalized to varying degrees, and self-stigma is a process that can occur for various stigmatized groups, including transgender individuals.

Why Come Out at All?

Given the risks and barriers discussed above, one might wonder why individuals come out at all. A diverse and growing body of literature suggests that the ongoing process of concealing and the accompanying cognitive and emotional demands can come with a heavy cost to psychological and physical health. Concealment can impact people directly, as well as indirectly by interfering with close relationships. We also note the potential benefits that can follow from disclosure. It is important to highlight these potential gains as more than just avoiding the risks of concealment. Coming out can be an empowering experience, helping people to integrate their private and public lives.

Problems of the Closet

Diverse research on cognition, emotion, and identity finds that concealment is costly to mental and physical health (e.g., Gross & Levenson, 1993; Pennebaker & Chung, 2011; Smart & Wegner, 2000). Specifically, concealment of sexual or gender orientation inhibits the expression of identity (Bosson, Weaver, & Prewitt-Freilino, 2011), as well as the expression of significant social and behavioral impulses including public displays of affection and openness about one's personal life in daily conversation. In work settings, those that conceal evidence more negative job attitudes and fewer promotions (Ragins, Singh, & Cornwell, 2007) and more burnout (Sandfort, Bos, & Vet, 2006). One poignant study reveals the potential physical health costs of concealment: among gay men, HIV infection progressed more rapidly in those who concealed their sexual identity compared to those who do not (Cole, Kemeny, Taylor, & Visscher, 1996). Ullrich, Lutgendorf, and Stapleton (2003) found that gay men who concealed their identity reported greater depression and lower overall psychological well-being than those who disclosed. Concealment can also lead to a more negative evaluation of whatever is being concealed (Fishbein & Laird, 1979), suggesting that concealment can actually exacerbate feelings of self-stigma.

Experimental work by Critcher and Ferguson (2011) found that concealment of sexual orientation produces significant decrements in performance on both cognitive and physical tasks. This study and other work suggest that concealment appears to take its toll on physical and psychological health by consuming cognitive and self-regulatory resources (e.g. Baumeister, Vohs, & Tice, 2007). To remain concealed requires ongoing self-monitoring. Another reason that concealment can be costly is through the isolation from similar or supportive others (Pachankis, 2007). Thus, concealment can prevent people from experiencing some of the personal and relationship benefits of coming out.

Benefits of Disclosure

It is important to frame the question of why people come out as more just than avoiding the negative consequences of concealment. The evidence reviewed above suggests that disclosure can free up cognitive and emotional resources, increase positive self-evaluation, promote integration, and boost well-being and relationship satisfaction. Indeed, disclosing one's LGBT identity is important for developing a stable identity, coming to self-acceptance, and ameliorating some of the psychological harm caused by stigma (e.g., Cain, 1991; Ragins, 2004; Wells & Kline, 1987). Ideally, the coming out process can facilitate self-acceptance and integration of people's sexual minority identity with the whole of who they are. Cass (1979) referred to this as *identity synthesis*, the last stage of sexual minority identity development, whereby one's public and private sexual identity are integrated. Coming out can also help people connect to supports in the LGBT community and affiliate with others who can understand and validate experiences with stigmatization and rejection (Meyer, 2003). Similarly, Beals (2004) found that on days when sexual orientation was disclosed, individuals experienced greater well-being and this was mediated by experiences of social support.

Coming out can have important social and political benefits as well. Increasing visibility of those who are LGBT can help reduce sexual prejudice, as contact with an out-group member is one of the most effective ways to reduce prejudice (referred to as the *contact hypothesis*; Brown & Hewstone, 2005; Herek & Glunt, 1993). Coming out can reduce sexual prejudice with one's immediate social relationships, such as with one's family members or coworkers, as well as at a broader societal level to impact policy. Andersen Cooper, a famous reporter who came out to the public in July, 2012 said the following on why he chose to come out: "I've also been reminded recently that while as a society we are moving toward greater inclusion and equality for all people, the tide of history only advances when people make themselves fully visible (Sullivan, 2012, para. 7)."

Beyond the issue of coming out, research shows that being more authentic in one's relationships relates to higher relationship satisfaction and better relationship functioning (Brunell et al., 2010; Lopez & Rice, 2006). Research by Uysal and colleagues (2010, 2012) found that concealing information about oneself from others related to lower overall well-being and lower relationship well-being. Conversely, those who concealed less self-relevant information experienced better well-being overall and in their romantic relationship. This pattern was found both cross-sectionally and at the daily-diary level. Interestingly, concealment not only adversely impacted one's own well-being but it adversely impacted one's partner's well-being, thus illustrating the far-reaching effects of concealing parts of oneself in a relationship.

Coming out and being authentic in one's relationships has a high potential to benefit LGBT individuals. It allows them to be themselves with others, as well as develop a healthy identity that incorporates their sexuality (Meyer, 2003). Coherence and integration around all aspects of identity help people experience a full and healthy life (e.g., Rogers, 1961; Weinstein, Deci, & Ryan, 2011). We thus turn to exploring qualities of relationships that promote positive and meaningful coming out experiences that can help people come to greater coherence and self-acceptance around their LGBT identity.

Assessing Supports and Threats in the Environment

Given these potential risks and benefits of coming out, LGBT individuals often choose to selectively disclose their sexual or gender identity to others (Cole, 2006; Legate et al., 2012). Individuals across the life span vary in how much they come out to different people. D'Augelli (2006) found that only 23 % of LGB youth were completely out to everyone in their life. A similar rate was found among LGB adults over the age of 60 (D'Augelli & Grossman, 2001). It is thus the case that many LGBT individuals are selective in disclosure, and vary in their level of disclosure across important relationships. Supportive others are presumably critical in that they permit self-disclosure when doing so is otherwise felt to be unsafe.

The fear of rejection, discrimination, and even violence from important people in one's life arguably represents one of the biggest risks of coming out. Assessing the risk can be difficult. Some workplaces, schools, friends or family members subtly convey to LGBT individuals that they would be rejected or lose social support if they were to come out. Others make it very clear that they will be bullied or harassed for being LGBT. Thus, important relationships and the broader structural context in which they occur vary in terms of how risky or safe they feel to LGBT persons. This feeling of safety vs. risk in turn influences decisions about whether disclosure is a desirable option in these relationships.

To understand how relationships can make people feel more or less safe to disclose, we apply a self-determination theory (SDT; Deci & Ryan, 1985, 2000; Ryan & Deci, 2000) perspective. We look specifically at *autonomy support* as an aspect of relationships that may make people feel safer to come out, reducing the perceived risks. We propose that perceiving autonomy support from important people in one's life can provide safety for the coming out process and play a powerful role in mitigating the negative impacts of holding a stigmatized identity.

Autonomy Defined

Before discussing how relationships support autonomy and facilitate the coming out process, it is important to establish what autonomy is and why it is so important for people. Within self-determination theory, *autonomy* refers to the extent that people are behaving authentically and acting in accord with their beliefs and feelings. When people are being autonomous they are being themselves, and experience a sense of choicefulness in their behavior. The opposite of autonomy is feeling *controlled*, or a sense of pressure to act in certain ways that might please others. When someone is acting on the basis of controlled motivations, they are behaving as they "ought" to, in line with expectations that they perceive from others.

Autonomy plays an important role in how one behaves and responds to others in relationships as well as how one conceives of one's self. Broadly speaking, autonomy has been linked with positive intrapersonal and interpersonal functioning. Autonomy is associated with better mental health (e.g., Ryan & Deci, 2000), physical health (e.g., Williams, Grow, Freedman, Ryan, & Deci, 1996), greater persistence on tasks (e.g., Deci, Koestner, & Ryan, 1999), more creativity (Amabile, 1983), and greater satisfaction at work (e.g., Richer, Blanchard, & Vallerand, 2002). In other words, the more individuals can act autonomously, the better their functioning and wellness.

As a note, any behavior can be more or less autonomous (Chirkov, Ryan, Kim, & Kaplan, 2003; Ryan, 1995). Applied to the issue of coming out, someone may disclose an LGBT identity (or conceal it) for autonomous or for controlled reasons. For example, people who come out for autonomous reasons do so because disclosing this aspect of their identity to close others fits with their values and beliefs. On the other hand, some may come out because they feel pressure from others to do so, and they might feel guilty if they did not. SDT would posit that those who come out for more autonomous reasons would have a more positive experience and better outcomes, though this has yet to be empirically tested.

Autonomy Support in Relationships

According to SDT, important others can either support or thwart one's autonomy (Lynch, La Guardia, & Ryan, 2009; Ryan, La Guardia, Solky-Butzel, Chirkov, & Kim, 2005). When others are being autonomy supportive, they are conveying a message that they accept and support people for who they are. This would naturally encompass accepting people for their sexual and gender identity. Autonomy support helps people to express themselves authentically and behave in ways that are consistent with deeply held values (La Guardia & Ryan, 2007; Lynch et al., 2009; Sheldon, Ryan, Rawsthorne, & Ilardi, 1997). Lynch and Ryan (2004) argue that autonomy support is necessary for people to 'be themselves.' When people perceive autonomy support, they tend to express themselves more authentically (Lynch et al., 2009), an especially poignant finding when the challenges of LGBT self-disclosure are considered.

Just as relationships can support one's need for autonomy, they can thwart or interfere with satisfaction of this need as well. One way that a parent, teacher, romantic partner or friend can thwart autonomy is through *conditional regard*, or conveying that someone is only loveable under certain conditions. Perceiving conditional regard from parents can lead to feelings of internal compulsion to comply with parents' expectations, unstable self-esteem, lower well-being, and a tendency to suppress emotions (Roth, Assor, Niemiec, Ryan, & Deci, 2009). The conditionally regarding message that being LGBT is unacceptable or unlovable is, unfortunately, all too common. As discussed earlier in this chapter, this message of non-acceptance exists at an institutional level, in schools, workplaces and homes, and it can also exist within a LGBT person in the form of self-stigma. Autonomy support, therefore, seems crucial to help an LGBT individual feel safe enough to come out.

Autonomy Support Fosters Interpersonal Safety

Perceiving autonomy support from others is recognizing the message that one is accepted for who one is, thereby minimizing the threat of being evaluated or rejected. This dynamic of autonomy support and safety starts in infancy. Recent work has found that maternal autonomy support fosters a secure attachment in

15 month-old infants (Whipple, Bernier, & Mageau, 2011). In adults, La Guardia, Ryan, Couchman, and Deci (2000) found that when close others (e.g., parents, best friends) are seen as supporting an individual's autonomy, he or she has a more secure attachment with that relationship partner. Similarly, other work has found that people report feeling closer to, more attached, and happier in relationships in which their autonomy is supported, a finding supported across cultures (e.g. Lynch et al., 2009). This is true for the giver as well as the receiver of autonomy support (Deci, La Guardia, Moller, Scheiner, & Ryan, 2006).

Experimental work by Hodgins and colleagues (2010) looked at how enhancing people's sense of autonomy through a priming manipulation impacted their level of openness versus defensiveness in relationships. They found that priming autonomy facilitated people's openness and decreased their physiological threat response in an interpersonal interaction task. This finding suggests that perceiving autonomy support from someone might facilitate greater openness regarding one's LGBT identity. Related research by Weinstein, Hodgins, and Ryan (2010) found that dyads primed with autonomy interacted more constructively than those primed with control. Specifically, these dyads felt closer, were more emotionally and cognitively attuned to their partners, provided empathy and encouragement to partners, and performed more effectively than dyads who were primed with control. Similarly, work by Niemiec and Deci (2012) found that contextual supports for autonomy facilitated self-disclosure and relationship closeness in strangers. Thus, relationships function more smoothly and with more openness and trust when autonomy is supported.

Taken together, this work suggests that experiencing support for autonomy helps people to be themselves, increasing feelings of interpersonal safety and acceptance. For LGBT individuals who run the risk of being rejected or discriminated against by others on the basis of their sexual or gender identity, perceiving autonomy support from important others may thus signal safety in a sometimes not-so-safe world. Free from judgment, LGBT individuals might feel more inclined to reveal part of their identity that they might otherwise conceal.

Autonomy Support Makes It Safe to Come Out

Recent work has examined the importance of autonomy support for LGB individuals making decisions to come out. Examining various relationship contexts (i.e., family, friends, coworkers, school peers, and religious communities), Legate et al. (2012) found that, at both between- and within-person levels of analysis, autonomy support was a strong predictor of LGB identity disclosure, or *outness*. In addition, results showed that autonomy support was also an important moderator of the relation between outness and wellness such that the benefits of coming out were limited to autonomy-supportive relationship contexts (see Fig. 9.1). Specifically, greater outness was linked to lower levels of anger and depression and greater self-esteem when the context was autonomy-supportive. Yet, there were no mental-health benefits when disclosing to controlling, or low autonomy-supportive, others.

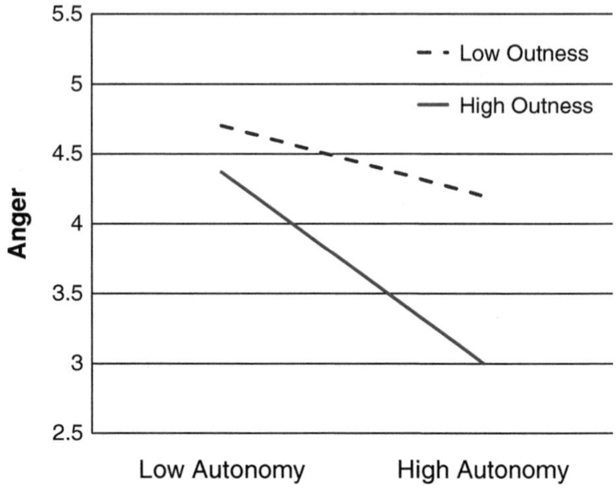

Fig. 9.1 Relationship-specific anger predicted by autonomy support and outness. Patterns are similar for depression and self-esteem

This study has important implications for individuals who face stigma: Identifying people in their day-to-day lives who can facilitate beneficial coming out experiences may help buffer against the deleterious effects of prejudice, discrimination, and violence that sexual minorities often face. As LGBT individuals often anticipate stigmatization, rejection, and judgments from others when disclosing their sexual or gender identity, it seems then that an autonomy-supportive friend or family member can reduce the perceived risks of disclosing. A controlling relationship, on the other hand, might make the risk of rejection or negative judgments salient, making it less likely that someone would disclose this aspect of their identity with high potential for stigmatization. Further, disclosing in safe, accepting environments helps people feel better, suggesting that autonomy support may catalyze well-being processes within individuals.

Autonomy Support and Becoming Oneself

Receiving autonomy support in close relationships can help people feel more security and safety in these relationships, but it can also facilitate integration, congruence and well-being *within* the individual (Ryan, 1995; Ryan & Deci, 2000). A substantial body of evidence suggests that *congruence*, or behaving in line with one's true self, relates to psychological adjustment (e.g., Diehl, Hastings, & Stanton, 2001; Diehl & Hay, 2007, 2010; Rogers, 1961; Sheldon et al., 1997; Sherman, Nave, & Funder, 2010). Authenticity, a related construct, has also been shown to relate to better self-esteem and well-being (Kernis, 2003). Therefore, when people receive autonomy support and feel accepted by others, it can help them accept and feel good about themselves.

Weinstein and colleagues (2011) conducted five studies looking at acceptance and integration of positive and negative aspects of the self. Specifically, they investigated how primed autonomy, or autonomy that is enhanced by the environment, influences people's tendencies to integrate positive and negative aspects of themselves and life events. They found that people who were primed with autonomy were more able to accept and integrate positive and negative aspects of themselves into their self-concept, including aspects of themselves and memories that they may regret or judge as shameful. Yet, people primed with control were only able to accept parts of themselves that they considered positive; they did not allow the integration of negative memories or events into their self-concept. The authors further showed that distancing from negative life events diminished well-being.

Importantly, defensive processes mediated these effects: when autonomy was enhanced, people felt less threatened by negative characteristics and events, allowing fuller integration than that evidenced by control-primed participants. Stated differently, when experiencing autonomy, people were able to accept parts of themselves that they regretted or considered shameful. Thus enhancing autonomy, whether primed experimentally or through the support of others (e.g., Soenens & Vanstinkiste, 2005), can help people grow in self-acceptance.

These findings, especially the finding that defending against aspects of oneself lowers well-being, have implications for understanding internalized homophobia. Many people high in internalized homophobia consider their sexual identity a shameful aspect of who they are, and struggle against integrating it with the rest of their self-concept. This difficulty with integrating sexual identity may help explain the poor mental-health outcomes consistently associated with internalized homophobia.

Parental Autonomy Support and Integrating Sexual Identity

Two sets of studies examined this issue of sexual identity integration, focusing on the role of parental autonomy support in childhood. Parent-child relationships are crucial to identity formation, since parents shape their children across critical periods of development (Grolnick & Ryan, 1989; Joussemet, Landry, & Koestner, 2008). Autonomy-supportive parents convey the message that their children will be accepted and loved "no matter what", whereas autonomy-thwarting parents can send messages that their children will be loved only if they act in ways that the parents want. These messages set the stage for negotiating different aspects of identity. When faced with an identity that has high potential for censure (such as being LGBT), individuals with autonomy-thwarting parents may defend against these impulses because they threaten the relationship (Rogers, 1961; Roth et al., 2009). Because their relationship is not on the line, those with autonomy-supportive parents should be better able to integrate a potentially stigmatized identity.

Studies by Weinstein and colleagues (2012) investigated these dynamics in the context of sexual orientation. They assessed sexual identity using both explicit (self-report) and implicit (reaction-time based) measures. Results showed that when parents were autonomy-thwarting, people developed an incongruent sexual identity whereby self-reported sexual orientation was discrepant from implicit indicators. Yet when people recalled that their parents were autonomy-supportive during childhood, they showed greater correspondence between implicit and explicit assessments of sexual identity.

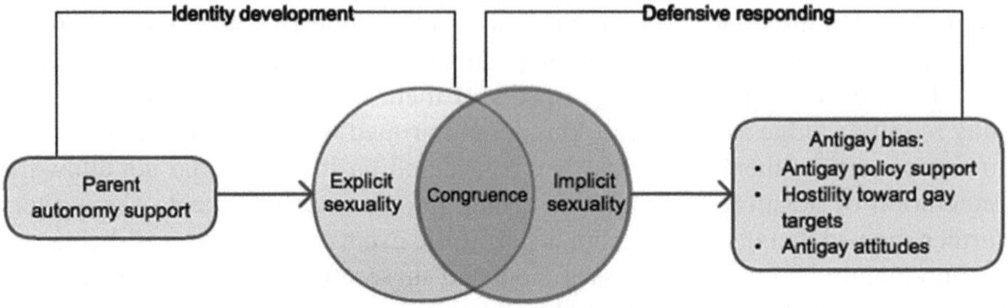

Fig. 9.2 Theoretical model of how parent autonomy support impacts integration of sexual identity and protects against defensive responding

Interestingly, this study also found evidence for *reaction formation*, a defense whereby individuals adopt beliefs that directly oppose socially unacceptable inner impulses or desires that they identify in themselves (Freud, 1915). Those who had parents who were autonomy-thwarting evinced less congruence between self-reported and implicitly measured sexual orientation, which in turn predicted greater antigay attitudes, hostility, and policy support (see Fig. 9.2). Those with autonomy-supportive parents did not show this pattern of defensive responding. These data suggest that autonomy support can facilitate the integration of sexual identity into the rest of an individual's self-concept. They also have implications beyond the self for social problems such as bullying in schools and antigay violence, suggesting that parental autonomy support can buffer against hostile, defensive responding toward vulnerable out-groups. Research employing autonomy-enhancing interventions to reduce prejudice provides additional support for this idea (see Legault, Gutsell, & Inzlicht, 2011).

Three recent studies tested similar dynamics in a LGB sample in order understand the developmental antecedents of internalized homophobia (Legate, Ryan, DeHaan, Weinstein, & Ryan, 2012). It was hypothesized that parental autonomy support during childhood would lead to better self-concept integration (less shame, internalized homophobia and emotional suppression, and more outness) and better mental health (less depression and more self-esteem) in adulthood. Results supported this model: those who described their parents as more autonomy-supportive reported less internalized homophobia and emotional suppression, more outness, and better mental health. These relations were mediated by shame proneness, such that parental autonomy support buffered against a general tendency to feel ashamed of oneself, thus rendering an individual less vulnerable to feeling ashamed of his or her sexual orientation. Otherwise stated, parent autonomy support appeared to protect against the development of internalized homophobia by protecting against a general tendency to feel ashamed of oneself. These results have important implications for LGB wellness, as internalized homophobia is a potent risk factor for mental health problems, self-harm and HIV-risk-taking behavior (e.g., Meyer, 2003; Williamson, 2000).

Acceptance and LGBT Wellness

Taken together, this research underscores the importance of accepting, autonomy-supportive relationships for LGBT wellness. Autonomy support can buffer against the deleterious effects of stigma and discrimination. Research outside of self-determination theory also highlights the importance of acceptance in relationships to LGBT well-being. Research conducted by the Human Rights Campaign (2012) surveying more than 10,000 LGBT youth found that the biggest problem facing these youths' lives is having non-accepting families – one third reported feeling a lack of family acceptance. Receiving family acceptance has been shown to promote LGBT health and wellness, whereas family rejection appears to have the opposite effect. For example, a sense of acceptance from parents and caregivers relates to lower depression and suicide attempts among LGB adolescents (Ryan, Russell, Huebner, Diaz, & Sanchez, 2010). Moreover, rejecting behaviors from parents during adolescence have been related to poorer health of LGB young adults (Ryan, Huebner, Diaz, & Sanchez, 2009). Specifically, having rejecting parents predicted illegal drug use, depression, suicide attempts, and sexual health risk. Another study similarly found that LGB teens who felt rejected after they came out to different people such as family members, coaches, teachers, and friends had higher rates of substance abuse (Rosario, Schrimshaw, & Hunter, 2009). It seems, then, that perceiving acceptance from important others is associated with LGBT wellness directly, and indirectly by helping people to come to self-acceptance.

Summary and Future Directions

In this chapter, we provided an account of how social relationships are critical for decisions surrounding coming out as LGBT, and the experiences that follow. We reviewed research finding that autonomy support helps people to be more accepting of themselves and less prejudiced against others who might express stigmatized identities. Perceiving autonomy support allows people to express themselves more fully, even when they might worry that some aspects of themselves might be viewed as shameful. Autonomy support makes the decision to come out feel less risky than it would be with others who tend to be judgmental or critical of their behavior. Not only does autonomy support help people to be more themselves with others and disclose more with them, it helps people to grow and come to greater personality integration. Further, autonomy support from parents appears to be particularly important for coherence and integration of one's sexual identity, leading to less internalized homophobia and defensiveness.

Although promising and consistent so far, research examining how autonomy support impacts processes related to coming out and internalized homophobia is novel and still sparse. More scientific inquiry is needed to explain important unanswered questions. We have identified three main issues that should be the focus of future research: mechanisms, costs, and causality.

What is the mechanism through which autonomy support facilitates the coming out process? A likely mediator we have pointed to throughout this chapter for the link between autonomy support and coming out is perceived safety in the relationship. When relationship partners convey the message that "you are loveable no matter what," as opposed to "you are loved if…," it fosters a sense of security, or safety that they will not lose love and affection if they disclose or embrace their sexual or gender identity. On the other hand, controlling contexts may inhibit disclosure because of the perceived risk in revealing part of one's identity that may be rejected or judged negatively. In other words, in a controlling relationship one may feel that the relationship is "on the line" when revealing a LGBT identity, which one would be less likely to feel if the relationship is autonomy supportive. As of yet, however, these explanations are speculative and need to be tested and refined.

Also regarding the question of mechanism, research is needed to answer the question of why autonomy support leads to beneficial coming out experiences and controlling relationships do not. A potential candidate is psychological need satisfaction, especially the needs for autonomy and relatedness. Feeling like one can be authentic with a close other fulfills the need for autonomy, as well as a sense of relatedness, which in turn enhances well-being. In contrast, coming out to controlling others likely does not promote either autonomy or relatedness need satisfactions, and may even thwart these needs.

Considering the risks of coming out as a sexual or gender minority, a second question we have concerns the costs of being in controlling contexts. Specifically, what are the relative costs and benefits of concealing, or conversely, coming out in controlling contexts? To answer this, researchers will likely need to employ more sophisticated methods than cross-sectional self-report surveys. Using psychophysiological indicators of stress could point to the potential moment-to-moment costs of making decisions regarding coming out in controlling contexts. Observing fluctuations in mood and physiological activation (e.g., blood pressure, heart rate variability, and skin conductance response) as a function of relational autonomy support or control will provide compelling evidence for the role that environments play in affecting minority mental and physical health. Such a model might also be applied to understand the lack of congruence that leads to sexual prejudice, both directed towards others and directed towards the self. Examining other potential psychological and physiological consequences of autonomy-supporting or autonomy-thwarting environments for LGBT individuals represents an important future direction for this line of research.

Finally, to address the issue of causality, longitudinal and experimental studies will need to be employed. Following LGBT individuals over time as they make decisions about coming out is necessary to show the [presumed] benefits of having autonomy-supportive others, and the consequences of having autonomy-thwarting others, in their lives. This method could also potentially reveal both short- and long-term outcomes of differential coming out experiences, and might lead to further questions about the impact of relationships on an individual's first coming out experience, versus subsequent coming out experiences. Additionally, experimental paradigms would also allow us to better infer causality. For example, randomly assigning people to interact with either real or virtual autonomy-supportive or controlling strangers and observing whether people come out more and/or have different feelings when they are with these people, would be enlightening and lend additional support to our claims. Both of these methods would allow for causal statements about the role of autonomy support in coming out, and represent a crucial future direction of this research.

Given the history of oppression suffered by LGBT individuals that still endures today, and the consequent high rates of stress and psychological disorders found in this population (Sandfort, de Graaf, Bijl, & Schnabel, 2001), research on processes that can facilitate both their social and self-acceptance is a critical agenda. Such research has implications for both clinical interventions and policy formation regarding people who identify as LGBT, as well as interventions targeting the majority population to reduce antigay prejudice and hostility (for example, in schools with children and adolescents who bully). Specifically, better understanding the role of autonomy in ameliorating the effects of stigma is critical for designing interventions to increase the quality of social support given to LGBT individuals. Identifying ways that important relationships can best support LGBT youth and adults, as well as buffer against the development of antigay prejudice in the majority population, represents essential steps in promoting LGBT health and wellness.

References

Amabile, T. M. (1983). *The social psychology of creativity*. New York: Springer.

Balsam, K. F., & Mohr, J. J. (2007). Adaptation to sexual orientation stigma: A comparison of bisexual and lesbian/gay adults. *Journal of Counseling Psychology, 54*, 306–319. doi:10.1037/0022-0167.54.3.306.

Baumeister, R. F., Vohs, K. D., & Tice, D. M. (2007). The strength model of self-control. *Current Directions in Psychological Science, 16*, 351–355. doi:10.1111/j.1467-8721.2007.00534.x.

Beals, K. (2004). Stigma management and well-being: The role of social support, emotional processing, and suppression (Doctoral dissertation, University of California, Los Angeles, 2003). *Dissertation Abstracts International, 65*, 1070.

Beals, K. P., Peplau, L. A., & Gable, S. L. (2009). Stigma management and well-being: The role of perceived social support, emotional processing, and suppression. *Personality and Social Psychology Bulletin, 35*, 867–879. doi:10.1177/0146167209334783.

Bohan, J. S. (1996). *Psychology and sexual orientation: Coming to terms*. New York: Routledge.

Bosson, J. K., Weaver, J. R., & Prewitt-Freilino, J. L. (2011). Concealing to belong, revealing to be known: Classification expectations and self-threats among persons with concealable stigmas. *Self and Identity, 11*, 114–135. doi:10.1080/15298868.2010.513508.

Brown, R., & Hewstone, M. (2005). An integrative theory of intergroup contact. In M. P. Zanna (Ed.), *Advances in experimental social psychology* (Vol. 37, pp. 255–343). San Diego, CA: Elsevier Academic Press.

Brunell, A. B., Kernis, M. H., Goldman, B. M., Heppner, W., Davis, P., Cascio, E. V., et al. (2010). Dispositional authenticity and romantic relationship functioning. *Personality and Individual Differences, 48*, 900–905. doi:10.1016/j.paid.2010.02.018.

Cain, R. (1991). Stigma management and gay identity development. *Social Work & Society, 36*, 67–73.

Cass, V. C. (1979). Homosexual identity formation: A theoretical model. *Journal of Homosexuality, 4*, 219–235. doi:10.1080/00224498409551214.

Chirkov, K., Ryan, R. M., Kim, Y., & Kaplan, U. (2003). Differentiating autonomy from individualism and independence: A self-determination theory perspective on internalization of cultural orientations and well-being. *Journal of Personality and Social Psychology, 84*, 97–110. doi:10.1037/0022-3514.84.1.97.

Cole, S. W. (2006). Social threat, personal identity, and physical health in closeted gay men. In A. M. Omoto & H. S. Kurtzman (Eds.), *Sexual orientation and mental health: Examining identity and development in lesbian, gay, and bisexual people* (pp. 245–267). Washington, DC: American Psychological Association.

Cole, S. W., Kemeny, M. E., Taylor, S. E., & Visscher, B. R. (1996). Elevated physical health risk among gay men who conceal their homosexual identity. *Health Psychology, 15*, 243–251. doi:10.1037//0278-6133.15.4.243.

Critcher, C. R., & Ferguson, M. J. (2011, January). *Concealment and ego depletion: Does "Don't Ask, Don't Tell" hinder performance?* Paper presented at the meeting of the Society for Personality and Social Psychology, San Antonio, TX.

D'Augelli, A. R. (2006). Developmental and contextual factors and mental health among lesbian, gay, and bisexual youths. In A. M. Omoto & H. S. Kurtzman (Eds.), *Sexual orientation and mental health: Examining identity and development in lesbian, gay, and bisexual people* (pp. 37–53). Washington, DC: American Psychological Association.

D'Augelli, A. R., & Grossman, A. H. (2001). Disclosure of sexual orientation, victimization, and mental health among lesbian, gay, and bisexual older adults. *Journal of Interpersonal Violence, 16*, 1008–1027. doi:10.1177/088626001016010003.

D'Augelli, A. R., Hershberger, S. L., & Pilkington, N. W. (1998). Lesbian, gay, and bisexual youth and their families: Disclosure of sexual orientation and its consequences. *American Journal of Orthopsychiatry, 68*, 361–371. doi:10.1037/h0080345.

Deci, E. L., Koestner, R., & Ryan, R. M. (1999). A meta-analytic review of experiments examining the effects of extrinsic rewards on intrinsic motivation. *Psychological Bulletin, 125*, 627–668. doi:10.1037//0033-2909.125.6.627.

Deci, E. L., La Guardia, J. G., Moller, A. C., Scheiner, M. J., & Ryan, R. M. (2006). On the benefits of giving as well as receiving autonomy support: Mutuality in close friendships. *Personality and Social Psychology Bulletin, 32*, 313–327. doi:10.1177/0146167205282148.

Deci, E. L., & Ryan, R. M. (1985). *Intrinsic motivation and self-determination in human behavior*. New York: Plenum.

Deci, E. L., & Ryan, R. M. (2000). The "what" and "why" of goal pursuits: Human needs and the self-determination of behavior. *Psychological Inquiry, 11*, 227–268. doi:10.1207/S15327965PLI1104_01.

Diehl, M., Hastings, C. T., & Stanton, J. M. (2001). Self-concept differentiation across the adult life span. *Psychology and Aging, 16*, 643–654. doi:10.1037//0882-7974.16.4.643.

Diehl, M., & Hay, E. L. (2007). Contextualized self-representations in adulthood. *Journal of Personality, 75*, 1255–1284. doi:10.1111/j.1467-6494.2007.00475.x.

Diehl, M., & Hay, E. L. (2010). Risk and resilience factors in coping with daily stress in adulthood: The role of age, self-concept incoherence, and personal control. *Developmental Psychology, 46*, 1132–1146. doi:10.1037/a0019937.

Faulkner, A. H., & Cranston, K. (1998). Correlates of same-sex sexual behavior in a random sample of Massachusetts high school students. *American Journal of Public Health, 88*, 262–266. doi:10.2105/AJPH.88.2.262.

Fishbein, M. J., & Laird, J. D. (1979). Concealment and disclosure: Some effects of information control on the person who controls. *Journal of Experimental Social Psychology, 15*, 114–121. doi:10.1016/0022-1031(79)90023-4.

Frable, D. E. S., Platt, L., & Hoey, S. (1998). Concealable stigmas and positive self-perceptions: Feeling better around similar others. *Journal of Personality and Social Psychology, 74*, 909–922. doi:10.1037/0022-3514.74.4.909.

Freeman, J. B., Johnson, K. L., Ambady, N., & Rule, N. O. (2010). Sexual orientation perception involves gendered facial cues. *Personality and Social Psychology Bulletin, 36*, 1318–1331. doi:10.1177/0146167210378755.

Freud, S. (1915). Further recommendations in the technique of psychoanalysis: Observations on transference-love. *Collected Papers, 2*, 377–391.

Grolnick, W. S., & Ryan, R. M. (1989). Parent styles associated with children's self-regulation and competence in school. *Journal of Educational Psychology, 81*, 143–154. doi:10.1037/0022-0663.81.2.143.

Gross, J. J., & Levenson, R. W. (1993). Emotional suppression: Physiology, self-report, and expressive behavior. *Journal of Personality and Social Psychology, 64*, 970–986. doi:10.1037//0022-3514.64.6.970.

Hatzenbuehler, M. L., Dovidio, J. F., Nolen-Hoeksema, S., & Phills, C. E. (2009). An implicit measure of anti-gay attitudes: Prospective associations with emotion regulation strategies and psychological distress. *Journal of Experimental Social Psychology, 45*, 1316–1320. doi:10.1016/j.jesp.2009.08.005.

Hatzenbuehler, M. L., Keyes, K. M., & Hasin, D. S. (2009). State-level policies and psychiatric morbidity in lesbian, gay, and bisexual populations. *American Journal of Public Health, 99*, 2275–2281. doi:10.2105/AJPH.2008.153510.

Hatzenbuehler, M. L., McLaughlin, K. A., Keyes, K. M., & Hasin, D. S. (2010). The impact of institutional discrimination on psychiatric disorders in lesbian, gay, and bisexual populations: A prospective study. *American Journal of Public Health, 100*, 452–459. doi:10.2105/AJPH.2009.168815.

Herek, G. M. (2009). Hate crimes and stigma-related experiences among sexual minority adults in the United States: Prevalence estimates form a national probability sample. *Journal of Interpersonal Violence, 24*, 54–74. doi:10.1177/0886260508316477.

Herek, G. M., & Berrill, K. T. (1992). *Hate crimes: Confronting violence against lesbians and gay men*. London: Sage.

Herek, G. M., Cogan, J. C., Gillis, J. R., & Glunt, E. K. (1998). Correlates of internalized homophobia in a community sample of lesbians and gay men. *Journal of the Gay and Lesbian Medical Association, 2*, 17–25.

Herek, G. M., Gillis, J. R., & Cogan, J. C. (2009). Internalized stigma among sexual minority adults: Insights from a social psychological perspective. *Journal of Counseling Psychology, 56*, 32–41. doi:10.1037/a0014672.

Herek, G. M., & Glunt, E. K. (1993). Interpersonal contact and heterosexuals' attitudes toward gay men: Results from a national survey. *Journal of Sex Research, 30*, 239–244. doi:10.1080/00224499309551707.

Hodgins, H. S., Weisbust, K. S., Weinstein, N., Shiffman, S., Miller, A., Coombs, G., et al. (2010). The cost of self-protection: Threat response and performance as a function of autonomous and controlled motivations. *Personality and Social Psychology Bulletin, 36*, 1101–1114. doi:10.1177/0146167210375618.

Human Rights Campaign. (2010). *Demanding equality face to face: 2010 annual report*. Washington, D.C.

Human Rights Campaign. (2012). *Growing up LGBT in America: HRC youth survey report key findings*. Washington, D.C.

Joussemet, M., Landry, R., & Koestner, R. (2008). A self-determination theory perspective on parenting. *Canadian Psychology, 49*, 194–200. doi:10.1037/a0012754.

Kaufman, G., & Raphael, L. (1996). *Coming out of shame: Transforming gay and lesbian lives*. New York: Doubleday.

Kernis, M. H. (2003). Optimal self-esteem and authenticity: Separating fantasy from reality: Reply. *Psychological Inquiry, 14*, 83–89. doi:10.1207/S15327965PLI1401_03.

Kleck, R. (1968). Physical stigma and nonverbal cues emitted in face-to-face interaction. *Human Relations, 21*, 19–28. doi:10.1177//001872676802100102.

La Guardia, J. G., & Ryan, R. M. (2007). Why identities fluctuate: Variability in traits as a function of situational variations in autonomy support. *Journal of Personality, 75*, 1205–1228. doi:10.1111/j.1467-6494.2007.00473.x.

La Guardia, J. G., Ryan, R. M., Couchman, C. E., & Deci, E. L. (2000). Within-person variation in security of attachment: A self-determination theory perspective on attachment, need

fulfillment, and well-being. *Journal of Personality and Social Psychology, 79*, 367–384. doi:10.1037//0022-3514.79.3.367.
Legate, N., Ryan, R. M., & Weinstein, N. (2012). Is coming out always a "good thing"? Exploring the relations of autonomy support, outness, and wellness for lesbian, gay, and bisexual individuals. *Social Psychological and Personality Science, 3*, 145–152. doi:10.1177/1948550611411929.
Legate, N., Ryan, W., DeHaan, C. R., Weinstein, N., & Ryan, R. M. (2012). *Growing up gay: How parental autonomy support impacts self-concept and wellness of gay, lesbian and bisexual adults*. Unpublished manuscript. University of Rochester, Rochester, NY.
Legault, L., Gutsell, J. N., & Inzlicht, M. (2011). Ironic effects of anti-prejudice messages: How motivational interventions can reduce (but also increase) prejudice. *Psychological Science, 22*, 1472–1477. doi:10.1177/0956797611427918.
Lopez, F. G., & Rice, K. G. (2006). Preliminary development and validation of a measure of relationship authenticity. *Journal of Counseling Psychology, 53*, 362–371. doi:10.1037/0022-0167.53.3.362.
Lynch, M. F., La Guardia, J. G., & Ryan, R. M. (2009). On being yourself in different cultures: Ideal and actual self-concept, autonomy support, and well-being in China, Russia, and the United States. *The Journal of Positive Psychology, 4*, 290–304. doi:10.1080/17439760902933765.
Lynch, M. F., & Ryan, R. M. (2004). On being yourself: Consistency versus authenticity of self-concept in cultural and interpersonal contexts. In H. W. Marsh, J. Baumert, G. E. Richards, & U. Trautwein (Eds.), *Self-concept, motivation and identity: Where to from here? Proceedings of the third international biennial SELF research conference*, Berlin. SELF Research Centre, University of Western Sydney, Australia.
Major, B., & Gramzow, R. H. (1999). Abortion as stigma: Cognitive and emotional implications of concealment. *Journal of Personality and Social Psychology, 77*, 735–745. doi:10.1037/0022-3514.77.4.735.
Meyer, I. H. (2003). Prejudice, social stress, and mental health in lesbian, gay, and bisexual populations: Conceptual issues and research evidence. *Psychological Bulletin, 129*, 674–697. doi:10.1037/0033-2909.129.5.674.
Mohr, J. J., & Fassinger, R. E. (2000). Measuring dimensions of lesbian and gay male experience. *Measurement and Evaluation in Counseling and Development, 33*, 66–90.
Mohr, J. J., & Fassinger, R. E. (2003). Adaptation to sexual orientation stigma: A comparison of bisexual and lesbian/gay adults. *Journal of Counseling Psychology, 50*, 482–495. doi:10.1037/0022-0167.50.4.482.
Niemiec, C. P., & Deci, E. L. (2012). *The effects of provision and deprivation of autonomy on interaction quality between strangers*. Unpublished manuscript. University of Rochester, Rochester, NY.
Pachankis, J. E. (2007). The psychological implications of concealing a stigma: A cognitive-affective-behavioral model. *Psychological Bulletin, 133*, 328–345. doi:10.1037/0033-2909.133.2.328.
Pennebaker, J. W., & Chung, C. K. (2011). Expressive writing, emotional upheavals, and health. In H. S. Friedman (Ed.), *The Oxford handbook of health psychology*. New York: Oxford University Press.
Quinn, D. M., Kahng, S. K., & Crocker, J. (2004). Discreditable: Stigma effects of revealing a mental illness history on test performance. *Personality and Social Psychology Bulletin, 30*, 803–815. doi:10.1177/0146167204264088.
Ragins, B. R. (2004). Sexual orientation in the workplace: The unique work and career experiences of gay, lesbian and bisexual workers. *Research in Personnel and Human Resources Management, 23*, 35–120. doi:10.1016/S0742-7301(04)23002-X.
Ragins, B. R., Singh, R., & Cornwell, J. M. (2007). Making the invisible visible: Fear and disclosure of sexual orientation at work. *Journal of Applied Psychology, 92*, 1103–1118. doi:10.1037/0021-9010.92.4.1103.
Richer, S. F., Blanchard, C., & Vallerand, R. J. (2002). A motivational model of work turnover. *Journal of Applied Social Psychology, 32*, 2089–2113. doi:10.1111/j.1559-1816.2002.tb02065.x.
Rogers, C. R. (1961). *On becoming a person*. Boston: Houghton–Mifflin.

Rosario, M., Schrimshaw, E. W., & Hunter, J. (2009). Disclosure of sexual orientation and subsequent substance use and abuse among lesbian, gay, and bisexual youths: Critical role of disclosure reactions. *Psychology of Addictive Behaviors, 23*, 175–184. doi:10.1037/a0014284.

Roth, G., Assor, A., Niemiec, C. P., Ryan, R. M., & Deci, E. L. (2009). The emotional and academic consequences of parental conditional regard: Comparing conditional positive regard, conditional negative regard, and autonomy support as parenting practices. *Developmental Psychology, 45*, 1119–1142. doi:10.1037/a0015272.

Rule, N. O., Ambady, N., Adams, R. B., & Macrae, C. N. (2008). Accuracy and awareness in the perception and categorization of male sexual orientation. *Journal of Personality and Social Psychology, 95*, 1019–1028. doi:10.1037/a0013194.

Ryan, C., Huebner, D., Diaz, R. M., & Sanchez, J. (2009). Family rejection as a predictor of negative health outcomes in white and Latino lesbian, gay and bisexual young adults. *Pediatrics, 123*, 346–352. doi:10.1542/peds.2007-3524.

Ryan, C., Russell, S. T., Huebner, D., Diaz, R., & Sanchez, J. (2010). Family acceptance in adolescence and the health of LGBT young adults. *Journal of Child and Adolescent Psychiatric Nursing, 23*, 205–213. doi:10.1111/j.1744-6171.2010.00246.x.

Ryan, R. M. (1995). Psychological needs and the facilitation of integrative processes. *Journal of Personality, 63*, 397–427. doi:10.1111/j.1467-6494.1995.tb00501.x.

Ryan, R. M., & Deci, E. L. (2000). Self-determination theory and the facilitation of intrinsic motivation, social development, and well-being. *American Psychologist, 55*, 68–78. doi:10.1037//0003-066X.55.1.68.

Ryan, R. M., La Guardia, J. G., Solky-Butzel, J., Chirkov, V., & Kim, Y. (2005). On the interpersonal regulation of emotions: Emotional reliance across gender, relationships, and cultures. *Personal Relationships, 12*, 145–163. doi:10.1111/j.1350-4126.2005.00106.x.

Sandfort, T. G., Bos, H., & Vet, R. (2006). Lesbians and gay men at work: Consequences of being out. In A. M. Omoto & H. S. Kurtzman (Eds.), *Sexual orientation and mental health: Examining identity and development in lesbian, gay, and bisexual people* (pp. 225–244). Washington, DC: American Psychological Association.

Sandfort, T. G., de Graaf, R., Bijl, R. V., & Schnabel, P. (2001). Same-sex sexual behavior and psychiatric disorders: Findings from the Netherlands Mental Health Survey and Incidence Study (NEMESIS). *Archives of General Psychiatry, 58*, 85–91. doi:10.1001/archpsyc.58.1.85.

Sheldon, K. M., Ryan, R. M., Rawsthorne, L., & Ilardi, B. (1997). Trait self and true self: Cross-role variation in the Big Five traits and its relations with authenticity and subjective well-being. *Journal of Personality and Social Psychology, 73*, 1380–1393. doi:10.1037//0022-3514.73.6.1380.

Sherman, R. A., Nave, C. S., & Funder, D. C. (2010). Situational similarity and personality predict behavioral consistency. *Journal of Personality and Social Psychology, 99*, 330–343. doi:10.1037/a0019796.

Smart, L., & Wegner, D. M. (2000). The hidden costs of stigma. In T. F. Heatherton, R. E. Kleck, M. R. Hebl, & J. G. Hull (Eds.), *The social psychology of stigma* (pp. 220–242). New York: Guilford Press.

Soenens, B., & Vanstinkiste, M. (2005). Antecedents and outcomes of self-determination in 3 life domains: The role of parents' and teachers' autonomy support. *Journal of Youth and Adolescence, 34*, 589–604. doi:10.1007/s10964-005-8948-y.

Sullivan, A. (2012). Andersen Cooper: "The fact is, I'm gay." *The Daily Beast*. Retrieved from http://andrewsullivan.thedailybeast.com/2012/07/anderson-cooper-the-fact-is-im-gay.html

Szymanski, D. M., Chung, Y., & Balsam, K. F. (2001). Psychosocial correlates of internalized homophobia in lesbians. *Measurement and Evaluation in Counseling and Development, 34*, 27–38.

Ullrich, P. M., Lutgendorf, S. K., & Stapleton, J. T. (2003). Concealment of homosexual identity, social support and CD4 cell count among HIV-seropositive gay men. *Journal of Psychosomatic Research, 54*, 205–212. doi:10.1016/S0022-3999(02)00481-6.

Uysal, A., Lin, H. L., & Knee, C. R. (2010). The role of need satisfaction in self-concealment and well-being. *Personality and Social Psychology Bulletin, 36*, 187–199. doi:10.1177/0146167209354518.

Uysal, A., Lin, H. L., & Knee, C. R. (2012). The association between self-concealment from one's partner and relationship well-being. *Personality and Social Psychology Bulletin, 38*, 39–51. doi:10.1177/0146167211429331.

Weinstein, N., Deci, E. L., & Ryan, R. M. (2011). Motivational determinants of integrating positive and negative past identities. *Journal of Personality and Social Psychology, 100*, 527–544. doi:10.1037/a0022150.

Weinstein, N., Hodgins, H. S., & Ryan, R. M. (2010). Autonomy and control in dyads: Effects on interaction quality and joint creative performance. *Personality and Social Psychology Bulletin, 36*, 1603–1617. doi:10.1177/0146167210386385.

Weinstein, N., Ryan, W. S., DeHaan, C. R., Przybylski, A. K., Legate, N., & Ryan, R. M. (2012). Parental autonomy support and discrepancies between implicit and explicit sexual identities: Dynamics of self-acceptance and defense. *Journal of Personality & Social Psychology, 102*, 815–832. doi:10.1037/n0026854.

Wells, J. W., & Kline, W. B. (1987). Self-disclosure of homosexual orientation. *Journal of Social Psychology, 127*, 191–197. doi:10.1080/00224545.1987.9713679.

Whipple, N., Bernier, A., & Mageau, G. A. (2011). Broadening the study of infant security of attachment: Maternal autonomy-support in the context of infant exploration. *Social Development, 20*, 17–32. doi:10.1111/j.1467-9507.2010.00574.x.

Williams, G. C., Grow, V. M., Freedman, Z., Ryan, R. M., & Deci, E. L. (1996). Motivational predictors of weight loss and weight-loss maintenance. *Journal of Personality and Social Psychology, 70*, 115–126. doi:10.1037//0022-3514.70.1.115.

Williamson, I. (2000). Internalized homophobia and health issues affecting lesbians and gay men. *Health Education Research, 15*, 97–107. doi:10.1093/her/15.1.97.

Part III
Applications of Motivation Research

Chapter 10
Parental Conditional Regard: Psychological Costs and Antecedents

Avi Assor, Yaniv Kanat-Maymon, and Guy Roth

> Still today I ask myself… if I did not spend so many days and so many nights, if I did not cover with ink so many pages, if I did not throw into the book market so many books that nobody cared for – only out of the crazy hope to please my grandfather
>
> Jean Paul Sartre (1981): The Words

The experience Sartre describes in this quote refers to his feeling that his revered grandfather's regard and respect were contingent on Sartre's intellectual excellence and public acclaim. Sartre's father died when he was 15 months old and for the first 11 years of his life he lived in his grandfather's home and was in continual contact with him. In the present article we refer to the experience Sartre describes as perceived conditional regard. Although Sartre's quote refers to his grandfather patriarchal figure, it appears to apply to parents as well; namely, the unsettling experience that parents' regard is conditional and contingent on compliance with parents' specific expectations. In this chapter we examine some of the consequences, correlates and potential antecedents of the phenomenon of parental conditional regard (PCR).

Parental Conditional Regard and Its Hypothesized Effects

Parental conditional regard (PCR) as defined and measured by Assor, Roth, and Deci (2004) is a socializing practice in which parents make their affection and appreciation contingent on the child's display of parentally desired behaviors. It is

Note: Much of the research reported in this chapter was supported by grants from the Israel-US Bi-National Science foundation and from the Israel Science Foundation.

A. Assor (✉) • G. Roth
Department of Education, Ben-Gurion University of The Negev

Y. Kanat-Maymon
Department of Psychology, Interdisciplinary Center, Hertzlia, Israel

N. Weinstein (ed.), *Human Motivation and Interpersonal Relationships: Theory, Research, and Applications*, DOI 10.1007/978-94-017-8542-6_10,

useful to further distinguish between: (a) Parental conditional positive regard (PCPR)-giving more affection when the child complies with parents' expectations, and (b) Parental conditional negative regard (PCNR)-giving less affection when the child complies with parents' expectations. In our research (e.g., Assor & Tal, 2012; Roth, Assor, Niemiec, Ryan, & Deci, 2009), we treat both as harmful or at least non-optimal qualities of relating to others. It is also important to note that we treat parental conditional regard as being domain-specific. For example, a child may receive a great deal of affection only if s/he does well in school, but this does not necessitate that parents' affection is contingent on his/her behavior in other domains, for example in relation to sports performance.

Specifically with regard to parental conditional positive regard (PCPR), it is important to note that this practice is not identical to positive feedback. Children may report that their parents frequently provide positive feedback, and still do not feel conditionally regarded because they do not experience the feedback as implying that their value as a person or their parents' love depends on their attainment of specific outcomes or enactment of specific behaviors. The notion that feedback does not necessarily entail conditional regard is endorsed by Dweck (1999) and Ginott (1969); both state that positive feedback is likely to be harmful or perceived as conditional regarding only to the extent that it is character- or trait- focused; in contrast, these authors claim that when positive feedback is accomplishment- or effort- oriented, it is not likely to create an experience of conditional regard.

From a behaviorist perspective, conditional regard might represent the contingent administration of reinforcements and punishments, which are expected to improve discrimination between desired and undesired behaviors and to increase the likelihood of desired behaviors that are emitted (Gewirtz & Pelaez-Nogueras, 1991; McDowell, 1988). However, other psychological theorists have presented a quite different view of conditional regard as a socializing strategy. Rogers (1951) proposed that parents' conditional regard undermines children's self-esteem and interferes with personal exploration. Object relations theorists (e.g., Miller, 1981) have suggested that children, when they learn they are loved conditionally, behave in ways they imagine will yield the desired love. The instrumental behaviors thus persist, but the satisfaction the children experience when they successfully execute the behaviors is fleeting because the behaviors never yield the unconditional regard the children truly desire.

Although the concept of PCR is close to the widely examined construct of psychological control (Barber, Stolz, & Olsen, 2005), there are also some important differences. PCR differs from psychological control in that it refers to ways of controlling children via both contingent *positive* regard (e.g., giving more affection and esteem when the child complies) and contingent negative regard (i.e., giving less affection and esteem when the child fails to comply). Psychological control only refers to contingent negative regard. In addition, psychological control differs from PCR in that it includes components of intrusiveness and blame which children cannot affect by their behavior (e.g., "blames me for other family members' problems"), thus making it a particularly aversive parenting style. A more minor difference

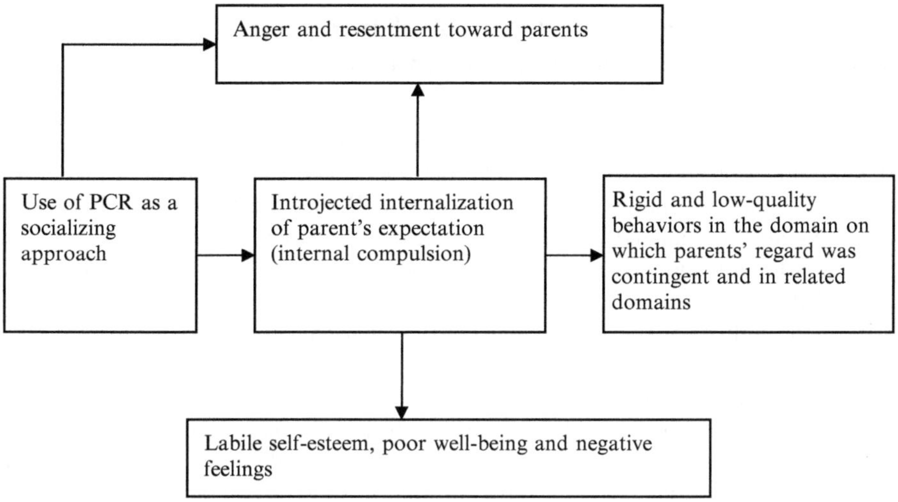

Fig. 10.1 Expected effects of parental conditional regard

is that PCR usually refers to a general parental style, whereas PCPR and PCNR usually refer to specific behavioral domains.

The practice of domain-specific conditional parental regard, unlike psychological control, was hardly examined empirically, except perhaps for the recent work of Soenens and his colleagues (e.g., Soenens, Vansteenkiste, & Luyten, 2010).[1] In view of the lack of sufficient research on conditional parental regard and the divergent theoretical views on the desirability of this practice, we set up a program of research to investigate the correlates and effects of parental conditional regard, and to compare it to other practices that we consider more desirable. This research is guided, mainly, by Self Determination Theory (SDT; Ryan & Deci, 2000).

We hypothesized that parents' conditional regard leads to (1) a stressful type of internalization of the parent's expectations, referred to as introjection, which then leads to the following three additional types of negative outcomes: (2) pressured, anxious, rigid and low-quality performance in the domains on which parents' regard was contingent, (3) negative effects on one's well-being and self-esteem dynamics, and (4) negative affect toward the parent who uses PCR. These effects are summarized in Fig. 10.1, and will be discussed in the following sections.

[1] Recently, Soenens and his colleagues (e.g., Soenens et al., 2010) have introduced the concept of dependency-oriented and achievement-oriented psychological control. These concepts are very close to the concept of domain-specific conditional regard, although they include a guilt arousal component that is not included in our construct and scales, and they also do not separate between positive and negative parental regard. Future research may attempt to examine the relations between the concepts and the scales, and perhaps integrate them.

Conditional Regard as a Predictor of Introjected Internalization of Parents' Expectations

According to Self Determination Theory (SDT; Ryan & Deci, 2000), in this type of internalization, behaviors and goals that are valued by parents are "taken in" without the child accepting them as truly valuable. Rather, the reason those behaviors and goals are internalized is that they prevent loss of parental regard or enhance parental affection and appreciation (see Assor et al., 2004). As a result, behavior is controlled by the desire to avoid feeling guilty, ashamed or unworthy, as well as the striving for highly positive evaluations (self-evaluation and others' evaluations).

The pressure of avoiding loss of self-regard or gaining more self-regard causes the motivation resulting from introjected internalization to feel controlling and not autonomous. Thus, according to SDT, introjection-based motivation involves feelings of internal and inner compulsion, and often people may also be aware that they are doing a certain behavior in order to feel love-worthy and proud of themselves or in order to avoid feeling unworthy, ashamed or guilty (see Assor, Vansteenkiste, & Kaplan, 2009). Overall, then, we assume that parental conditional regard represents a prototypic social context for promoting introjection, because the contingent esteem from parents can be readily transformed into the contingent self-esteem that underlies introjected regulation (see Assor, 2011; Assor et al., 2004; Ryan, Deci, & Grolnick, 1995). As a result, the driving force behind behaviors rooted in parental regard is to minimize shame and guilt and/or to increase self-esteem.

Empirical evidence supporting our formulation concerning the effects of PCR on internalization comes from five studies. Assor et al. (2004) found that American college students who perceived their parents as hinging their regard on academic success, achievement in sport, pro-social behavior or suppression of negative emotions reported feeling internally compelled to act in ways that would attain those parentally valued attributes. They described their sense of internal compulsion and pressure with phrases such as: "Sometimes I feel like there is a something inside me which, in a way, drives and compels me to suppress my negative emotions and not show them", "Sometimes I feel that, no matter how hard I practice for sport, it is never enough". In addition, PCR was either not linked, or negatively linked to sense of choice or identification with parents' expected behaviors.

Assor, Cohen-Melayev, Kaplan, and Friedman (2005) identified a similar pattern in the domain of religious socialization, finding that in the domain of religious practice, parents' use of conditional regard to promote a child's observance of religious practices was associated with introjected internalization of the religious practices by students attending a modern orthodox Jewish school.

Roth (2008) examined the relations of perceptions of parents as using conditional regard versus autonomy-support to promote internalization of pro-social behavior, among north American college students. It was found that perceptions of parental conditional regard correlated positively with introjected internalization of the tendency to behave pro-socially, whereas autonomy support correlated positively with a more autonomous internalization of this tendency.

A fourth study examining conditional regard as a predictor of internalization was carried out by Roth et al. (2009), who studied Jewish-Israeli high school students. These researchers differentiated between the effects of (a) conditional positive regard: giving more affection and esteem when the child complies with parental expectations, and (b) conditional negative regard: giving less affection and esteem when the child does not meet parental expectations. The study focused on the use of conditional positive regard, conditional negative regard, and autonomy support to promote two parentally desired child attributes: academic achievement and regulation of negative emotions of fear and anger. Conditional positive regard predicted introjected internalization of the motivation for academic achievement and regulation of negative emotions. Introjected motivation was indicated by a sense of compulsion to enact the relevant behaviors (e.g., "I feel that my need to study hard controls me and leads me to give up things I really want to do", "I feel like there is something inside me that, in a way, drives and compels me to suppress my anger and not show it"). Conditional negative regard predicted resentment toward parents, and sense of choice (e.g., "I feel a real sense of choice about my attempts to study hard", "I feel a real sense of choice about my tendency to suppress my anger and not show it").

The fifth study was conducted by Israeli, Roth, and Assor (2012; and see also Assor, Roth, Israeli-Halevi, Freed, & Deci, 2007), and focuses specifically on conditional positive regard. We believe that it is particularly important to study PCPR because unlike other types of parental control such as psychological control (Barber et al., 2005) or conditional negative regard, it appears benign (that is, giving more affection rather than withdrawing love seems like a beneficial act). Moreover, it is recommended by many researchers and parenting books (e.g., Frost, 2005; Gewirtz & Pelaez-Nogueras, 1991; Latham, 1994; McDowell, 1988; Patterson & Gullion, 1976; Steinberg, 2004). However, Self Determination Theory (Assor et al., 2004; Ryan & Deci, 2012), in contrast to the above views, conceives of PCPR as *another harmful type of parental control, despite its seemingly benign nature.* Uncovering the harmful effects of conditional positive regard is therefore particularly important exactly because it might be perceived as an alluring strategy that parents and educators in distress might opt for without realizing its hidden and not so hidden psychological costs.

Israeli et al. (2012; and see also Assor et al., 2007) studied Israeli children in grades 7–8 and their mothers, and focused specifically on the strategy of using parental conditional positive regard (PCPR) to promote children's suppression of anxiety. In this strategy, parents provide more affection and appreciation when children suppress their anxiety. They found that mothers' self-reported PCPR predicted children's perceptions of mothers' use of PCPR, which in turn predicted adolescents' introjected motivation to suppress anxiety. These effects were obtained also when controlling for the effects of mothers' use of maternal conditional negative regard (i.e., providing less affection and appreciation when the child expresses anxiety).

An important strength of this study was the correlation between mothers and child's reports of the extent to which mothers' actually use conditional positive and negative regard, suggesting that previous findings based mainly on children's reports cannot be viewed as children's construal that have little to do with the mothers' actual behaviors. The correlations between mothers' and children's reports were also found in a study focusing on parental conditional regard in the academic domain to be reported later.

Together, the research findings suggest that using conditional regard as a socializing practice may lead to an introjected pattern of internalization and motivation that is associated with feeling of internal pressure and compulsion. Advocates of the use of conditional regard might argue that the process of introjection is simply a step toward a more integrated regulation. However, the research results provide no support for this position. Most of the participants in the studies reviewed here were university students who recalled examples of conditional regard from their childhood and adolescence, yet they continued to display a pressured form of introjected regulation years later. Moreover, the effects of conditional regard were always accompanied by negative emotional states, suggesting that behaviors regulated by conditional regard had not been integrated in a growth-enhancing way.

Conditional Regard as a Predictor of Rigid Behavior

If a parental value is internalized, regardless of the type of internalization, one would expect some degree of subsequent enactment of behavior reflecting that value. Thus, to the degree that parental conditional regard promotes introjection, it is expected to promote enactment of the behaviors on which parental affection depends. However, the feelings of pressure, anxiety and ambivalence accompanying the introjected value are likely to result in a constricted and uncreative enactment of the parentally valued behaviors (e.g., Assor & Roth, 2005; Roth et al., 2009). The anxiety children experience may cause them to stick to known methods rather than taking a chance on creative or personally suitable methods. In addition, the weight placed on success may cause needless practicing (repeated training even though one knows the drill), which Covington (1992) described as over-striving.

Finally, the ambivalence, and sometime anger, experienced with regard to the introjected parental value may, subconsciously, undermine the motivation for high quality performance. What is important is not the action or the subject itself, but getting the expected regard following the enactment of that behavior. Moreover, if this regard is attained with less than optimal performance, this is satisfactory, perhaps even providing a sense of freedom in that one feels that she/he is not enslaved by an act he/she does not really identify with. The relations between parental conditional regard and rigid, low-quality performance has been examined in multiple domains, as we now describe.

Academic Engagement

Roth et al. (2009) found that Israeli high school students who perceived their parents as using the practice of PCPR to promote academic achievement were described by their teachers as showing grade-focused academic engagement. This type of engagement is characterized by a tendency to study only what appears in the test, feeling deeply hurt when one does not succeed in an assignment or test, and arguing forcefully with the teacher about grades. Importantly, CPR was negatively related to a higher quality of academic involvement termed interest-focused engagement. This deeper type of intellectual engagement was also measured via teacher ratings and refers to students' tendency to show interest and invest effort and time also in materials that might not appear in the test. Consistent with our theory, the effect of positive conditional regard on grade-focused studying was mediated by the feeling that one is internally compelled to study hard (i.e., introjected internalization of the value of academic work). It appears then that while conditional positive regard did promote academic effort, this engagement was rather narrow and shallow.

PCNR in the academic domain was related to lack of academic achievement, and was unrelated to grade-focused engagement and interest-focused engagement. Interestingly, Assor, Kaplan, Roth, and Kanat-Maymon (2005) described a similar pattern of lack of academic engagement that is associated with highly controlling teacher behavior. Thus, conditional negative regard appears particularly problematic since it does not promote any kind of effortful investment, not even a rigid, low-quality, engagement.

The stressful and rigid engagement associated with parental conditional positive regard was further explored by Assor and Tal (2012). These authors found that PCPR predicted compulsive academic over-striving. Over-striving is characterized by the tendency to invest a lot of time in studying what is already known about the subject, which causes students to unnecessarily give up activities they really enjoy. The relation between PCPR and over-striving was mediated by self-aggrandizement (grandiose and narcissistic feelings) following success and to a lesser degree by self-derogation and shame following failure. Assor and Tal also found that PCNR in the academic domain predicted self-derogation and shame after failure, which in turn predicted avoidance of academic challenges.

Pro-social Behavior

In line with our general model, we expected that children who perceive parental regard as contingent on helping others would indeed help but would also show relatively little empathy and sensitivity toward those they assist. Assor et al. (2004) found that offspring's perceptions of parents' regard as being contingent on helping others were associated with introjected motivation for helping others (indicated mainly by a sense of internal compulsion to help), which in turn predicted frequent (self-reported) helping. Roth (2008) studied the association between parental conditional regard and self-versus other-oriented prosocial tendencies among Israeli college students. Self-oriented prosocial helping was defined as helping behavior enacted for the sake of others' approval and appreciation, whereas other-oriented helping was defined as helping done while focusing on others' needs and preferences. Parental conditional regard was associated with self-oriented behavior but not with other-oriented helping behavior.

Regulation of Fear, Anger and Sadness

Children who perceive parental regard as contingent on suppressing or hiding negative emotions are inclined to feel compelled to suppress and hide these emotions. In addition, avoiding one's own negative emotions tends to restrict a person's ability to identify emotions in other people. Moreover, the ability to listen and show empathy in the face of painful emotional disclosures in close relationships may be compromised. Roth et al. (2009) found that children who perceived their parent as making positive regard contingent on successful suppression of fear or anger reported that they often felt flooded and overwhelmed by negative emotions, making it difficult for them to engage in daily tasks when feeling angry or fearful. In other words, this kind of emotion regulation is actually conducive to dysregulation. PCPR was also associated with a suppressive regulatory style, which involves suppressing and concealing one's negative emotions.

Assor, Eilot, and Roth (2009) studied Israeli high school students and found a positive correlation between perceptions of parents as using conditional positive regard to promote anger suppression in children, and children's reports of suppressive anger regulation and anger dysregulation. Another study by Roth and Assor (2003) yielded similar results. Although they did not distinguish between conditional positive and conditional negative regard, they still found that perceived parental conditional regard was associated with emotion suppression and dysregulation. In addition, Roth and Assor found that parental conditional regard was negatively associated with the ability to recognize feelings in facial expressions of emotions and in stories. Furthermore, parental conditional regard predicted poor ability to support a romantic partner, and this association was mediated by poor emotion recognition.

In another study, Roth and Assor (2010) explored the association between parental conditional regard and empathy among kindergarten children. This study was based on parental reports on their own practice of conditional regard toward their child and an emotion regulation task completed by the children. The findings revealed negative associations between both negative and positive parental conditional regard and children's ability to feel sadness, recognize sadness in others, and empathize with and help a child who looked sad. The findings of Roth and Assor (2010) are particularly important because they are not based on retrospective children's self-reports, use a measure of PCR based on parents' reports, and include a performance measure of emotion recognition by children. These features suggest that the relations found in previous studies of PCR cannot be attributed only to children's retrospective reporting biases.

Identity Exploration

The identity-formation process involves attempts to explore the possibility of integrating childhood and contemporaneous identifications into a larger, self-determined, and relatively coherent set of self-identified ideals that feels authentic and meaningful (Erikson, 1968; Schwartz, 2001). Exploration, which Grotevant (1987) argued to be the "work" of identity-formation, describes a core process of finding and processing self-relevant information and attempting to integrate such knowledge into a comprehensive set of values and commitments. Assor and Shavit (2012, and see also Shavit, 2009) showed that college students who perceived their parents' regard as dependent on their compliance with parents' expectations were less inclined to engage in deep identity exploration. Apparently, the guilt experienced when starting to raise questions about parents' expectations prevented a serious exploration of parents' values.

Further findings supporting this interpretation come from the qualitative and quantitative studies presented in Assor et al. (2005). Participants were modern orthodox Jewish students in Israel, coming from religious homes who also embraced modern technology and ways of life, and were therefore exposed to views and materials disseminated by the secular mass media. Moreover, these students also studied in a non-religious and fairly secular institution. Because the norms and values of the secular contexts and of Orthodox Judaism often differ widely, modern orthodox Jewish students face a rather demanding task of forming values and goals that integrate contradictory religious and secular viewpoints in ways that feel coherent, authentic and autonomous.

Based on both qualitative and quantitative analyses, the authors identified two styles of exploration that religiously raised youth employ when they cope with the religion-modernity conflict: *Radical Exploration* and *Revisionist. Radical exploration* is characterized by a highly emotional, and at times oppositional, questioning of one's personal-emotional relations with the religion's core beliefs and life-style. This type of exploration revolves around the personal costs involved in maintaining a religious way of life and the extent to which a religious life-style conflicts with personal dispositions and beliefs (e.g., an assertive feminist woman who opposes what may seem to be gender discriminatory religious practices). It also includes a concern with the sense of authenticity and level of internalization of one's religious involvement (e.g., "why is it that I am religious? Does it reflect the real me?"). The term "radical exploration" highlights the emotional intensity and the grappling with deep and fundamental personal issues that are associated with this process. Although radical exploration often involves questioning of the merits of conducting a religious way of life, it is usually not sophisticated, thorough, or cognitively complex. In fact, because of its highly emotional nature and its commonly oppositional quality, *radical exploration often may be quite unsystematic, simplistic, and rigid.* This type of exploration seems to be focused more on raising difficult questions and on making extreme and quick decisions than on the process of resolving the conflict through synthesis and integration.

In comparison, revisionist exploration focuses mainly on synthesis and integration: the question is not whether to maintain the religion of origin, but how to do it in ways that are coherent with various beliefs already endorsed? Thus, in this style of exploration, fundamental religious tenets and the merits of maintaining a religious way of life are not questioned. Revisionist exploration involves little preoccupation with the personal emotional costs of maintaining a religious life-style or the extent to which one's religiosity feels authentic and self-chosen. Rather, such exploration involves serious reflection and decision-making concerning the *kind* of religious life one wants to lead, ability to examine various options also when this takes considerable time, and an ability to think critically in response to solutions offered by various religious authorities. In the Jewish and Christian religions, revisionist exploration may involve, for example, grappling with questions concerning the role of women in religion, sexual relations before and after marriage, issues pertaining to human rights (e.g., abortion, euthanasia, and homosexual relations), and the meaning of scientific theories and findings to religion. Although these are serious and often emotionally-laden issues, their examination is not dominated by intense emotional reactions involving personal costs, and therefore is relatively balanced and cognitively complex.

Qualitative analysis of the participants' responses to open response questionnaires showed that youth whose parents were described as using conditional regard to promote observance of religious practices were much more inclined to adopt a radical rather than a revisionist style of religious identity formation. For example, one of the participants showing a radical style wrote that when at the seventh grade she developed serious religious doubts, she felt a tremendous sense of guilt and did not share her any of her doubts or feelings with her parents. From her description. it appeared that one possible reason for feeling guilt and not sharing her doubts was that her parents failed to value reflection and critical thinking, and in fact did not appreciate others who raise serious questions concerning religious tenets. Overall, then, parental conditional regard appears to be promote a more rigid, simplistic and less systematic type of identity exploration.

Conditional Regard as a Predictor of Poor Well-Being and Fluctuations in Self-Esteem

Parental conditional regard causes children's self-esteem to depend on fulfillment of parental expectations. The dependence of self-esteem on performing desired behaviors may result in fluctuations in self-esteem, or unstable self-esteem (Kernis & Paradise, 2002), because satisfaction is likely to be fragile and short-lived. That is, satisfaction lasts only until the pressure of the next demand (actual or imagined), and failure to attain a particular outcome may lead to feelings of guilt and shame because failure is interpreted as implying unworthiness.

A number of studies have supported the hypothesis that conditional regard is associated with fluctuations in self-esteem, negative feelings and diminished well-being. Assor et al. (2004) found that successful fulfillment of parental expectations in the domains of academic achievement, sports, and negative emotion suppression was followed by short-lived satisfaction and then feelings of disappointment or emptiness. Furthermore, when conditionally regarded participants did not achieve athletic success or were unable to suppress negative affect, they felt guilty and ashamed. The idea that fluctuating self-worth results from parental conditional regard was supported by Assor et al. in four different domains. In the analysis that focused on the academic domain, the authors found that parental conditional regard was related to poor self-esteem.

Assor and Tal (2012) showed that self derogation and shame following academic failure was linked to both positive and negative parental conditional regard in the academic domain. Self-derogation also mediated the effects of conditional positive and negative regard on less adaptive modes of academic coping. In addition, parental conditional positive regard also predicted self-aggrandizement following success which in turn predicted over striving. Interestingly, self-derogation and self-aggrandizement were moderately correlated ($r = .50$). Importantly the effects of parental conditional positive regard emerged also when controlling for the effects of parental psychological control and conditional negative regard.

Results were replicated in a study conducted by Shapira, Ezra, Assor, Gabay-Elegy, and Shapira (2012), which showed that conditional positive regard predicted both self-derogation following failure and self-aggrandizement following success. Similarly, Assor et al. (2007, and see also Freed, 2010) found that parents and 13–14 year old children's reports of mothers' use of conditional positive regard to promote children's academic achievement predicted children's self derogation and shame following failure. Finally, Baron et al. (2010) found that perceived PCR predicted contigent self-worth (Crocker & Wolfe, 2001; Kernis, 2003).

The fact that parental conditional positive regard (PCPR) was found by Assor and Tal (2012) to have unique maladaptive correlates that cannot be accounted for by parental conditional negative regard or psychological control suggests that PCPR differs from other types of parental control in its psychological dynamics. Specifically, we assume that perceptions that parents are using conditional positive regard promote the development of a fragile, contingent (e.g., Crocker & Wolfe, 2001; Kernis, Brown, & Brody, 2000) and unstable sense of self (Kernis, Cornell, Sun, Berry, & Harlow, 1993), vacillating between feeling of worth, competence and pride on one hand and feelings of worthlessness, incompetence and shame on the other hand (see also Assor et al., 2004 on this issue). The present studies did not assess stability or fluctuations of self-esteem, nor did it assess contingent self worth. Yet, the fact that PCPR was related to both self-aggrandizement following success and shame following failure, as well as the fairly sizable correlation between shame and self-aggrandizement suggest that PCPR indeed is likely to contribute to an unstable self-esteem that is contingent on one's performance and others' feedback.

The notion that parental positive conditional regard is likely to promote an unstable sense of self is consistent with Kernis et al. (1998) views concerning the antecedents of unstable and fragile self-esteem. Kernis et al. highlighted the role of over-reliance on significant others' love and approval in promoting unstable self-esteem, which then leads to the feeling that one's self worth is fragile and vulnerable. Research by Kernis et al. (2000) has shown that children's perceptions of parents as using love withdrawal and guilt induction were associated with unstable self-esteem, as well as generally low level self-esteem. Similar findings were obtained by Assor et al. (2004) with regard to general perceptions of parental conditional regard, consisting mostly of conditional negative regard. Our analysis of PCPR, suggests that this specific practice is likely to be associated with unstable self-esteem, but, unlike PCNR or love withdrawal, it should not be associated with a generally low level of self-esteem. Further research may test this prediction.

Another aspect of self-esteem dynamics which might be related to PCPR involves narcissistic tendencies. The studies surveyed showed that PCPR was associated with feelings of self-aggrandizement and superiority following academic success. Such feelings are key components of a narcissistic personality disposition (Raskin, Novacek, & Hogan, 1991; Rhodewalt & Morf, 1998). Thus, it is possible that the self-aggrandizing responses after success reflect a more enduring narcissistic tendency, and PCPR promotes not only temporary feelings of grandiosity, but also a more chronic narcissistic inclination, which in turn provides the basis of temporary grandiose responses. A link between a narcissistic disposition and self-aggrandizing response after success was detected in research by Rhodewalt and Morf (1998). These researchers showed that people scoring high on narcissism made more self-aggrandizing attributions for success than did people scoring low on narcissism. However, Rhodewalt and Morf did not examine perceptions of parental practices or actual parental practices. Future research may examine the possibility that the impact of PCPR on self-aggrandizement following success is mediated by an enduring narcissistic disposition. That is, PCPR might promote narcissistic strivings, which in turn might lay the foundation for self-aggrandizing responses in specific situations.

But, why would PCPR lead to self-aggrandizing response following success? The studies surveyed obviously cannot answer this question. However, it is possible to speculate that PCPR creates a continual longing for the missing unconditional parental appreciation and affection. Against this background, self-aggrandizing responses reinforce the belief in one's potential greatness and superiority, which in turn allows one to nurture a hope or a fantasy that one can attain high achievements which would bring the missing unconditional parental love and a great deal of parental affection. Interestingly, the link between missing parental love and the development of narcissistic aspirations aimed at attaining the missing maternal love was articulated earlier by Freud in his article "The Ego and the Id" (Freud, 1923).

Of course, the flip side of the hope based on self-aggrandizing beliefs is the fear that failure to achieve would lead to shame and loss of parental regard. And indeed research on people with self-aggrandizing narcissistic tendencies shows that these tendencies are often associated with shame and avoidance or self handicapping in response to difficult tasks or possible failure (e.g. Broucek, 1991; Morrison, 1989; Rhodewalt, Tragakis, & Finnerty, 2001).

The last two studies described in this section focus on the link between PCR and susceptibility to negative affect. In a lexical decision study (see Kanat-Maymon, Roth, Assor, & Reizer, 2012), we found that participants who perceived their mothers as high, compared to low, on academic conditional regard were quicker to perceive stress-related words (e.g., anxiety, shame) but not other kinds of negative words when they were subliminally primed with the word "mother". This suggests that when facing an academic task, children who experienced conditional regard are more anxious and perturbed by the thought of shamefully failing. Another study by Shavit-Miller and Assor (2003, and see also Assor & Shavit-Miller, 2012) found that students whose parents practiced conditional regard confusion often experience feelings of guilt, low self-worth, meaninglessness, and confusion about their purpose in life.

Conditional Regard as a Predictor of Poor Relations with Parents and Romantic Partners

Parents' use of conditional regard to pressure children to behave in specific ways can arouse strong negative feelings in relation to parents. Specifically, such pressure can cause anger and resentment toward parents because it undermines children's sense of autonomy or because it indicates that the parents do not trust their children and do not believe that they will behave in desirable ways out of their own choice. Moreover, the strong linkage of the parent's affection to specific child behaviors can easily be construed by children as indicating an underlying parental rejection or disapproval. Empirical evidence supporting the link between PCR and negative affect toward parents comes from three studies.

Assor et al. (2004) found that American college students' perception of parental conditional regard in four different domains was related to perception of their parents as disapproving and to resentment toward the parents. In a subsequent study, Roth et al. (2009) studied Jewish Israeli high school students and found that perceptions of parental conditional negative regard in the domains of academic achievement and emotion regulation were associated with resentment toward the parent.

A third set of findings bearing on the relations between PCR and affect toward parents is reported in a study by Shavit-Miller and Assor (2003). In that study, it was found that women (and to a lesser extent men) who described their parents as using the practice of conditional regard tended to feel resentful or angry in relation to their parents. While men were more inclined to express their resentment and to openly voice their disagreements with parents, women often did not express their anger, yet, internally were often preoccupied with strong negative emotions and thoughts pertaining to unjust or harmful parental behavior.

Importantly, there is now evidence that the experience of conditional regard by one's parents or partner also undermines the quality of relations with romantic partners or peers. Specifically, Roth and Assor (2012) found that college students' experience of their parents as using conditional regard to promote suppression or expression of negative feelings by the adolescent predicted poor intimacy capacity in the offspring relations with romantic partners. In a recent project conducted with married couples (Kanat-Maymon et al., 2012), it was found that perceived conditional negative regard by a romantic partner was associated with relationship dissatisfaction, as indicated by lower levels of directly assessed relationship satisfaction and less direct measures such as inclusion of other in the self, doubts regarding the relationship, and a sense of entrapment. Moreover, participants who perceived their partners as providing conditional regard reported that they were less inclined to disclose personal information and listen empathically to their partner, and more inclined to avoid conflicts with their partner.

Antecedents and Moderators of Parents' Use of Conditional Regard as a Socializing Practice

We assume that there are a number of potential antecedents of parents' use of conditional regard as a socializing practice. One source of parents' use of PCR as a socializing practice maybe a relatively simple social learning or modeling process whereby parents emulate their own parents' practices. So, that if the parents' own parents used PCR, they will also use this practice with their children. Assor et al. (2004) presented data supporting this simple model of inter-generational transmission of the practice of PCR.

However, the experience of one's own parents' as providing regard only if one complies with their demands may generate additional, psychologically more complex processes, which in turn may lead to re-enactment of the PCR practice with parents' children. We have investigated two such mediators of the effects of parents' experience of their parents as using PCR in the academic domain: contingent self-esteem (in the academic domain) and perception of the world as highly competitive. Figure 10.2 presents the model.

The construct of academically-contingent self-esteem (Crocker, Sommers, & Luhtanen, 2002) refers to people's experience of their self-esteem as dependent on their academic achievements. The construct of a competitive worldview refers to

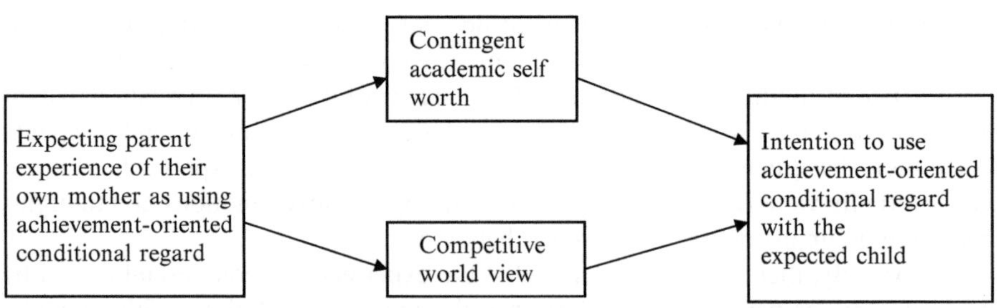

Fig. 10.2 Expecting parents' experiences of PCR with their own parents as predictors of personal attributes and intentions to use PCR with the future child

parents' perception of the world as highly competitive and ruthless (Gurland & Grolnick, 2005). In a study conducted with expecting parents (Baron et al., 2010), we hypothesized that the experience of one's parents as linking their love to academic achievements causes the self-esteem of expecting parents to depend on their academic achievements (academically-contingent self-esteem). Furthermore, we also hypothesized that expecting parents' experience of their self-esteem as dependent on academic achievements leads them to endorse the practice of conditional regard with regard to their expected children. The rationale underlying this prediction was that parents with contingent self-esteem expect to use PCR with their future children in order to ensure that children will indeed achieve, and children achievement will serve to protect parents' fragile self-esteem. To secure such achievements, parents then use PCR to pressure their children to achieve.

As for a competitive and ruthless world view, when parents use a controlling and insensitive achievement-oriented practice such academically oriented PCR, expecting parents are likely to adopt a competitive-ruthless world view. Once such a view is formed, these future parents may feel that they need to push their children to achieve so they could compete successfully in difficult environments. Moreover, they may also feel that they cannot afford to be sensitive and accommodating, because they have to toughen and harden their children and educate them to withstand the pressures of a tough world.

Mediation analyses based on the responses of 149 couples 2–4 months before the birth of their first child clearly supported the hypothesized model. Thus, academically-contingent self-esteem and a competitive world view were found to mediate the effect of expecting parents' perceptions of their own parents' use of PCR on expecting parents' endorsement of PCR as a preferred practice with their future child.

Using data from the same project, Assor et al. (2013) followed 73 couples for 2 years following the child birth. They found that expecting parents' intention to use the practice of PCR with their future child had a sizable correlation ($r = .60$) with parents self-reported enactment of the practice of PCR 2 years later, when children were in the second half of the second year. Moreover, regression analyses indicated that infants' temperament (as measured at 8 month) moderated the relations between pre-natal endorsement of PCR and post-natal enactment of PCR with one's child. Thus, the infant's temperament disposition to be easily distressed and frustrated (distress to limitations) enhanced parents' pre-natal tendency to use conditional regard, and reduced the pre-natal tendency to act in autonomy supportive ways.

Two additional studies further supported the role of parents' contingent self-esteem as an antecedent of parents' use of PCR with early adolescents. Israeli Halevi et al. (2012) showed that mother's contingent self-esteem predicted mothers' use of both conditional negative regard and conditional positive regard to promote children's suppression of anxiety and fear. Similarly, Assor et al. (2007) found that mother's contingent self-esteem predicted mothers' use of conditional positive regard to promote children's academic achievements. Importantly, in both studies mothers' use of conditional regard practices was assessed via both mother and child reports.

Overall, then, the studies surveyed suggest that parents' tendency to use the practice of PCR originates, at least in part, from parents' own experience of being subjected to the practice of PCR as children, and from parents' contingent self-esteem and competitive world view. In addition, it appears that children's temperament disposition to be easily frustrated amplifies parents' inclination to use the practice of PCR.

New Directions: Gender Differences, Innovations in Assessment and Vicarious Conditional Regard

In this last section, we present three studies exploring new directions in PCR research.

Gender Differences

Shavit-Miller (2009) and Assor and Shavit-Miller (2012) explored, in three studies, associations between parental conditional regard and the quality of offspring's internalization of parents' expectations, mainly in the academic domain, among college students in Israel and the United States. A qualitative analysis of open-ended questionnaire responses revealed that perception of parents as using conditional regard to promote academic achievement promoted introjected internalization of these expectations. The response of Sagit, a second year psychology student, provides a good example of introjected motivation driven by a great deal of conditional parental regard:

> "I see myself as very perfectionist. Everything has to be exactly as I planned… I believe this has to do with the home I grew up in, which always emphasized that one has to succeed….I always felt a duty to succeed. A strong will to succeed in something, even before I considered by myself why it is good or what it would give me….It was very important to me to prove to myself and maybe to my parents too that I am "worthy", I simply felt a duty to succeed in my studies

Sagit's response illustrates central aspects of introjected internalization and motivation: The feeling that one has no choice but to succeed, the feeling that one's sense of self-worth depends on one's success, the perception that one adopts a certain goal (success) not because one really understands or identifies with its value or utility but in order to gain parental appreciation, and the rigid nature of actions driven by this kind internalization ("everything has to be exactly as I planned" because there is "a duty to succeed").

A major thesis and finding of Shavit-Miller and Assor (2003, 2012) was that parental conditional regard is associated with more intense introjected internalization in women (daughters) than in men (sons). Moreover, the intense introjected internalization characterizing women was associated with fears of hurting parents and losing their approval, as well as feelings of anger toward parents, shame and embarrassment. Importantly, there were also feelings of anger toward parents and ambivalence toward parental goals. Yet, these feelings were nevertheless associated with a sense of obligation to pursue the goals in order to procure parental love.

Shavit-Miller and Assor (2003); Assor and Shavit (2012) also examined an alternative explanation, according to which the stronger vulnerability of females to the experience of PCR reflects a general gender-difference in the level of sensitivity to negative events, regardless of their content. Results did not support the alternative explanation, and showed instead that the same women who were sensitive to parental conditional regard were not more sensitive than men to frustration of social influence and achievement needs. Evidence also suggested that offspring experiencing high levels of parental conditional regard engaged in little reflection on the goals and values that parents attempted to promote and transmit.

Young women's vulnerability to parental conditional regard may be due to early gender socialization, with women's sense of self-worth and well-being being heavily dependent on the satisfaction of relatedness needs. As a result, they might be less able to tolerate parental love withdrawal and might also feel more responsible for their parents' suffering when they refuse to accept parental expectations. These processes may then lead many women to introject parental expectations that they do not identify with, while at the same time feeling angrier and more conflicted concerning the introjected parental expectations.

Towards a More Rigorous Assessment of the Effects of Parental Conditional Positive Regard

Assor, Shapira, Johnson, and Kanat-Maymon (2012) focused specifically on the phenomenon of PCPR, and examined if this practice is harmful also when defined and assessed in ways that are more consistent with traditional reinforcement theories (e.g., Skinner, 1969). In past studies we assessed conditional positive regard by examining the extent to which parents gave more affection than usual when the child complied with expectations. However, traditional reinforcement notions do not really claim that parents should give more affection in response to compliance in a valued domain relative to other domains or some general baseline. Similarly, they do not recommend that parents would limit the affection they generally give in order to increase the reinforcement value of the valued domain. Rather, proponents of reinforcement recommend showing high levels of affection and esteem when children comply, and to respond considerably less positively or not respond at all when they do not comply.

Another limitation of past research on conditional positive regard was that this construct was assessed by items such as: "my father gave me more affection than usual when I worked hard at school". With this type of questions, it is was difficult to know if reports of increased affection as a function of a specific behavior do not actually involve a shift from a cold and rejecting response to a warm response.

To address the latter problem and to provide a measure that is closer to traditional concepts of reinforcement, we devised a new measure. When completing this measure, participants are asked to indicate (on a nine point scale) the extent to which their parents responded to them warmly versus coldly following compliance with parents' expectations in the academic domain. They are then asked to indicate (again on a nine point scale) the extent to which parents respond warmly or coldly following breach of parents' expectations in the academic domain. Results using this measure show that for parents described as responding non-warmly to breach of expectations (being neither cold not really warm), increased warmth in response to compliance was associated with an increased sense of compulsion to achieve. Thus, it appears that conditional positive regard is associated with introjected internalization also when assessed in ways that are closer to reinforcement theories and in "purer" way (not capturing any shift from a cold to a warm response).

Vicarious PCR: Another Channel Through Which PCR Is Conveyed in Families

The last study to be surveyed in this section focused on a new type of conditional positive regard termed "implicit or vicarious conditional regard". The conception of conditional positive regard as an antecedent of introjected motivation assumes a direct dyadic process between parent and child. However, parents also respond to other people, and these responses can promote indirect (vicarious) learning processes that can have considerable impact on children (e.g., Kazdin, 1973). One such process may be parents' valuation of other people's attainment of academic achievements (i.e., high grades, prizes).

We view such valuation as an implicit type of conditional regard. In this vicarious process, children may perceive the increased esteem given to others who achieve as implying that their parents would value them more deeply and fully if they also attain such achievements. Experiences of implicit conditional parental regard can be aroused by parents' valuing achievements inside and outside one's families. However, it is likely that parents' valuation of siblings' achievements can arouse particularly strong feelings of jealousy and concerns of differential treatment by parents (e.g., Richmond, Stocker, & Rienks, 2005). These feelings and concerns can then trigger intense introjected academic motivation aimed at securing one's status within the family via outstanding academic achievements.

To examine these hypotheses we conducted two studies with Israeli university students. We found that direct experiences of PCPR in the academic achievement domain (measured via a scale adapted from Roth et al., 2009) indeed predicted introjected academic motivation (indicated via sense of compulsion as we as via introjected reasons to invest in studying). Also as expected, perceiving one's mother as valuing siblings or others because of their high achievements was associated with introjected academic motivation. Moreover, and of special interest, both explicit (direct) and implicit (vicarious) conditional regard served as unique predictors of introjected academic motivation.

The two studies expand our understanding regarding the scope and different appearances of PCPR. Specifically, they suggest that the phenomenon of PCPR has different forms, some of them not examined in past studies. Thus, even parents who do not use direct conditional positive regard in relation to their child may nevertheless promote negative motivational and self-esteem outcomes in their child through vicarious conditional regard processes in which they provide siblings or other people outside the family positive regard when these people achieve academically. The present findings, then, suggest that the negative effects of conditional positive regard might be even more widespread than suggested by past research because these effects operate both directly and indirectly through vicarious learning. Because the implicit forms of conditional positive regard are less direct and perhaps less detectable, parents may be less aware of its existence and of its negative effects.

A possible implication of these findings is that parents should be more aware of the way they demonstrate appreciation of academic achievements within and outside the family. Moreover, parents who would like to enhance learning and intellectual development in their children, may do well to focus more on the process, personal relevance and interest of their children in academic activities rather than show admiration for the high grades of other people or doing achievement-level comparisons.

Limitations

Most of the studies reported in this article assessed PCR and offspring's outcomes using mainly offspring's reports. Although many of the studies focused on adolescents and one has focused on kindergarten children, we have no prospective longitudinal data, which can support more reliable causal inferences. To address these limitations, future research might assess the various variables (particularly PCR) using methods which do not rely only on offspring's reports and using longitudinal prospective designs.

A particularly controversial aspect of our approach is the claim that positive PCR is harmful. That is, the idea that verbal praise and conditional provision of attention might be almost as problematic as love withdrawal. Although the correlational research presented in this article supports this claim, there is a need for research that can provide more direct causal evidence.

Conclusion

The findings from the various studies presented in this chapter suggest that while the use of conditional regard as a socializing practice might sometimes lead to the enactment of parentally expected behaviors, this practice has great psychological costs for both children and parents. Advocates of the use of conditional regard as a socializing strategy might argue that the process of introjection is simply a step toward integration. However, the results of the studies surveyed in this chapter provide no support for that position. Specifically, participants in several studies were university students who displayed a pressured introjected pattern many years after the parental conditional regard experiences they were recalling from their years as children and adolescents. Moreover, the effects of PCR on behavior were always accompanied by negative emotional states, suggesting that these behaviors have never been integrated in a comfortable, growth-enhancing, way. Together, then, the findings suggest that although the use of conditional regard may be an effortless and relatively convenient socialization approach, the negative psychological and relational consequences associated with it argue for the use of less controlling and more autonomy-supportive methods.

References

Assor, A. (2011). Autonomous moral motivation: Consequences, socializing antecedents, and the unique role of integrated moral principles. In M. Mikulincer & P. R. Shaver (Eds.), *The social psychology of morality*. Washington, DC: American Psychological Association.

Assor, A., Cohen-Melayev, M., Kaplan, A., & Friedman, D. (2005). Choosing to stay religious in a modern world: Socialization and exploration processes leading to an integrated internalization of religion among Israeli Jewish youth. In M. L. Maehr & S. Karabenick (Eds.), *Advances in motivation and achievement* (Religion and motivation, Vol. 14, pp. 105–150). Amsterdam: Elsevier.

Assor, A., Eilot, K., & Roth, A. (2009). *In search of an optimal style of negative emotion regulation: Correlates and potential parental antecedents of integrated regulation*. Paper presented at the Society for Research in Child Development (SRCD), Denver, CO, USA.

Assor, A., Ezra, O., Kanat-Maymon, Y., Gabay-Elegy, P., Iluz-Cohen, M., & Shapira, D. (2013). *Infant's distress to limitation amplifies the use of conditional regard and reduces autonomy support among first time parents*. Paper to be presented at the 5th International Conference on Self-Determination Theory, Rochester, NY.

Assor, A., Kaplan, H., Kanat-Maymon, Y., & Roth, G. (2005). Directly controlling teacher behaviors as predictors of poor motivation and engagement in girls and boys: The role of anger and anxiety. *Learning and Instruction, 15*, 397–413.

Assor, A., & Roth, G. (2005). Conditional love as a socializing approach: Costs and alternatives. *Scientific Annals of the Psychological Society of Northern Greece, 7*, 17–34.

Assor, A., Roth, G., & Deci, E. L. (2004). The emotional costs of perceived parents' conditional regard: A self-determination theory analysis. *Journal of Personality, 72*, 47–89.

Assor, A., Roth, G., Israeli-Halevi, M., Freed, A., & Deci, E. L. (2007). Parental conditional positive regard: Another harmful type of parental control. In A. Assor & W. S. Grolnick (Chairs), *Disentangling the construct of parental control: Conceptual and measurement issues*. Symposium conducted at the Biennial Meeting of the Society for Research on Child Development (SRCD), Boston, MA.

Assor, A., Shapira, D., Johnson, G., & Kanat-Maymon, Y. (2012). *Parental conditional positive regard has negative correlates also when assessed in ways that are consistent with behavioral approaches*. Unpublished manuscript. Ben Gurion University.

Assor, A., & Shavit-Miller, A. (2012). *Vulnerability to the experience of negative conditional parental regard in the academic domain: Gender differences and possible mechanisms*. Paper presented at the conference of the Society for Research on Adolescence (SRA), Vancouver, BC, Canada.

Assor, A., & Tal, K. (2012). When parents' affection depends on child's achievement: Parental conditional positive regard, self-aggrandizement, shame and coping in adolescents. *Journal of Adolescence, 35*, 249–260. doi:10.1016/j.adolescence.2011.10.004.

Assor, A., Vansteenkiste, M., & Kaplan, A. (2009). Identified versus introjected-approach and introjected-avoidance motivations in school and in sports: The limited benefits of self-worth strivings. *Journal of Educational Psychology, 2*, 482–497.

Barber, B., Stolz, H., & Olsen, J. (2005). Parental support, psychological control and behavioral control: Assessing relevance across time, culture and method. *Monographs of the Society for Research in Child Development, 70*, 1–151.

Baron, I., Kanat-Maymon, Y., Assor, A., Gabay-Elegy, P., Iluz-Cohen, M., & Moed, A. (2010). *Expecting parents' beliefs in conditional regard and autonomy support as socializing practices: Parental, self-esteem and world-view determinants*. Paper presented in the Fourth International Conference on Self Determination Theory, Ghent, Belgium.

Broucek, F. J. (1991). *Shame and the self*. New York: The Guilford Press.

Covington, M. (1992). *Making the grade: A self-worth perspective on motivation and school reform*. New York: Cambridge University Press.

Crocker, J. (2002). The costs of seeking self-esteem. *Journal of Social Issues, 58*(3), 597–615.

Crocker, J., Sommers, S., & Luhtanen, R. (2002). Hopes dashed and dreams fulfilled: Contingencies of self-worth in the graduate school admissions process. *Personality and Social Psychology Bulletin, 28*, 1275–1286.

Crocker, J., & Wolfe, C. T. (2001). Contingencies of self-worth. *Psychological Review, 108*(3), 593.

Dweck, C. S. (1999). *Self-theories: Their role in motivation, personality, and development*. Philadelphia, PA: Psychology Press.

Erikson, E. H. (1968). *Identity, youth, and crisis*. New York: W.W. Norton & Co., Inc.

Freud, S. (1923/1962). *The Ego and the Id*. New York: Norton.

Frost, J. (2005). *Supernanny: How to get the best from your children*. New York: Hyperion.

Gewirtz, J. L., & Pelaez-Nogueras, M. (1991). Proximal mechanisms underlying the acquisition of moral behavior patterns. In W. M. Kurtines & J. L. Gewirtz (Eds.), *Handbook of moral behavior and development* (Theory, Vol. 1, pp. 153–182). Hillsdale, NJ: Erlbaum.

Ginott, H. (1969). *Between parent and child*. New York: Avon Books.

Grotevant, H. D. (1987). Toward a process model of identity formation. *Journal of Adolescent Research, 2*, 203–222.

Gurland, S. T., & Grolnick, W. S. (2005). Perceived threat, controlling parenting, and children's achievement orientations. *Motivation and Emotion, 29*, 103–121.

Israeli-Halevi, M., Assor, A., & Roth, G. (2012). *Mothers' use of conditional positive regard to promote anxiety suppression in children: A problematic emotion socializing strategy*. Manuscript under review. Ben Gurion University, Israel.

Kanat Maymon, Y., Roth, G., Assor, A., & Reizer, A. (2012). Conditional regard in close relationships. In P. E. Shaver & M. Mikulincer (Eds.), *Meaning, mortality, and choice: The social psychology of existential concerns*. Washington, DC: American Psychological Association.

Kazdin, E. A. (1973). The effect of vicarious reinforcement on attentive behavior in the classroom. *Journal of Applied Behavior Analysis, 63*, 71–78.

Kernis, M. H. (2003). Toward a conceptualization of optimal self-esteem. *Psychological Inquiry, 14*, 1–26.

Kernis, M. H., Brown, A. C., & Brody, G. H. (2000). Fragile self-esteem in children and its associations with perceived patterns of parent-child communication. *Journal of Personality, 68*, 225–252.

Kernis, M. H., Cornell, D. P., Sun, C. R., Berry, A., & Harlow, T. (1993). There's more to self-esteem than whether it is high or low: The importance of stability of self-esteem. *Journal of Personality and Social Psychology, 65*, 1190–1204.

Kernis, M. H., & Paradise, A. W. (2002). Distinguishing between fragile and secure forms of high self-esteem. In E. L. Deci & R. M. Ryan (Eds.), *Handbook of self-determination research* (pp. 339–360). Rochester, NY: University of Rochester Press.

Kernis, M. H., Whisenhunt, C. R., Waschull, S. B., Greenier, K. D., Berry, A. J., Herlocker, C. E., et al. (1998). Multiple facets of self-esteem and their relations to depressive symptoms. *Personality and Social Psychology Bulletin, 24*, 657–668.

Latham, G. I. (1994). *The power of positive parenting: A wonderful way to raise children.* Logan, UT: P&T Ink.

McDowell, J. J. (1988). Matching theory in natural environments. *The Behavior Analyst, 11*, 95–109.

Miller, A. (1981). *Prisoners of childhood.* New York: Basic Books.

Morrison, A. P. (1989). *Shame: The underside of Narcissism*. Hillsdale, NJ: The Analytic Press.

Patterson, G. R., & Gullion, M. E. (1976). *Living with children: New methods for parents and teachers*. Champaign, IL: Research Press.

Raskin, R., Novacek, J., & Hogan, R. (1991). Narcissistic self-esteem management. *Journal of Personality and Social Psychology, 60*, 911–918.

Rhodewalt, F., & Morf, C. C. (1998). On self-aggrandizement and anger: A temporal analysis of narcissism and affective reactions to success and failure. *Journal of Personality and Social Psychology, 74*, 672–685.

Rhodewalt, F., Tragakis, M. W., & Finnerty, J. (2001). Narcissism and self-handicapping: Linking self-aggrandizement to behavior. *Journal of Research in Personality, 40*, 573–597.

Richmond, M. K., Stocker, C. M., & Rienks, S. L. (2005). Longitudinal associations between sibling relationship quality, parental differential treatment, and children's adjustment. *Journal of Family Psychology, 19*, 550–559.

Rogers, C. R. (1951). *Client centered therapy*. Boston: Houghton-Mifflin.

Roth, G. (2008). Perceived parental conditional regard and autonomy support as predictors of young adults' self- versus other-oriented prosocial tendencies. *Journal of Personality, 76*, 513–534.

Roth, G., & Assor, A. (2003, April). *Autonomy supporting and suppressing parental practices as predictors of flexible versus rigid emotion regulation in children.* Paper presented at the biennial meeting of the Society for Research in Child Development (SRCD), Tampa, FL.

Roth, G., & Assor, A. (2010). Parental conditional regard as a predictor of deficiencies in young children's capacities to respond to sad feelings. *Infant and Child Development, 19*, 465–477.

Roth, G., & Assor, A. (2012). The costs of parental pressure to express emotions: Conditional regard and autonomy support as predictors of emotion regulation and intimacy. *Journal of Adolescence, 35*, 799–808.

Roth, G., Assor, A., Niemiec, C. P., Ryan, R. M., & Deci, E. L. (2009). The negative emotional and behavioral consequences of parental conditional regard: comparing positive conditional regard, negative conditional regard, and autonomy support as parenting practices. *Developmental Psychology, 45*, 1119–1142.

Ryan, M. R., Deci, E. L., & Grolnick, W. S. (1995). Autonomy, relatedness, and the self: Their relation to development and psychopathology. In D. Chicchetti & D. J. Cohen (Eds.), *Developmental psychopathology: Theory and methods* (pp. 618–655). New York: Wiley.

Ryan, R. M., & Deci, E. L. (2000). Self-determination theory and the facilitation of intrinsic motivation, social development and well-being. *American Psychologist, 55*, 68–78.

Sartre, J. (1981). *The words: The autobiography of Jean-Paul Sartre*. New York: Knopf Doubleday Publishing Group.

Schwartz, S. J. (2001). The evolution of Eriksonian and neo-Eriksonian identity theory and research: A review and integration. *Identity, 1*, 7–58.

Shapira, M., Ezra, O., Gabay-Elegy, P., Shapira, D., & Assor, A. (2012). *The multiple appearances of parental conditional positive regard: Direct and vicarious conditional regard as predictors of labile self-esteem dynamics*. Paper presented in the International Conference on Motivation (ICM), Frankfurt, Germany.

Shavit-Miller. (2009). *Vulnerability to the experience of conditional parental regard in the academic domain: Gender differences and possible mechanisms*. Doctoral dissertation submitted to Ben Gurion University, Israel.

Shavit-Miller, A., & Assor, A. (2003). *The experience of conditional parental regard and its effects on development: A study of gender differences*. Paper presented at the 10th European Association for Research on Learning and Instruction (EARLI), Padua, Italy.

Skinner, B. F. (1969). *Contingencies of reinforcement: A theoretical analysis*. New York: Appleton.

Soenens, B., Vansteenkiste, M., & Luyten, P. (2010). Towards a domain-specific approach to the study of parental psychological control: Distinguishing between dependency-oriented and achievement-oriented psychological control. *Journal of Personality, 78*, 217–256.

Steinberg, L. (2004). *The ten basic principles of good parenting*. New York: Simon & Schuster.

Chapter 11
Relationships Within Physical Activity Settings

Martyn Standage and Lydia G. Emm

Introduction

Physical activity behaviors occur within social contexts that afford countless opportunities for individuals to establish and maintain meaningful and close relationships. Akin with other life contexts, the interpersonal interactions between individuals and key social agents such as their peers, coaches, exercise instructors, and parents serve to shape and determine the quality of their physical activity engagement and experiences. As people have an innate propensity to feel related, connected, and to establish and maintain meaningful bonds with others (cf. Baumeister & Leary, 1995; Deci & Ryan, 2000; Sullivan, 1953), examining the dynamics and qualities of differing social interactions and affiliations that occur within physical activity settings represents an important avenue of research. Indeed, and via such research endeavors, we can better understand how people influence our, and we their, motivation, well-being, and behavior.

Although to date there has been considerable research pertaining to characteristics of relationships within and across physical activity settings (see Carr, 2012; Jowett, 2007; Smith, 2007; for reviews), Relationships Motivation Theory (RMT; Deci & Ryan, Chap. 3, this volume) provides a much needed systematic and coherent theoretical perspective to integrate relational aspects with broader contemporary motivation phenomena (e.g., issues pertaining to competence, autonomy, differing motivation types, diverging goals/aspirations, and varying social contexts). Representing the sixth mini-theory within the broader Self-Determination Theory (SDT; see Deci & Ryan, 2012 for a review), RMT provides a motivational account of the dynamics underpinning high quality relationships. To this end, within RMT it is proposed that a person's innate need to satisfy their need for relatedness (viz., the need to feel close, connected, and cared for with important others) will activate

M. Standage (✉) • L.G. Emm
Department for Health, University of Bath, Bath, UK
e-mail: M.Standage@bath.ac.uk

N. Weinstein (ed.), *Human Motivation and Interpersonal Relationships: Theory, Research, and Applications*, DOI 10.1007/978-94-017-8542-6_11,

the perusal of relationships and predict well-being and relational experiences, but alone such feelings of belongingness are not sufficient to ensure high quality relational bonds (Deci & Ryan, Chap. 3, this volume). Indeed, RMT specifies that relationships will be of the highest quality when the needs for autonomy (i.e., the need to experience activities as self-endorsed and choicefully enacted) and competence (i.e., the need to interact effectively within the environment) are also supported. Moreover, and even within warm relationships, Deci and Ryan argue that only those within which both partners experience autonomy and provide autonomy support will be of high quality. In a similar vein, the frustration of these basic needs by interpersonal elements (i.e., need-thwarting contexts/factors) such as conditional regard, control, and objectification impede an individuals need satisfaction and lead to poor quality relationships (see Deci & Ryan, Chap. 3, this volume for a discussion).

The purpose of this chapter is to review and critique past relationship-related research within a number of different physical activity settings (viz., sport, exercise, PE classes, and active play). Although RMT is a new mini-theory and the tenets espoused within this theory not directly tested in physical activity settings, we will review key empirical findings and associated phenomena, providing insight from both a RMT and broader SDT perspective. In view of the wide variety of physical activity settings (e.g., sport, exercise, active play) and diverse nature of relationships within these (e.g., exercise buddies, sport coaches, parents, peers, teachers, and volunteers), we suggest some pertinent practical applications and specific examples of future avenues following a review of each sub-context (viz., active play, school physical education, exercise, community/volunteering schemes, and sport). Finally, we conclude by highlighting a number of generic suggestions for future research across physical activity domains.

Relationships Motivation Theory in Physical Activity Contexts

To date, research addressing tenets central within RMT has somewhat naturally focused on close personal relationships such as between romantic partners and among friends as these dyadic relational interactions offer unique dynamics of interdependence such that they have the highest potential for reciprocal, mutual exchange (La Guardia & Patrick, 2008). Collectively, this empirical body of work documents that (i) relationship quality as well as better phenomenological and functional outcomes are related to the satisfaction of autonomy and competence in addition to experiencing relatedness satisfaction (e.g., La Guardia, Ryan, Couchman, & Deci, 2000; Patrick, Knee, Canavello, & Lonsbury, 2007; Reis, Sheldon, Gable, Roscoe, & Ryan, 2000); (ii) being autonomously motivated to engage in relationships supports higher relationship satisfaction and better indices of well-being (e.g., Blais, Sabourin, Boucher, & Vallerand, 1990), (iii) inductions of contextual supports for autonomy (as opposed to controlling elements such as ego involvement) support high quality relational interactions (e.g., Niemiec & Deci, 2013), and (iv) mutuality in which each partner provides, as well as receives, high levels of autonomy support are facilitative of relationship quality and adjustment as well as partner well-being and need satisfaction (e.g., Deci, La Guardia, Moller, Scheiner, & Ryan, 2006).

Extending insight from this growing body of RMT-related research to physical activity settings has vast theoretical and applied implication. Indeed, the complexity of numerous reciprocal and non-reciprocal relationships/partnerships differing in terms of the authority, degree of mutuality, structure (being structured/unstructured), as well as the developmental stage of individuals in within and across physical activity settings provide the basis for some intriguing and potentially impactful empirical contributions. Physical activity settings also provide scholars with a diverse range of differing relational bonds (e.g., relationships among peers, coaches and athletes, and instructors and clients) as well as numerous physical activity settings (e.g., active play, school physical education, exercise, community/volunteering initiatives, recreational sport, and elite sport) to couch their work. It is to a number of these settings that our attention now turns.

Extant Research Within Specific Physical Activity Contexts

Young Children and Active Play

Within SDT, humans are considered to be growth-oriented organisms who actively seek optimal challenges and new experiences to master and integrate (Ryan & Deci, 2000). Intertwined with the notion of active and spontaneous activity, the term *intrinsic motivation* is used within SDT to describe when people are fully self-regulated and volitionally engage in activities out of interest and enjoyment without the aid of external rewards and/or constraints (Deci & Ryan, 2012). An enchanting example of intrinsic motivation is that of children at play, wherein they actively seek out challenge, fun, learning, and exercise their capabilities as they explore their environments because they are absorbed in activities for inherent interest and enjoyment as opposed to instrumental gain (Deci & Ryan). From the perspective of SDT, the maintenance of the vitality expressed via interest, enjoyment and curiosity, derives from the inherent satisfaction of the basic needs for autonomy, competence, and relatedness. At this juncture it is worth noting that, although the need for relatedness is considered to be more distal in supporting intrinsic motivation, intrinsically motivated behaviors are more likely to occur and thrive in contexts supportive of a sense of connectedness and belonging (Standage & Ryan, 2012).

Despite it being commonly assumed that young children are inherently active via their play, data show that 73–84 % of their waking day is made up of sedentary time (e.g., Reilly et al., 2004; Vale, Silva, Sontos, Soares-Miranda, & Mota, 2010). Key to reductions in time spent as being active rest predominantly with shifts in modern lifestyles (e.g., technologies, professionalization of parenthood, and increased reliance of structured activities), which have somewhat engineered play out of the lives of children. Declines in the provision for children to engage in play is somewhat alarming as such activities are central to the development of key skills such as creativity, motor function, decision making, emotional well-being, and social skills (cf. Ginsburg, 2007). Active play also serves as a natural tool for children to meet recommended levels of physical activity for health and has been linked to a reduction in markers of obesity (Campbell & Hesketh, 2007).

The relationship between the child and parent/caregiver is at the heart of the child's socialization and provides the social context that can either support or hinder a child's opportunity to engage in play. According to SDT, parents can socialize their children to be active agents in their learning, play, development, and functioning by providing supports for their autonomy, competence, and relatedness (e.g., taking on board the child's inner frame of reference, and providing clear rules, structure, and expectations within a caring and supportive environ). In contrast, directive, cold, and controlling parental practices can serve to hinder a child's natural propensity towards play and learning by frustrating their innate needs for autonomy, competence, and relatedness (see Grolnick, Deci, & Ryan, 1997; Soenens & Vansteenkiste, 2010 for discussions regarding parental practices). To date, data from observational, cross-sectional, and interview studies support the notion that when parents provide autonomy-support (i.e., social contexts that support choice, initiation, and understanding) as opposed to being perceived as being controlling (i.e., social contexts that are authoritarian, pressuring, and dictating), their children report/show greater levels of autonomous motivation, task engagement, social and academic adjustment, well-being, and persistence (cf. Joussemet, Landry, & Koestner, 2008).

Although active play has not been examined explicitly from an SDT perspective, insight can be gleaned from motivational work focusing on other types of child's play. Indeed, Grolnick, Frodi, and Bridges (1984) conducted an observational study with 41 mothers and their infants to (i) examine the associations between infant mastery-related behavior and maternal control style, attitudes, and sensitivity, and (ii) assess the bond among infant and mother attachment and mastery behavior in the infants second year of life. The authors quantified maternal autonomy support during a play session within which mothers were asked to demonstrate the use of three toys to their 1-year-old children and to sit next to them as they played. Each session was video- and audio-taped and analyzed in terms of mothers' vocalizations, task-oriented behavior, and affect, with ratings reflecting the degree to which the mothers' behavior was supportive of autonomy versus control. Results showed that infants with autonomy-supportive mothers were more task-oriented and competent during play 8 months later. Extending similar methods to need-supportive and need-thwarting parental styles and how these transfer to components of active play would be an intriguing direction for work couched in RMT to take. Similarly, as rewards are commonly employed by parents to entice, direct, control, and prompt behaviors of young children such work could examine how it may be possible to provide rewards that are non-salient, non-evaluative, and non-pressuring (e.g., informational in nature). The importance of this work reinforced by the meta-analytical findings of Deci, Koestner, and Ryan (1999) in which the authors reported that rewards on self-reported and behavioral indicators of intrinsic motivation were significantly more negative for children when compared with data from work carried out with college-aged participants.

In terms of applied implications, a recent systematic review showed that the applications of parent or family physical activity interventions have been few in comparison to school-based efforts (cf. O'Connor, Jago, & Baronowski, 2009). This is somewhat surprising in view of children spending considerable time with their parents/guardians, with these socializing agents key to the physical activity experiences of children during family time. There is clear need for research examining how parents can create need-supportive contexts for their children in helping to shape environments that support active play as well as reducing sedentary time (e.g., screen-viewing time such as watching TV, playing computer/video games, etc.). Drawing from a rich body of work across domains, applied work would do well to examine how parents can use motivational strategies to best support and nurture children in optimally engaging in an important domain which is indeed part of their human nature. Such strategies could include how the family promotes fun, enjoyment, and satisfaction within activities, how do they promote the internalization of values and practices, how as gatekeepers do they set appropriate limits for the child for use (e.g., not removing screen-time, but providing structure), to what extent to do they acknowledge their child's perspectives, how do they best use effective reward structures (e.g., information feedback as opposed to engagement-contingent), and how do they administer praise (cf. Ryan, Deci, Grolnick, & La Gaurdia, 2006). From a research perspective, it would also be interesting to examine how need-thwarting practices such as conditional regard, control, and objectification impede a child's need satisfaction and relate to maladaptive relational and well-being outcomes (see Deci & Ryan, Chap. 3, this volume for a discussion). For example, do need-thwarting environments lead children to become compulsively compliant in their exercise-related behaviors?

Interestingly, parents of young children have also been identified as a demographic group at high risk of low levels of physical activity (or high levels of inactivity) (Bellows-Riecken & Rhodes, 2008). As such, there are many relationship-related dynamics for researchers to explore in terms of the interaction of their provision and receipt of need support. Via the use of a multilevel approach and diary methods, it would be interesting to explore the mutuality of need-supports and need-satisfaction of children and their caregivers and whether this manifests in increased activity via supports for volitional and enjoyable engagement. Longitudinal work would also identify whether relationship quality is enhanced via mutual engagement in active play and physical activity pursuits. As aptly pointed out by Rhodes, Naylor & McKay (2010), work focusing on parents/families and children would seemingly serve to increase the energy expenditure of two identified at-risk segments of society.

School Physical Education

Although young children are spending less time engaged in play, it is when children enter their adolescent years that marked decrements in their levels of physical activity have been reported (e.g., Biddle, Gorely, & Stensel, 2004; Sallis, 2000).

Moreover, there is some evidence to suggest that amounts of school-age physical activity influences adult levels of physical activity (e.g., Telema et al., 2005). Taking such data collectively, it is not therefore surprising that the setting of school physical education (PE) has been advanced as a vehicle by which to counter the reported reductions in physical activity participation (e.g., Shephard & Trudeau, 2000). Akin with such reasoning, one line of SDT-related investigations has been for researchers to focus on the role that school physical education (PE) plays in supporting students' motivation experiences, well-being, and physical activity behavior (cf. Standage, Gillison, & Treasure, 2007).

As with more traditional classroom settings (cf. Ryan & Deci, 2009), the interpersonal style of PE teachers have been shown to be influential in predicting student motivation, engagement, and experiences of school PE (Ntoumanis & Standage, 2009a; Standage et al., 2007). Akin with the majority of SDT-related work to examine social contexts, research conducted within PE settings has examined the degree to which school pupils perceive PE teachers to be autonomy-supportive (i.e., PE environments which support choice, initiation, and understanding). Numerous empirical investigations have shown pupil perceptions of the PE teacher as being autonomy supportive to positively predict the satisfaction of the innate needs for autonomy, competence, and relatedness (see Standage et al., 2007). Moreover, perceptions of autonomy support have been shown to positively predict levels of autonomous motivation, both directly (e.g., Hagger et al., 2007) and via the satisfaction of autonomy, competence, and relatedness (e.g., Standage, Duda, & Ntoumanis, 2006; Standage, Gillison, Ntoumanis, & Treasure, 2012). Similarly, perceptions of autonomy support from PE teachers have also been shown to positively predict adaptive outcomes such as physical self-worth, health-related quality of life, self-reported activity levels, greater pedometer step-counts, attitudes and/or intentions as they relate to exercise activity (cf. Ntoumanis, 2012; Standage et al., 2007).

Research has also taken a broader examination of social contexts that are predictive of need satisfaction (e.g., Standage, Duda, & Ntoumanis, 2005). For example, Standage et al. (2005) conducted a cross-sectional study of 950 secondary school children to (i) test a model of motivation that theorized that perceptions need supports for autonomy, competence and relatedness would facilitate autonomous motivation and adaptive PE experiences by fulfilling pupil need satisfaction, and (ii) examine the invariance of the motivation model across male and female pupils. Results of their study showed that supports for autonomy, competence, and relatedness positively predicted the pupils' overall need satisfaction. Indirect effects also showed a need supportive context to positively predict intrinsic motivation and positive motivational consequences (viz., positive affect, task challenge, and concentration).

One key question regarding application relates to how the choice of motivational strategies employed by PE teachers affects pupils' motivation and PE-related experiences. To this end, Taylor and Ntoumanis (2007) addressed this issue in a study of 787 British PE pupils taught by 51 PE teachers. Employing multilevel modeling analyses, the authors found that the pupils' perceptions of the use of autonomy support, structure, and involvement by their PE teacher positively predicted their own autonomous motivation toward PE. This relationship was mediated by their reported satisfaction of autonomy and competence. As one would be expect, the PE teachers' reports of their use of the three motivational strategies, relative to students' reports, were not as strongly related to students' need satisfaction and autonomous motivation. Taylor and Ntoumanis' work also reported some interesting perceptional discrepancies between teachers and pupils. First, PE teachers' perceptions of pupils' motivation related only moderately to pupils' own reports of their motivation. This finding raises some concern given that teachers' perceptions of pupils' motivation have been shown to be related to teachers' use of autonomy-supportive motivational strategies (e.g., Taylor, Ntoumanis, & Smith, 2008). Second, the relations between PE teachers' and pupils' reports of autonomy support, structure, and involvement were small-to-moderate in magnitude, which may, in part, be explained by teachers' social desirability bias, teaching experience, and/or experience within a particular class. Accordingly, the more objective measures (e.g., independent observers) of the teaching environment might be useful in evaluating the plausibility of teachers' reports (Ntoumanis & Standage, 2009a). Similar to the work of Taylor, Ntoumanis, and Standage (2008), extending this research to also better understand the antecedents of controlling and need-thwarting teaching practices on need frustration, motivation, and the pupils' PE experiences would also be insightful (e.g., do controlling practices come from a lack of teacher competence, such that control is the style adopted? Are experienced teachers' teaching styles more difficult to change? What are the multilevel determinants such as organizational and curriculum effects?).

In addition to understanding the choice of strategies used by PE students, an important line of work in PE has drawn from past work in research in classroom-based education (cf. Reeve, Jang, Carrell, Jeon, & Barch, 2004) to examine whether their teaching styles are malleable (e.g., Chatzisarantis & Hagger, 2009; Cheon, Reeve, & Moon, 2012). For example, in one study Chatzisarantis and Hagger employed a cluster-randomized design to target 215 pupils from ten schools over a period of 5 weeks. Schools were allocated to either autonomy supportive versus a control condition (neutral modal operators). Results of this intervention study showed that pupils in the autonomy-supportive condition reported stronger intentions to exercise during their leisure-time and participated more frequently in leisure-time physical activities, compared to students in the neutral condition. Research has also supported that teachers' interpersonal styles are malleable to intervention. For example, Reeve (1998) used a sample of pre-service teachers to show that participants exposed to just an 80-min training session reported significant and enduring changes in their interpersonal teaching style when compared with a control group (i.e., they became more autonomy-supportive).

Commenting on such findings, Ntoumanis and Standage (2009a) alluded to the promise of such intervention studies, yet called for larger scale and truly-randomized interventions that also manipulate other adaptive facets of the teaching environment (i.e., supports for competence and relatedness such as structure and involvement, respectively) and obtain long-term follow-up data to provide stronger evidence for the feasibility, fidelity, and effectiveness of such an approach. It would also be interesting to extend this work to techniques and behaviors targeting competence and relatedness to broaden the focus on need-supportive interpersonal climates. Indeed, it would be intriguing to build on past work (cf. Standage & Ryan, 2012) to identify the key supports (or "active ingredients") for the satisfaction of each need and the techniques and teacher behaviors that best support these.

Peer Influence and Relationships

Although there has been a focus on the effects of adults' (e.g., parents and teachers) social influence within physical activity settings, there has also been increasing attention paid to peer relationships over the past two decades. In the English language, the term "peer" refers to a person of equal standing/rank and being within the same age social-set group of the person in question. Commensurate with increasing age, there are shifting priorities for the child in terms of the importance and developmental needs of their peer relations (see Buhrmester & Furman, 1986; Sullivan, 1953). Coupled with these developmental changes is the somewhat purposeful flight away from parents and other attachment figures so as to establish independence in the face of what many adolescents consider to be restrain and ties (Allen & Land, 1999). At this juncture, we would argue that these developmental adjustments would be best supported by a secure backdrop of need supports from proximal and significant social agents such as parents and teachers. Within SDT autonomy does not equate to independence (likewise being independent does not ensure autonomy; Ryan et al., 2006), rather need supports provide the basis for secure and high quality inner resources as children face challenges and experience good mental well-being, both immediate and well beyond adolescence. That is, need supports provide the basis for what is sometimes labeled 'secure and autonomous patterns of attachment' and the myriad of psychological and adjustment outcomes that are associated with this modal style (cf. Howe, Brandon, Hinings, & Schofield, 1999).

Research examining peer relationships in the physical activity domain have typically been conducted within youth sport settings. The origins of such work derive from a number of descriptive motives studies conducted in the 1980s in which "affiliation" was identified as a central motive towards participation in youth sports (cf. Weiss & Petlichkoff, 1989). Yet, it was not until the past 15 years that recent years that peers began to be studied via the use of guiding theoretical frameworks within the context of sport (e.g., Attachment Theory, Interpersonal Theory of Psychiatry, and Competence Motivation Theory). Recent peer-related research has taken a number of avenues and the effort by researchers to ground their work in theory has helped to enhance understanding of peer-related processes (see Smith, 2007; Weiss, Amorose, & Kipp, 2012, for reviews).

A growing body of empirical work has documented the importance of peers as key social agents. Within this chapter we focus on just a few examples of peer influence (see Smith & McDonough, 2008 for a review of differing dimensions). From the perspective of SDT and RMT, the peer-created social context and the dyadic interactions experienced within represents an interesting avenue of work.

Specifically, insight into receipts of, and supports for, autonomy, competence, and relatedness would provide valuable and rich information that holds strong theoretical and practical relevance.

At the social context level, content analytic findings from interviews with young athletes suggests the peer-created climate to encompass a number of facets that may support (e.g., improvement, relatedness-support, cooperation, autonomy-support) or undermine (e.g., intra-team competition, intra-team conflict) sport participants' needs for autonomy, competence, and relatedness (Vazou, Ntoumanis, & Duda, 2005). Following the development and validation of a questionnaire to assess perceptions of the peer-related climate using two higher order factors of task-involving (lower order factors being: improvement, relatedness support, and effort) and ego-involving perceptions (lower order factors being: intrateam competition/ability, intrateam conflict) (see Ntouamnis & Vazou, 2005), Vazou, Ntoumanis, and Duda (2006) assessed the additive and interactive influence of young athletes' perceptions of coach-created and peer-created climates on affective responses (i.e., physical self-worth, enjoyment, trait anxiety) and effort as rated by their coach. Results of this work showed perceptions of a task-involving peer climate to positively predict young athletes' perceptions of physical self-worth and enjoyment. Similarly, the coach-created social context also showed perceptions of a task-involving climate to positively predict enjoyment and coach ratings of effort, whereas an ego-involving climate positively predicted trait anxiety. Commenting on their findings, Vazou et al. suggested that future research examining young athletes' self-perceptions and motivation-related variables in sport should consider both coach and peer influences. This said, and as suggested by Standage and Vallerand (2008), work would also do well to include other social agents (e.g., mother, father, organizing structures) in unison with these important social influences to allow us to tease out which characteristics of each social agent best supports levels of need-satisfaction (and subsequently indices of motivation and well-being).

Similarly, Smith, Gustafsson, and Hassmén (2010) examined the role of the peer social context in regard to athlete burnout in a sample of adolescent athletes while controlling for weekly training hours and perceived stress. Results showed peer motivational climate variables, stress, and training hours to predict components of athlete burnout. Specifically, canonical loadings showed lower scores on weekly training hours, higher perceived stress and perceptions of peer-created social context (higher intra-team conflict and lower improvement, relatedness support, and effort scores) to be associated with higher scores on all components of athlete burnout. The results also showed perceptions of the peer-created social context to predict a modest amount of variance, above and beyond the control variables. Interestingly, stronger prediction was found for individual, as opposed to team, athletes.

In another example, Jõesaar, Hein, and Hagger (2011) used a 1-year prospective design to examine a motivational model that specified that the peer-related social context (task versus ego) would impact on adolescent athletes' levels of intrinsic motivation via the satisfaction of the basic needs for autonomy, competence, and relatedness. Results of structural equation modeling provided support for a model of motivation in which perceptions of a task-involving peer social context indirectly influenced intrinsic motivation by providing support for the basic psychological needs specified within SDT. Moreover, perceptions of a task-involving peer social context emerged as the only distal predictor of intrinsic motivation and sport persistence. Collectively, such findings reinforce the important role that the peer-created social context plays in supporting sustained engagement in youth sport.

Past work has also provided support for the notion that being accepted and/or sharing close friendships has important implications for the physical activity experiences of individuals. For instance, Smith, Ullrich-French, Walker, and Hurley (2006) found that being accepted by peers and having positive friendship quality was positively related to perceived competence, autonomous motivation, and enjoyment. Further, cluster analyses showed that even if a child reported a high conflict with a friend, if they reported relatively high perceptions of quality of friendships and peer acceptance then they were able to preserve their reported levels of perceived competence, autonomous motivation, and enjoyment. Similarly, Cox and Ullrich-French (2010) reported that pupils within PE classes who reported higher peer acceptance also reported higher levels of perceived relatedness and autonomy need satisfactions, autonomous motivation, enjoyment, and physical activity engagement than their counterparts who perceived lower peer acceptance. Via the use of cluster analysis, Smith et al. (2006) also reported variations in adaptive and maladaptive motivational profiles to be a function of peer-relationship profiles in a sample of youth sport participants aged 10–14 years. Specifically, youth sport camp participants categorized as having adaptive peer relationship profiles (i.e., based on peer acceptance, positive friendship quality, and friendship conflict scores) demonstrated higher scores for enjoyment, autonomous motivation, and competence and reported lower anxiety and self-presentational concerns than those with low scores on the categorizing variables.

Sport

There has been vast research attention applying an SDT perspective to the sport domain (e.g., see Hagger & Chatzisarantis, 2007 for reviews). Collectively, this body of work has provided a better understanding of the factors and processes that support, as opposed to forestall, high quality forms of motivation as well as athlete well-being, engagement performance, and persistence (cf. Ntoumanis, 2012; Standage, 2012). Indeed, dozens of studies encompassing a range of methodologies have supported the advantages of athletes engaging in sport for autonomous reasons with data showing such motives to link with better well-being and vitality (Gagné, Ryan, & Bargmann, 2003), higher levels of flow (Kowal & Fortier 2000), greater reported effort, interest, and persistence (Pelletier, Fortier, Vallerand, & Brière, 2001; Pelletier et al., 1995), and positive sportspersonship orientations (Ntoumanis & Standage, 2009b).

As we have already alluded, a key premise within SDT is that for individuals to be optimally motivated, experience psychological well-being, and function and perform effectively, they must satisfy their needs for autonomy, competence, and relatedness (Deci & Ryan, 2012). Empirical support for this key tenet has emerged with basic needs shown in extant work to positively predict autonomous forms of motivation (both independently and when combined; e.g., Blanchard et al., 2007; McDonough & Crocker, 2007), well-being (e.g., Gagné, Ryan, & Bargmann, 2003), and vitality (e.g., Adie, Ntoumanis, & Duda, 2008). In contrast, the thwarting of people's basic needs has been shown to be a positive predictor of exhaustion, disordered eating, depression, negative affect, burnout, and perturbed physiological arousal (as indexed by elevated levels of secretory 'immunoglobulin A' prior to training) (e.g., Bartholomew, Ntoumanis, Bosch, Ryan, & Thøgersen-Ntoumani, 2011; Bartholomew, Ntoumanis, Ryan, & Thogersen-Ntoumani, 2011).

With such findings in mind, understanding the social contexts and interpersonal interactions that are supportive of the basic needs of the provider and recipient within sport-related dyads becomes an important agenda from the perspective of RMT. To date, past work couched within SDT has shown that the social contexts that are promoted by significant others such as coaches and teammates play an important role in supporting or undermining the motivational strivings, well-being, engagement, and development of individuals. Understandably, much of this work has focused on the coach-created social context and akin with other life domains, the interpersonal climate that has received the most attention has been that of *autonomy support* (environs that support choice, initiation, and understanding, while minimizing the need to perform and act in a prescribed manner; Deci & Ryan, 2012). Although labeled as "autonomy-support", such contexts actually enhance the likelihood of an individual satisfying all three needs (Ryan & Deci, 2000). Indeed, when a person's autonomy is supported, not only is the supporter likely to be attuned to other needs, but the individual will be more empowered and free to actively fulfill other needs (Standage & Ryan, 2012). Support for such associations has been provided in past SDT work within the sport domain (e.g., Adie et al., 2008). Similar to work within PE settings however (e.g., Standage et al., 2005), it would be interesting to extend the study on social contexts to those that can be classed as need-supportive (i.e., conducive to the satisfaction of competence and relatedness as well as autonomy).

Drawing from the approach of Reeve and colleagues (see the "School physical education" section of this chapter), Pelletier, Vallerand, Brière, and Blais (2006) developed an 18-month intervention program to assist swim coaches to create a more autonomy-supportive social context and with the view to facilitating their swimmers' autonomous motivation and engagement. Results of this work revealed the program to be highly effective in leading swimmers to perceive their coach as more autonomy-supportive and less controlling, and to experience greater levels of perceived competence and intrinsic motivation. Notably, attendance at practice also markedly increased whereas dropout was significantly reduced.

Exercise

Whereas participation in sport is often underpinned by intrinsic motives such as fun, challenge, and learning, engagement in exercise behaviors are more frequently instrumental in nature (e.g., Frederick & Ryan, 1993). This said, research within the exercise domain suggests that the integration of extrinsic motivation can concurrently occur alongside the development of intrinsic motivation, or sometimes independently of it (Standage & Ryan, 2012). For instance, the work of Ryan, Frederick, Lepes, Rubio, and Sheldon (1997) suggests that even though individuals may initially partake in exercise for extrinsic reasons (e.g., to improve their health, enhance their appearance, or increase their fitness), intrinsic motives are central to sustained persistence. Building on such work, there is now a cogent body of extant work that shows autonomous forms of motivation to be positively associated with adaptive outcomes such as greater psychological well-being, increased behavioral persistence, and indices reflective of more objectively assessed behavior/investment (see Standage & Ryan).

In view of the many positive concomitants associated with being autonomously motivated, an important line of empirical investigation has been to identify and test the social conditions and processes that support volitional and self-enacted exercise engagement. Work within the exercise domain has shown that environments that are conducive to the satisfaction of a person's basic needs form the basis for high quality exercise motivation, better psychological well-being, more adaptive self-perceptions, and greater engagement in exercise behavior (see Standage & Ryan, 2012, for a review).

At this point, it is worth noting that the need for relatedness is considered to be more distal in supporting intrinsic motivation than competence and autonomy; within SDT, relatedness is to a large extent the impetus for internalizing values and regulatory processes (Ryan & Deci, 2000). Indeed, people are more likely to accept and internalize the values, norms, and guidelines espoused by socializing agents for whom they feel a sense of connection and belonging (e.g., Roth, Assor, Niemiec, Ryan, & Deci, 2009). Indirect support for this tenet has been reported in the exercise domain wherein perceptions of relatedness have been shown to positively predict internalized forms of motivation, indices of well-being, and positive attitudes towards physical activity (e.g., Vierling, Standage, & Treasure, 2007; Wilson, Longley, Muon, Rodgers, & Murray, 2006).

With regards to the leisure time exercise domain, the importance of proximal relationships may not always be as obvious as in other contexts (i.e., exercise behaviors are often carried out in isolation – e.g., gym attendance, jogging, etc.). However, within SDT it is held that intrinsically motivated and well-internalized external regulations are more likely to occur and thrive in contexts supportive of a sense of connectedness and belonging. It would be interesting in future work to examine the effects of need-supports that are directly proximal (e.g., exercise buddy, exercise instructor), as well as those that are a little more distal (e.g., general support for exercise behaviors from a partner) on both the given exercise behavior and the exercise experiences of individuals.

Research within the context of an exercise referral scheme has shown that when the referred patient felt relatedness in the absence of autonomy support, their level of introjected regulation increased, though social assimilation reduced this effect (Markland & Tobin, 2010). Such findings support tenets of RMT in that relatedness alone was not sufficient for a relationship to be truly effective, rather the psychological needs for autonomy and competence must also be supported. The authors also reported that the satisfaction of all three basic psychological needs led to the promotion of identified regulation, further highlighting the importance of need support within autonomously endorsed relationships.

To date, much of the extant work examining interpersonal styles within the exercise domain have focused on autonomy support. To this end, empirical work has provided support for SDT in showing that exercise settings perceived by participants to be autonomy supportive positively predict adaptive outcomes such as greater autonomous motivation (e.g., Wilson & Rodgers, 2004), better need satisfaction (e.g., Edmunds, Ntoumanis, & Duda, 2006), and more positive exercise-related attitudes/experiences (e.g., Vierling et al., 2007).

Some experimental support also identifies the positive impact that autonomy-supportive contexts have on motivation-related outcomes. For example, Edmunds, Ntoumanis, and Duda (2008) studied the effects of instructional styles based on SDT (i.e., autonomy support, structure, and involvement) on participants' affect, psychological need-satisfaction, motivational regulations, behavioral intentions, and attendance. Female exercisers at a university were exposed to either a SDT-based ($n=22$) or typical ($n=31$) teaching style class for 10 weeks. Analyses revealed that participants in the SDT-based condition reported a significantly greater linear increase in interpersonal involvement, perceived competence, relatedness, and positive affect. Further, attendance rates were higher in the SDT-based intervention group. Similar findings were reported by Moustaka, Vlachopoulas, Kabitsis, and Theodorakis (2012) in their work with a sample of middle-aged women. These authors contrasted an 8 week autonomy-supportive exercise intervention (n = 19 classes) with a control group (n = 16 classes). Results showed that participants in the experimental group increased their levels of perceived autonomy support, fulfillment of the needs for autonomy and competence, identified regulation, intrinsic motivation, and subjective vitality. Collectively, such findings support the application of intervention strategies that manipulate exercise instructor behaviors such that the prevailing social context is perceived by participants to be more autonomy-supportive. However, it would be interesting in future work to extend the intervention content to also include interventional supports for competence and relatedness (i.e., in addition to autonomy support). In view of work showing an automated tele-health advice system being able to maintain physical activity increases at a similar level to that provided by human advisors (e.g., King et al., in press), future interventions using innovative delivery mechanisms (e.g., apps, interactive web-tools, interactive watch devices, etc.) represent an exciting and potentially cost-effective means by which to increase physical activity levels via need-supportive content.

Older Adults: An Example of an "At Risk" Group

Physical activity will long continue to be a vehicle of health promotion across strata's including those of groupings classed as being "high risk" (e.g., older adults, those overweight and obese, those suffering from cardiovascular risk, diabetes or cancer, etc.; cf. Taylor et al., 2004). Herein, we will focus only on one example in which a better understanding of relationships within the physical activity domain may have marked theoretical and practical importance; namely that of aging adults.

Research with older adults has provided support for the importance of perceived high-quality relationships with relatives and friends for psychological well-being (e.g., Kasser & Ryan, 1999). Keeping the importance of relational aspects in mind, commensurate with rising age is the risk of being socially isolated and as well as increased risk of experiencing feelings of loneliness (e.g., Theeke, 2009). Using data from the English Longitudinal Study of Ageing, Shankar, McMunn, Banks, and Steptoe (2011) reported social isolation and loneliness to be associated with an increased risk of being physically inactive, greater likelihood of smoking, as well as reporting multiple health-risk behaviors. The authors also found social isolation to be positively associated with blood pressure, C-reactive protein, and fibrinogen levels. Similarly, using data from the Third National Health and Nutrition Examination Survey (1988–1994), Reed, Crespo, Harvey, and Andersen (2011) reported that the incidence of engaging in no leisure-time physical activity increases with age across both male and females in US older adults. Moreover, in non-Hispanic whites, non-Hispanic blacks, and Mexican Americans, the incidence of engaging in no leisure-time physical activity was found to increase in older adults classed as being socially isolated (i.e., as compared with their more socially integrated counterparts).

Relationships and social interactions have been identified as being key motives for older adults to attend exercise classes and/or engage in physical activity (e.g., Ferrand, Nasarre, Hautier, & Bonnefoy, 2012). Older adults have also identified the need for an exercise group to be mutually supportive of their basic psychological needs, bringing warmth, affection, and peer acceptance in order to maximize the physical and psychological benefits (Ferrand et al., 2012). Another possible means of intervention that may suit this segment of society is the use of volunteers. Given that the "volunteer – health benefits" relationship is dependent on a positive social interaction (Poulin, 2013), much could be gleaned from past SDT work. Specifically, research adopting this approach could directly draw from work out of the SDT tradition that shows that when people volitionally help others, not only do the recipients experience better well-being, but the provider also experiences greater well-being; an effect that appears to be mediated by satisfactions for autonomy, competence, and relatedness (e.g., Weinstein & Ryan, 2010). Extending the mutuality-related work to physical activity settings to test whether high quality interactions support peoples' physical and psychological well-being as well as their physical activity engagement would represent an interesting line of inquiry.

Although SDT research involving older adults is not as prevalent in the extant physical activity literature, empirical findings mirror those in reported with younger participants (e.g., youth sport, college-aged participants). Indeed, and from an applied perspective, research has also supported the empirical effectiveness of providing need supportive advice/coaching to older adults so as to promote and foster their engagement in physical activity (Van Hoecke, Delecluse, Bogaerts, & Boen, in press).

Application

The practical applications from tenets within SDT may be best highlighted via the use of the basic psychological needs as an organizing structure. A broad and rich body of empirical research has shown that social conditions supportive of the needs serve to maintain or enhance intrinsic motivation, support the internalization and integration of extrinsic motivation, provide support for intrinsic goals (or aspirations), and directly impact an individuals' health and wellness. In view of the focus of the current chapter, we will focus on the qualities and nature of a number of environments and practices that are supportive of relatedness. As specified within RMT, however, provisions and supports for autonomy, competence, and relatedness are of particular import to practitioners (for practical examples of autonomy and competence supports in sport and exercise, see Standage, 2012 and Standage & Ryan, 2012, respectively).

Examples of Relational Supports in Physical Activity Settings

As key social agents introducing the values of various activities/tasks in exercise, sport, and PE settings; instructors, coaches and teachers would ideally seek to engage in close, caring, warm, and respectful interactions with their clients, athletes, and pupils. Examples of how people acting in these roles may foster secure attachments and perceptions of belonging include an expression of authentic value and interest in the individual as well as within their interactions with them. Such interactions include using a caring, respectful, and warm manner in which they express empathy, avoid blame, act in a non-judgmental way, and via showing concern and care when others are faced with challenges (LaGuardia & Patrick, 2008; Standage & Ryan, 2012).

In considering relatedness to entail a sense of being significant and cared for by others, one element of physical activity settings that can foster relatedness is involvement. Within the SDT tradition, involvement has been defined as the degree to which significant others devote time, energy, and interest to the other (Grolnick & Ryan, 1989). When social agents such as parents, coaches and teachers show interest and dedication, their involvement is more likely to foster relatedness and, in turn, the internalization of values and motives (Standage & Ryan, 2012). The use of involvement should also be characterized by autonomy support rather than pressure and control to effectively promote integration and true self-regulation. A further means to develop a sense of connection and belonging with others could be by pairing athletes with similar aims, objectives, and ability. In this instance, such an approach may provide provision for cooperation and relational support as well as supporting mutually beneficial training schedules and goals.

A further means of attempting to develop a sense of connection and belonging with others includes the use of "exercise buddy" schemes or via pairing athletes or pupils with similar goals, objectives, and/or abilities. This approach could yield provision for cooperation and relational support by offering people structure as they work together to develop and stick to mutually beneficial schedules and goals (Standage & Ryan, 2012).

Relatedness may also be facilitated by the organization or structure of activities. For example, relatedness satisfaction may be achieved if a coach/teacher/instructor uses small group activities and sets reward structures that support cooperation (e.g., group level outcomes). Not only would such an approach support relatedness, but learning within small groups also allows people to (i) perceive more control, ownership, and input regarding learning, (ii) interact, provide feedback, and promote and support each other's successes, and (iii) experience better psychological health (when contrasted against competing) (cf. Johnson & Johnson, 1989, 1998).

Future Research Directions

There are many directions for future research grounded in RMT and the broader SDT framework to take; indeed, far too many for us to attempt to comprehensively capture within this section. Herein we highlight just a few avenues of work that we consider important. We also draw from a key tenet within RMT that specifies that individuals also need to experience relationships and interactions within physical activity settings as being autonomy supportive and satisfying of their needs for autonomy and competence to experience the high quality relations and the well-being that these can offer. Moreover, we discuss the use of volunteering which provides an example of mutuality within physical activity contexts.

Dynamic Interplay and Relations Among the Basic Needs

Research from a RMT perspective would do well to extend the focus of relations within physical activity settings to relationship quality and the wellness and functional outcomes that are linked to the satisfaction of autonomy and competence in addition to experiencing relatedness satisfaction. Although not designed to test tenets within RMT, past work has often reported the needs for autonomy, competence, and relatedness to be moderately/highly correlated, especially within given settings (e.g., Véronneau, Koestner, & Abela, 2005). In the context of school PE, Standage and colleagues (2003) discussed a number of inter-relations among the need satisfaction variables that emerged within their data. Despite being cross-sectional findings, each relation has direct relevance to the discussion of the needs within the dynamic relationship among PE teachers and their pupils. This said, it is important to note that as the needs share reciprocal relationships, causality is not inferred from these findings, rather these results are used to refer to as a basis for a discussion regarding their interplay. First, Standage et al. found a path between competence and relatedness. This finding was akin with past work in the context of sport that has suggested that children who are physically competent are more likely to be accepted by their peers (e.g., Evans, 1985; Weiss & Duncan, 1992). In the event that some children in PE form relationships commensurate with perceptions of competence, an important avenue for future research is to address how the social context can be structured by PE teachers to support children of all levels of ability and through this parity, hopefully affiliations with others (see also section on "Peer relationships/friendships" in this chapter). A second path in this work was from autonomy to relatedness. This finding suggests that when pupils feel that they choicefully endorse their actions, they also feel more efficacious in initiating connections with others. Alternatively, it is equally plausible that feelings of "belongingness" allow for and foster a sense of autonomy, as the pupil feels supported in his/her actions. The third and final additional path to emerge in Standage et al.'s work was between autonomy and competence. Such findings are commensurate with the tenets of SDT as situational influences that enhance perceptions of competence only facilitate intrinsic motivation in the presence of some autonomy (i.e., to be "intrinsically motivated, one must feel that one's competent actions come from the self" Ryan, 1993, p. 22).

To address such questions, research would do well to adopt similar methodology that has been used in past work designed to examine the relation between basic need satisfaction and indices of well-being using within- and between-person designs (e.g., Reis et al., 2000). Such an approach would be particularly insightful to examine the ongoing and dynamic nature of how, when, and why the highly compatible need variables interact and how these are supported by temporal changes in the relationships between individuals and key social agents within their proximal environments (e.g., peers, coaches, teachers, exercise instructors, and parents). Work of this nature would provide the basis for a better understanding of the role that relationship characteristics play in shaping the quality and experiences of engagement within and across physical activity settings.

In addition to examining the dynamic interplay among the needs on a repeated basis, future work addressing tenets of RMT within physical activity settings would benefit greatly from incorporating actor-partner interdependence models (cf. Kashy & Donnellan, 2012). Employing this approach would allow researchers to look at individuals nested within dyadic relationships/friendships across time accounting for the interdependence among the *actor* and *partner* effects. This approach would be particularly adept to exploring mutuality effects within physical activity settings.

High and Poor Quality Relationships and/or Interpersonal Interactions

It is important to point out that as much as high quality relationships can support a person's to develop and improve, and to flourish; low quality interactions and the social context supported therein can serve to constrain, isolate, or objectify individuals (see Deci & Ryan, Chap. 3, this volume). Accordingly, not only would the relationship between need-supports and need-satisfaction be of interest to researchers, but complete models also examining the associations among need-thwarting contexts and need frustration within relationships and interpersonal interactions would provide valuable theoretical and applied information regarding the motivational predictors of adaptive and maladaptive engagement (see Vansteenkiste & Ryan, 2013, for a discussion of basic needs as a unifying principle for understanding psychological growth and vulnerability).

Effects of Multiple Social Agents

Future research would do well to also consider the simultaneous influences of multiple social agents on autonomy, competence, and relatedness (Standage & Vallerand, 2008). Indeed, the inclusion and study of the multifaceted social context as created by a number of key social agents (e.g., coachers, parents, peers, and policy-makers) would provide a more comprehensive insight into how various elements of these environs interact to predict the participants' need satisfaction (as well as need frustration). If such work encompasses parents, researchers would also do well to also tease out the unique contributions of mother and father as these socializing agents have been shown to have differing effects on the motivational responses of adolescents (Niemiec et al., 2006; Soenens & Vansteenkiste, 2005). To this end, it would be particularly intriguing to study the dynamic interplay among parents that adopt contrasting parenting styles (e.g., one parent who is high in provision of need support contrasted with another whom uses high levels of conditional regard).

Toward Intervention

As should be evident in this chapter as well as reviews published elsewhere (e.g., Hagger & Chatzisarantis, 2007; Ntoumanis, 2012; Standage & Ryan, 2012; Standage & Vallerand, 2008), there are many potential strategies based on the tenets of SDT that can be implemented and evaluated across different physical activity settings. As with work in other contexts (e.g., healthcare) researchers should systematically develop key elements (or intended 'active ingredients') prior to testing their effects in large scale projects (e.g., via randomized controlled trials). Indeed, several smaller (or pilot) studies may be required to progressively refine the design and procedures prior to empirically testing the effectiveness of such methods in and across different physical activity settings. Interventions may work best if they are tailored to specific contexts, so process and outcome evaluations should be nested in the work to help identify why interventions were successful or failed, e.g., assessments of fidelity, quality of implementation, contextual variables related to outcomes, etc. (see Craig et al., 2008 for a review). Lastly, Standage and Ryan (2012) recently suggested the use of simultaneous mixed-method approaches as being an effective addition to intervention trials. Extending this approach to sport-related research would glean in-depth accounts of the differing motivational experiences of particular groupings (i.e., those for whom an intervention was effective, those who changed little, if at all, and those for whom an intervention had unintended or negative effects).

Summary

Within this chapter we have provided a brief overview of some key relationship-related research findings within physical activity settings. Collectively, these empirical findings highlight the psychological benefits to individuals of interacting with others in a manner that is attuned to the satisfaction of their own and the other persons' basic psychological needs. We also reviewed a number of strategies and techniques to promote relatedness, both via contextual inducements and through interpersonal interactions. Drawing from existing wok and in view of potential application, the relevance of tenets advanced within RMT to physical activity settings is clear and herein we provide just a few examples of future work. We hope that the work reviewed and the identified areas for future directions will stimulate some thoughtful contemplation and encourage researchers to examine important relationship-related group variables from the perspective of RMT. It is our hope that this chapter has played a small role in encouraging such needed and meaningful lines of inquiry.

References

Adie, J. W., Duda, J. L., & Ntoumanis, N. (2008). Autonomy support, basic need satisfaction and the optimal functioning of adult male and female sport participants: A test of basic needs theory. *Motivation & Emotion, 32*, 189–199.

Allen, J. P., & Land, D. (1999). Attachment in adolescence. In J. Cassidy & P. R. Shaver (Eds.), *Handbook of attachment theory and research and clinical applications* (pp. 319–335). New York: Guilford.

Bartholomew, K. J., Ntoumanis, N., Bosch, J. A., Ryan, R. M., & Thøgersen-Ntoumani, C. (2011). Self-determination theory and diminished human functioning: The role of interpersonal control and psychological need thwarting. *Personality and Social Psychology Bulletin, 37*, 1459–1473.

Bartholomew, K. J., Ntoumanis, N., Ryan, R., & Thogersen-Ntoumani, C. (2011). Psychological need thwarting in the sport context: Development and initial validation of a psychometric scale. *Journal of Sport and Exercise Psychology, 33*, 75–102.

Baumeister, R., & Leary, M. R. (1995). The need to belong: Desire for interpersonal attachments as a fundamental human motivation. *Psychological Bulletin, 117*, 497–529.

Bellows-Riecken, K. H., & Rhodes, R. E. (2008). The birth of inactivity? A review of physical activity and parenthood. *Preventive Medicine, 46*, 99–110.

Biddle, S. J. H., Gorely, T., & Stensel, D. J. (2004). Health-enhancing physical activity and sedentary behaviour in children and adolescents. *Journal of Sports Sciences, 22*, 679–701.

Blais, M. R., Sabourm, S., Boucher, C., & Vallerand, R. J. (1990). Toward a motivational model of couple happiness. *Journal of Personality and Social Psychology, 59*, 1021–1031.

Blanchard, C. M., Mask, L., Vallerand, R. J., de la Sablonnière, R., & Provencher, P. (2007). Reciprocal relationships between contextual and situational motivation in a sport setting. *Psychology of Sport & Exercise, 8*, 854–873.

Buhrmester, D., & Furman, W. (1986). The changing function of friends in childhood. A eo-Sullivanian perspective. In V. Derlega & B. Winstead (Eds.), *Friendship and social interaction* (pp. 41–62). New York: Springer.

Campbell, K., & Hesketh, K. (2007). Strategies which aim to positively impact on weight, physical activity, diet and sedentary behaviors in children from zero to five years. A systematic review of the literature. *Obesity Reviews, 8*, 327–338.

Carr, S. (2012). Relationships and sport and performance. In S. Murphy (Ed.), *Handbook of sport and performance psychology* (pp. 400–417). New York: Oxford University Press.

Chatzisarantis, N. L. D., & Hagger, M. S. (2009). Effects of an intervention based on self-determination theory on leisure time physical activity. *Psychology and Health, 24*, 29–48.

Cheon, S. H., Reeve, J., & Moon, I. S. (2012). Experimentally based, longitudinally designed, teacher-focused intervention to help physical education teachers be more autonomy supportive toward their students. *Journal of Sport & Exercise Psychology, 34*, 365–396.

Cox, A. E., & Ullrich-French, S. (2010). The motivational relevance of peer and teacher relationships profiles in physical education. *Psychology of Sport and Exercise, 11*, 337–344.

Craig, P., Dieppe, P., Macintyre, S., Mitchie, S., Nazareth, I., & Petticrew, M. (2008). Developing and evaluating complex interventions: The new medical research council guidance. *BMJ, 337*, 979–983.

Deci, E. L., Koestner, R., & Ryan, R. M. (1999). A meta-analytic review of experiments examining the effects of extrinsic rewards on intrinsic motivation. *Psychological Bulletin, 125*, 627–668.

Deci, E. L., La Guardia, J. G., Moller, A. C., Scheiner, M. J., & Ryan, R. M. (2006). On the benefits of giving as well as receiving autonomy support: Mutuality in close friendships. *Personality and Social Psychology Bulletin, 32*, 313–327.

Deci, E. L., & Ryan, R. M. (2000). The "what" and "why" of goal pursuits: Human needs and the self-determination of behavior. *Psychological Inquiry, 11*, 227–268.

Deci, E. L., & Ryan, R. M. (2012). Motivation, personality, and development within embedded social contexts: An overview of self-determination theory. In R. M. Ryan (Ed.), *Oxford handbook of human motivation* (pp. 85–107). New York: Oxford University Press.

Edmunds, J., Ntoumanis, N., & Duda, J. L. (2006). A test of self-determination theory in the exercise domain. *Journal of Applied Social Psychology, 26*, 2240–2265.

Edmunds, J., Ntoumanis, N., & Duda, J. L. (2008). Testing a self-determination theory-based teaching style intervention in the exercise domain. *European Journal of Social Psychology, 38*, 375–388.

Evans, J. R. (1985). *The process of team selection in children's self-directed and adult directed games*. Unpublished doctoral dissertation. University of Illinois at Urbana-Champaign.

Ferrand, C., Nasaire, S., Hautier, C., & Bonnefoy, M. (2012). Aging and well-being in French older adults regularly practicing physical activity: A self-determination perspective. *Journal of Aging and Physical Activity, 20*, 215–230.

Frederick, C. M., & Ryan, R. M. (1993). Differences in motivation for sport and exercise and their relations with participation and mental health. *Journal of Sport Behavior, 16*, 124–146.

Gagné, M., Ryan, R. M., & Bargmann, K. (2003). Autonomy support and need satisfaction in the motivation and well-being of gymnasts. *Journal of Applied Sport Psychology, 15*, 372–390. doi:10.1080/10413200390238031.

Ginsburg, K. R. (2007). The importance of play in promoting healthy child development and maintaining strong parent-child bonds. *Pediatrics, 119*, 182–191.

Grolnick, W. S., Deci, E. L., & Ryan, R. M. (1997). Internalization within the family: The self-determination theory perspective. In J. E. Grusec & L. Kuczynski (Eds.), *Parenting and children's internalization of values: A handbook of contemporary theory* (pp. 135–161). New York: Wiley.

Grolnick, W. S., Frodi, A., & Bridges, L. (1984). Maternal control styles and the mastery motivation of one-year-olds. *Infant Mental Health Journal, 5*, 72–82.

Grolnick, W. S., & Ryan, R. M. (1989). Parent styles associated with children's self- z and competence in school. *Journal of Educational Psychology, 81*, 143–154.

Hagger, M. S., & Chatzisarantis, N. L. D. (2007). *Intrinsic motivation and self-determination in exercise and sport*. Champaign, IL: Human Kinetics.

Hagger, M. S., Chatzisarantis, N. L. D., Hein, V., Pihu, M., Soós, I., & Karsai, I. (2007). The perceived autonomy support scale for exercise settings (PASSES): Development, validity, and cross-cultural invariance in young people. *Psychology of Sport and Exercise, 8*, 632–653.

Howe, D., Brandon, M., Hinings, D., & Schofield, G. (1999). *Attachment theory, child maltreatment, and family support*. Mahwah, NJ: Macmillan Press.

Jõesaar, H., Hein, V., & Hagger, M. S. (2011). Peer influence on young athletes' need satisfaction, intrinsic motivation and persistence in sport: A 12-month prospective study. *Psychology of Sport & Exercise, 12*, 500–508.

Johnson, D. W., & Johnson, R. (1989). *Cooperation and competition: Theory and research*. Edina, MN: Interaction Book Company.

Johnson, D. W., & Johnson, R. (1998). Cooperative learning and social interdependence theory. In R. Tindale, L. Heath, J. Edwards, E. Posavac, F. Bryant, Y. Suzrez-Balcazar, E. Henderson-King, & J. Myers (Eds.), *Theory and research on small groups* (pp. 9–36). New York: Plenum.

Joussemet, M., Landry, R., & Koestner, R. (2008). A self-determination theory perspective on parenting. *Canadian Psychology, 49*, 194–200.

Jowett, S. (2007). Interdependence analysis and the 3 + 1Cs in the coach-athlete relationship. In S. Jowett & D. Lavallee (Eds.), *Social psychology in sport* (pp. 15–27). Champaign, IL: Human Kinetics.

Kashy, D. A., & Donnellan, M. B. (2012). Conceptual and methodological issues in the analysis of data from dyads and groups. In K. Deaux & M. Snyder (Eds.), *The Oxford handbook of personality and social psychology* (pp. 209–238). New York: Oxford University Press.

Kasser, V. M., & Ryan, R. M. (1999). The relation of psychological needs for autonomy and relatedness to health, vitality, well-being and mortality in a nursing home. *Journal of Applied Social Psychology, 29*, 935–954.

King, A. C., Hekler, E. B., Castro, C. M., Buman, M. P., Marcus, B. H., Friedman, R. H., et al. (2013). Exercise advice by humans versus computers: Maintenance effects at 18 months. *Health Psychology*, advance online publication. doi:10.1037/a0030646

Kowal, J., & Fortier, M. S. (2000). Testing relationships from the hierarchical model of intrinsic and extrinsic motivation using flow as a motivational consequence. *Research Quarterly for Exercise and Sport, 71*, 171–181.

La Guardia, J. G., & Patrick, H. (2008). Self-determination theory as a fundamental theory of close relationships. *Canadian Psychology, 49*, 201–209.

La Guardia, J. G., Ryan, R. M., Couchman, C. E., & Deci, E. L. (2000). Within-person variation in security of attachment: A self-determination theory perspective on attachment, need fulfillment, and well-being. *Journal of Personality and Social Psychology, 79*, 367–384.

Markland, D., & Tobin, V. J. (2010). Need support and behavioural regulations for exercise among exercise referral scheme clients: The mediating role of psychological need satisfaction. *Psychology of Sport and Exercise, 11*, 91–99.

McDonough, M. H., & Crocker, P. R. E. (2007). Testing self-determined motivation as a mediator of the relationship between psychological needs and affective and behavioral outcomes. *Journal of Sport & Exercise Psychology, 29*, 645–663.

Moustaka, F. C., Vlachopoulos, S. P., Kabitsis, C., & Theodorakis, Y. (2012). Effects of an autonomy-supportive exercise instructing style on exercise motivation, psychological well-being, and exercise attendance in middle-age women. *Journal of Physical Activity and Health, 9*, 138–150.

Niemiec, C. P., & Deci, E. L. (2013). *Effects of provision and deprivation of autonomy on interaction quality between strangers*. Unpublished manuscript, University of Rochester, Rochester, NY.

Niemiec, C. P., Lynch, M. F., Vansteenkiste, M., Bernstein, J., Deci, E. L., & Ryan, R. M. (2006). The antecedents and consequences of autonomous self-regulation for college: A self-determination theory perspective on socialization. *Journal of Adolescence, 29*, 761–775.

Ntoumanis, N. (2012). A self-determination theory perspective on motivation in sport and physical education: Current trends and possible future research directions. In G. C. Roberts & D. C. Treasure (Eds.), *Motivation in sport and exercise* (Vol. 3, pp. 91–128). Champaign, IL: Human Kinetics.

Ntoumanis, N., & Standage, M. (2009a). Motivation in physical education classes: A self-determination theory perspective. *Journal of Research and Theory in Education, 7*, 194–202.

Ntoumanis, N., & Standage, M. (2009b). Morality in sport: A self-determination theory perspective. *Journal of Applied Sport Psychology, 21*, 365–380.

Ntoumanis, N., & Vazou, S. (2005). Peer motivational climate in youth sport: Measurement development and validation. *Journal of Sport and Exercise Psychology, 27*, 432–455.

O'Connor, T. M., Jago, R., & Baronowski, T. (2009). Engaging parents to increase youth physical activity: A systematic review. *American Journal of Preventive Medicine, 37*, 141–149.

Patrick, H., Knee, C. R., Canevello, A., & Lonsbary, C. (2007). The role of need fulfilment in relationship functioning and well-being: A self-determination theory perspective. *Journal of Personality and Social Psychology, 92*, 434–457.

Pelletier, L. G., Fortier, M. S., Vallerand, R. J., & Brière, N. M. (2001). Associations among perceived autonomy support, forms of self-regulation, and persistence: A prospective study. *Motivation and Emotion, 25*, 279–306.

Pelletier, L. G., Fortier, M. S., Vallerand, R. J., Tuson, K. M., Briere, N. M., & Blais, M. R. (1995). The Sports Motivation Scale (SMS): A measure of intrinsic motivation, extrinsic motivation and amotivation in sports. *Journal of Sport & Exercise Psychology, 17*, 35–53.

Pelletier, L. G., Vallerand, R. J., Brière, N. M., & Blais, M. R. (2006). *When coaches become autonomy-supportive: Effects on intrinsic motivation, persistence, and performance.* Unpublished manuscript, University of Ottawa.

Poulin, M. J. (2013). Volunteering predicts health among those who value others: Two national studies. *Health Psychology*, advance online publication. doi:10.1037/a0031620

Reed, S. B., Crespo, C. J., Harvey, W., & Andersen, R. E. (2011). Social isolation and physical inactivity in older U.S. adults: Results from the Third National Health and Nutrition Examination Survey. *European Journal of Sports Sciences, 11*, 359–365.

Reeve, J. (1998). Autonomy support as an interpersonal motivating style: Is it teachable? *Contemporary Educational Psychology, 23*, 312–330.

Reeve, J., Jang, H., Carrell, D., Jeon, S., & Barch, J. (2004). Enhancing students' engagement by increasing teachers' autonomy support. *Motivation and Emotion, 28*, 147–169.

Reilly, J. J., Jackson, D. M., Montgomery, C., Kelly, L. A., Slater, C., Grant, S., et al. (2004). Total energy expenditure and physical activity in young Scottish children: Mixed longitudinal study. *Lancet, 362*, 211–212.

Reis, H. T., Sheldon, K. M., Gable, S. L., Roscoe, J., & Ryan, R. M. (2000). Daily well-being: The role of autonomy, competence, and relatedness. *Personality and Social Psychology Bulletin, 26*, 419–435.

Rhodes, R. E., Naylor, P. J., & McKay, H. A. (2010). Pilot study of a family physical activity planning intervention among parents and their children. *Journal of Behavioral Medicine, 33*(2), 91–100. doi:10.1007/s10865-009-9237-0.

Roth, G., Assor, A., Niemiec, C. P., Ryan, R. M., & Deci, E. L. (2009). The emotional and academic consequences of parental conditional regard: Comparing conditional positive regard, conditional negative regard, and autonomy support as parenting practices. *Developmental Psychology, 45*, 1119–1142.

Ryan, R. M. (1993). Agency and organization: Intrinsic motivation, autonomy and the self in psychological development. In J. Jacobs (Ed.), *Nebraska symposium on motivation: Developmental perspectives on motivation* (Vol. 40, pp. 1–56). Lincoln, NE: University of Nebraska Press.

Ryan, R. M., & Deci, E. L. (2000). Self-determination theory and the facilitation of intrinsic motivation, social development and well-being. *American Psychologist, 55*, 68–78.

Ryan, R. M., & Deci, E. L. (2009). Promoting self-determined school engagement: Motivation, learning, and well-being. In K. R. Wentzel & A. Wigfield (Eds.), *Handbook on motivation at school* (pp. 171–196). New York: Routledge.

Ryan, R. M., Deci, E. L., Grolnick, W. S., & La Guardia, J. G. (2006). The significance of autonomy and autonomy support in psychological development and psychopathology. In D. Cicchetti & D. J. Cohen (Eds.), *Developmental psychopathology: Theory and method* (2nd ed., Vol. 1, pp. 795–849). Hoboken, NJ: Wiley.

Ryan, R. M., Frederick, C. M., Lepes, D., Rubio, N., & Sheldon, K. M. (1997). Intrinsic motivation and exercise adherence. *International Journal of Sport Psychology, 28*, 335–354.

Sallis, J. F. (2000). Age-related decline in physical activity: A synthesis of human and animal studies. *Medicine and Science in Sports and Exercise, 32*, 1598–1600.

Shankar, A., McMunn, A., Banks, J., & Steptoe, A. (2011). Loneliness, social isolation, and behavioral and biological health indicators in older adults. *Health Psychology, 30*, 377–385.

Shephard, R. J., & Trudeau, F. (2000). The legacy of physical education: Influences on adult lifestyle. *Pediatric Exercise Science, 12*, 34–50.

Smith, A. L. (2007). Youth peer relationships in sport. In S. Jowett & D. Lavallee (Eds.), *Social psychology in sport* (pp. 41–54). Champaign, IL: Human Kinetics.

Smith, A. L., Gustafsson, H., & Hassmén, P. (2010). Peer motivational climate and burnout perceptions of intensively sport involved adolescents. *Psychology of Sport and Exercise, 11*, 453–460.

Smith, A. L., & McDonough, M. H. (2008). Peers. In A. L. Smith & S. J. H. Biddle (Eds.), *Youth physical activity and sedentary behavior: Challenges and solutions* (pp. 295–320). Champaign, IL: Human Kinetics.

Smith, A. L., Ullrich-French, S., Walker, E. G., & Hurley, K. S. (2006). Peer relationship profiles and motivation in youth sport. *Journal of Sport & Exercise Psychology, 28*, 362–382.

Soenens, B., & Vansteenkiste, M. (2010). A theoretical upgrade of the concept of parental psychological control: Proposing new insights on the basis of self-determination theory. *Developmental Review, 30*, 74–99.

Soenens, B., & Vansteenkiste, M. (2005). Antecedents and outcomes of self-determination in 3 life domains: The role of parents' and teachers' autonomy support. *Journal of Youth and Adolescence, 34*(6), 589–604. doi:10.1007/s10964-005-8948-y.

Standage, M. (2012). Motivation: Self-determination theory and performance in sport. In S. Murphy (Ed.), *Handbook of sport and performance psychology* (pp. 233–249). New York: Oxford University Press.

Standage, M., Duda, J. L., & Ntoumanis, N. (2003). A model of contextual motivation in physical education: Using constructs from self-determination and achievement goal theories to predict physical activity intentions. *Journal of Educational Psychology, 95*, 97–110.

Standage, M., Duda, J. L., & Ntoumanis, N. (2005). A test of self-determination theory in school physical education. *British Journal of Educational Psychology, 75*, 411–433.

Standage, M., Duda, J. L., & Ntoumanis, N. (2006). Students' motivational processes and their relationship to teacher ratings in school physical education: A self-determination theory approach. *Research Quarterly for Exercise and Sport, 77*, 100–110.

Standage, M., Gillison, F., Ntoumanis, N., & Treasure, D. C. (2012). Predicting students' physical activity and health-related well-being: A prospective cross-domain investigation of motivation across school physical education and exercise settings. *Journal of Sport & Exercise Psychology, 34*, 37–60.

Standage, M., Gillison, F., & Treasure, D. C. (2007). Self-determination and motivation in physical education. In M. S. Hagger & N. L. D. Chatzisarantis (Eds.), *Intrinsic motivation and self-determination in exercise and sport* (pp. 71–85). Champaign, IL: Human Kinetics.

Standage, M., & Ryan, R. M. (2012). Self-determination theory and exercise motivation: Facilitating self-regulatory processes to support and maintain health and well-being. In G. C. Roberts & D. C. Treasure (Eds.), *Advances in motivation in sport and exercise* (3rd ed., pp. 233–270). Champaign, IL: Human Kinetics.

Standage, M., & Vallerand, R. J. (2008). Self-determined motivation in sport and exercise groups. In M. R. Beauchamp & M. A. Eys (Eds.), *Group dynamics advances in sport and exercise psychology: Contemporary themes* (pp. 179–199). New York: Routledge.

Sullivan, H. S. (1953). *The interpersonal theory of psychiatry*. New York: Norton.

Taylor, A. H., Cable, N. T., Faulkner, G., Hillsdon, M., Narici, M., & Van Der Bij, A. K. (2004). Physical activity and older adults: A review of health benefits and the effectiveness of interventions. *Journal of Sports Sciences, 22*, 703–725.

Taylor, I. M., & Ntoumanis, N. (2007). Teacher motivational strategies and student self-determination in physical education. *Journal of Educational Psychology, 99*, 747–760.

Taylor, I. M., Ntoumanis, N., & Standage, M. (2008). A self-determination theory approach to antecedents of physical education teachers' motivational strategies. *Journal of Sport & Exercise Psychology, 30*, 75–94.

Telema, R., Yang, X., Viikari, J., Valimaki, I., Wanne, O., & Raitakari, O. (2005). Physical activity from childhood to adulthood. A 21-year tracking study. *American Journal of Preventive Medicine, 28*, 267–273.

Theeke, L. A. (2009). Predictors of loneliness in U.S. adults over age sixty-five. *Archives of Psychiatric Nursing, 23*(5), 387–396. doi:10.106/j.apnu.2008.11.002.

Vale, S., Silva, P., Santos, R., Soares-Miranda, L., & Mota, J. (2010). Compliance with physical activity guidelines in preschool children. *Journal of Sports Sciences, 28*, 603–608.

Van Hoecke, A. S., Delecluse, C., Bogaerts, A., & Boen, F. (in press). The long-term effectiveness of need-supportive physical activity counselling compared with a standard referral in sedentary older adults. *Journal of Aging and Physical Activity.*

Vansteenkiste, M., & Ryan, R. M. (2013). On psychological growth and vulnerability: Basic psychological need satisfaction and need frustration as a unifying principle. *Journal of Psychotherapy Integration, 23*(3), 263–280.

Vazou, S., Ntoumanis, N., & Duda, J. L. (2005). Peer motivational climate in youth sport: A qualitative inquiry. *Psychology of Sport & Exercise, 6*, 497–516.

Vazou, S., Ntoumanis, N., & Duda, J. L. (2006). Predicting young athletes' motivational indices as a function of their perceptions of the coach- and peer-created climate. *Psychology of Sport and Exercise, 7*, 215–233.

Veitch, J., Salmon, J., & Ball, K. (2008). Children's active free play in local neighborhoods: A behavioral mapping study. *Health Education Research, 23*, 870–879.

Véronneau, M. H., Koestner, R., & Abela, J. R. Z. (2005). Intrinsic need satisfaction and well-being in children and adolescents: An application of the self-determination theory. *Journal of Social and Clinical Psychology, 24*, 280–292.

Vierling, K. K., Standage, M., & Treasure, D. C. (2007). Predicting physical activity and attitudes toward physical activity in an "at-risk" youth sample: A test of self-determination theory. *Psychology of Sport and Exercise, 8*, 795–817.

Weinstein, N., & Ryan, R. M. (2010). When helping helps: Autonomous motivation for prosocial behavior and its influence on well-being for the helper and recipient. *Journal of Personality and Social Psychology, 98*, 222–244.

Weiss, M. R., Amorose, A. J., & Kipp, L. E. (2012). Youth motivation and participation in sport and physical activity. In R. M. Ryan (Ed.), *The Oxford handbook of human motivation* (pp. 520–553). New York: Oxford University Press.

Weiss, M. R., & Duncan, S. C. (1992). The relationship between physical competence and peer acceptance in the context of children's sports participation. *Journal of Sport & Exercise Psychology, 14*, 177–191.

Weiss, M. R., & Petlichkoff, L. M. (1989). Children's motivation for participation in and withdrawal from sport: Identifying the missing links. *Pediatric Exercise Science, 1*, 195–211.

Wilson, P. M., Longley, K., Muon, S., Rodgers, W. M., & Murray, T. C. (2006). Examining the contributions of perceived psychological need satisfaction to well-being in exercise. *Journal of Applied Biobehavioral Research, 11*, 243–264.

Wilson, P. M., & Rodgers, W. M. (2004). The relationship between perceived autonomy support, exercise regulations and behavioral intentions in women. *Psychology of Sport & Exercise, 5*, 229–242.

Chapter 12
The Importance of Need-Supportive Relationships for Motivation and Psychological Health at Work

Véronique Dagenais-Desmarais, Jacques Forest, Sarah Girouard, and Laurence Crevier-Braud

Work as a Social Context

Work is a life domain that involves specific parameters leading to unique experiences for individuals. It is distinct from other domains such as family, intimate relationships, friends and leisure. Notably, work is the only life domain that provides us with sustenance and decent living conditions (Morin, 2004). However, work is nowadays much more than a mean to paying bills. As put by Vallerand and Houlfort (2003):

> Work is probably the single most important activity in one's life. We spend considerable time in schooling and training so that we get the opportunity to work someday. Once we embark in the work force, we typically devote more than half of our waking time to work either directly on the job, or indirectly by thinking or talking about job-related matters. Even after retirement, people often continue to engage in activities related to their former job. This is because work serves to define us. Because work is so central to most of us, we are not only people who work in computers, management, or sales, we are computer analysts, managers, or salespersons. This self-definition serves an important intrapersonal function. While some people may not care that much about work as they merely see it as labor, others see it as part of who they are deep down, it becomes part of their identity. They love their work and it has become part of who they are. They can't wait to get to work in the morning and it seems that the day doesn't have enough hours to do the things they want to do at work. (p. 176).

Not only is work a social context particularly well suited to define who we are, but it is also a life domain offering great opportunities to use our full potential by

V. Dagenais-Desmarais (✉)
Department of Psychology, Université de Montréal, P.O. Box 6128,
Downtown Station, Montréal, QC, Canada, H3C 3J7
e-mail: v.dagenais.desmarais@umontreal.ca

J. Forest
École des Sciences de la Gestion, Université du Québec à Montréal, Montréal, QC, Canada

S. Girouard • L. Crevier-Braud
Department of Psychology, Université du Québec à Montréal, Montréal, QC, Canada

N. Weinstein (ed.), *Human Motivation and Interpersonal Relationships: Theory, Research, and Applications*, DOI 10.1007/978-94-017-8542-6_12,

seeking and overcoming challenging assignments and responsibilities. At the same time, it also constrains us to deal with imposed responsibilities and externally prescribed expectations, which in some case can lead to maladaptive behaviors and suboptimal functioning.

In addition to being crucial to intra-individual processes such as self-definition and thriving, work is also an essential vector of interpersonal relationships. By its very own nature, this life domain involves complex relational systems, in which formal hierarchical and peer-to-peer relationships coexist in parallel with informal, non-written social systems composed of informal groups, cliques, political games and social norms (Morin, Savoie, & Beaudin, 1994). These complex relational systems can be catalysts to flourish at work, or can alter our well-being and lead to maladaptive behaviors. Consequently, interpersonal relationships in the workplace must inevitably be taken into account and managed, as work is an inherently social life domain.

Why are some individuals highly motivated at work and flourish in their jobs, while others, in comparable situations, seem to be disengaged and depleted from their resources and strengths? A theoretical approach, self-determination theory (SDT), explains the process by which this phenomenon may occur. At its core lies the premise that nurturing and fulfilling relationships in the workplace are a crucial ingredient for having a motivated and healthy workforce. However, before presenting this theoretical framework, let us have a look at a common misconception among lay people, but also in organizational life, about what is thought to be the ultimate motivator for a happy workforce: money.

Why Work Is Not Only About Money

When it comes to explaining workers' optimal performance and functioning in organizational settings, money is often seen as the best lever for boosting employees' efforts on the job, as well as for making them happy. Given the popular belief that a happy worker is a productive worker (a belief that seems to be only a partial truth given to scientific evidence; see for example Wright & Cropanzano, 2007; Zelenski, Murphy, & Jenkins, 2008 for details), paying more the employees or offering them a bonus should have desirable consequences for the individuals as well as for the organization.

This belief takes its roots in the classical, and hence the most widely used, theories in organizational behavior – human resources management and economics – that stress the importance of external rewards, such as salary and monetary rewards (e.g., expectancy theory; Lawler, 1971, 1973; Vroom, 1964). In our opinion (as well as others'; see Heath, 1999) these theories overemphasize the importance of extrinsic sources of motivation (such as money) to work-related behavior. Do people work only for attaining money or are there other reasons for job involvement? Empirical findings suggest individuals are motivated by a variety of other reasons.

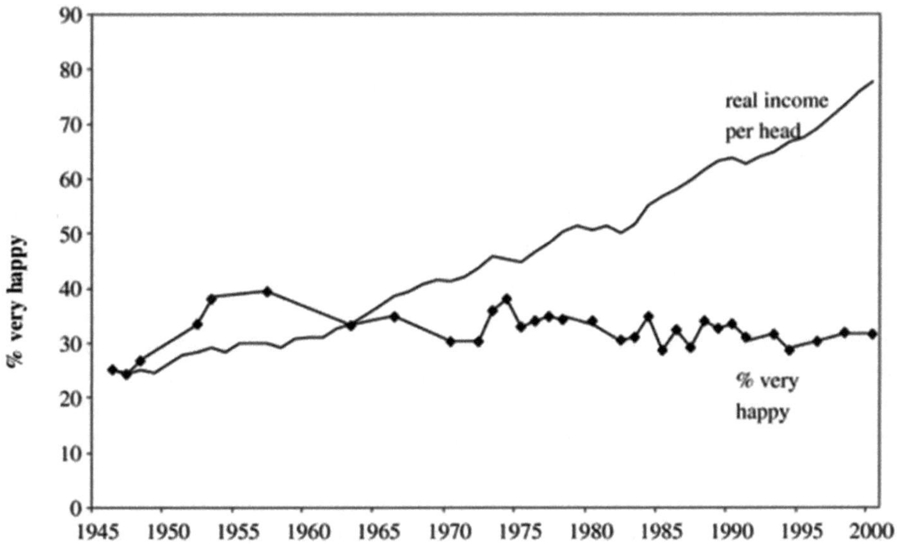

Fig. 12.1 Income and happiness in the United States (From Layard, 2005. Copyright 2005 by Richard Layard. Reprinted with permission)

First, it seems that most people would keep working even if they did not have to in order to survive. By using the lottery question that states: "Imagine that you won a lottery or inherited a large sum of money and could live comfortably for the rest of your life without working; what would you do about work?", researchers have explored what happens without the requirement for salary (e.g., Morse & Weiss, 1955; Paulsen, 2008). Four options were offered to participants: "I would stop working", "I would continue to work in the same job", "I would continue paid employment in a different job" or "I would continue to work, but under different conditions". In response to this question, between 6.5 and 39 % of people responded they would completely stop working (see Paulsen), but between 61 and 93.5 % of people responded they would continue to work despite not needing the money.

Studies also show that higher salaries do not make workers happier. A depiction of this is provided in the Fig. 12.1 above (reproduced from Layard, 2005; see also Brown, Kasser, Ryan, Linley, & Orzech, 2009; Csikszntmihalyi, 1999; Easterlin, 1995, 2005; Easterlin, Angelescu McVey, Switek, Sawangfa, & Smith Zweig, 2010 for other points of view on the same topic). In this graphic, it is possible to see that, over time, even though salaries are going up, the percentage of people who are very happy does not follow the same trend. The same result can be found in a meta-analysis conducted by Howell and Howell (2008) that showed that money is especially important for individuals with very low incomes. In other words, money can make a difference when one does not have a lot of it (in this case, getting access to money will shape one's cognitive evaluation of life, i.e. the assessment of his quality of life) but, above a certain threshold, it will have a negligible impact. Research done with lottery winners indeed shows that, a year after they won the lottery, people are no happier than they were before (Brickman, Coates, & Janoff-Bulman, 1978).

In a research using a sample representative of 96 % of the planet, Diener, Ng, Harter, and Arora (2010) showed that positive life evaluation relates to wealth; the more money individuals have, the more comfortable they perceive their lives to be. However, over and above satisfying perceived living conditions, this research showed that satisfaction of basic psychological needs was the most robust predictor of emotional well-being (i.e., more positive feelings and less negative feelings). Thus, according to these authors, there seems to be two types of prosperity. The *economic prosperity* relates to a more positive life evaluation and favorable life conditions, whereas *social psychological prosperity* is mostly influenced by conditions under which need satisfaction is made possible. Hence, organizations offering attractive salaries are at best only favoring positive life evaluation among their employees, but they are not raising morale and optimal functioning level among the workforce.

This is where the distinction between the economic function and expressive function of work is important (MOW International Research Team, 1987). Work indeed serves an economic purpose where salary helps to put in place satisfactory living conditions. However, as we mentioned previously, it is not its only function; it also serves as a basis for self-definition and perceived efficiency and, through organized and planned efforts, to create a sense of life meaning. These findings suggest that, although necessary to attain basic living conditions, money is not the best path for optimal well-being and satisfaction at work.

Organization and managers may be making a mistake by overly relying on the power of money for having a mobilized and healthy workforce. In addition to not being the only or the best path to happiness, money can be a double-edged sword, which may lead to detrimental consequences for mental health and motivation in the workplace. As many studies show, materialism, or wanting more money, leads to negative consequences (Brown et al., 2009; Kasser & Ryan, 1993, 1996; Kasser, Ryan, Zax, & Sameroff, 1995; Ryan, Chirkov, Little, Sheldon, Timoshina, & Deci, 1999; Ryan, Sheldon, Kasser, & Deci, 1996; Schmuck, Kasser, & Ryan, 2000; Sheldon & Kasser, 1998; Williams, Cox, Hedberg, & Deci, 2000). In one of our recent studies with 825 certified human resources specialists (Forest, Gagné, Girouard, Houlfort, & Crevier-Braud, 2011), we tested a theoretical model of compensation and motivation based on SDT (Gagné & Forest, 2008). Our results are consistent with previous studies: contingent-reward (that is, the perception of pay-for-performance in organizations) is related to more work efforts, but also more burnout, less performance (in the private sector), and more counterproductive work behaviors (in the public sector). Pay-for-performance incentives have also been shown to lead to negative physical health consequences such as heart problem (Manuck & Garland, 1979; Richter & Gendolla, 2007; Siegrist, 1996), a medical condition that is not without consequences for an organization. Even in terms of performance, research shows that paying for performance increases quantity (e.g., Lazear, 2000), but this is oftentimes done to the detriment of quality (e.g., Shearer, 2004). Thus, spending money in pay-for-performance programs to boost economic performance and work motivation could potentially lead to higher costs than profits.

These results directly challenge assumptions that the motivational power of money is unsurpassed: "No other incentive or motivational technique comes even close to money with respect to its instrumental value" (Locke, Feren, McCaleb, Shaw, & Denny, 1980, p. 340). The generally accepted wisdom in the literature on compensation, i.e., stating that if compensation packages are correctly designed they will inevitably lead to superior performance, may be erroneous or at least, overly simplified (e.g., Milkovich, Newman, & Gerhart, 2010; Rynes & Gerhart, 2000).

This section explained in great length why the workplace wrongly overemphasizes extrinsic incentives and monetary rewards to stimulate optimal functioning. One could be left wondering what indeed stimulates performance, motivation and optimal psychological health at work, after basic physiological and survival needs are met. In the next section, we review SDT (Deci & Ryan, 1985, 2000, 2008), a global framework that describes the psychological processes that contribute to happy and productive workplace environments.

SDT: An Integrative Approach to Workplace Motivation

SDT is a global framework that explains human motivation in various life contexts, including work (Gagné & Deci, 2005; Gagné & Forest, 2009; Sheldon, Turban, Brown, Barrick, & Judge, 2003). It is particularly relevant to the work setting because of its universality (it can be applied in any work setting) and broad range of antecedents – such as compensation (e.g., Gagné & Forest, 2008), leadership (e.g., Bono & Judge, 2003), and job design (e.g., Gagné, Senécal, & Koestner, 1997). But beyond explaining motivation, this theory can also predict a vast array of consequences: psychological health (e.g., well-being and psychological distress; Fernet, Gagné, & Austin, 2010), physical health (e.g., somatization; Blais, Hess, Bourbonnais, Saintonge, & Riddle, 1995), behaviors (e.g., creativity; Grant & Berry, 2011), and economic consequences (e.g., profit and costs due to employees effort and stress; Forest, Gilbert, Beaulieu, LeBrock, & Gagné, in press).

At the core of SDT lie two fundamental categories of concepts, namely different types of motivation, and basic psychological needs. We explain both in more detail below.

Different Types of Work Motivation

Motivation is usually defined as an energy that has a direction, intensity and persistence (Pinder, 1998). Motivation varies not only in quantity but, and more importantly for SDT, in quality. This is where SDT is differentiated from other work

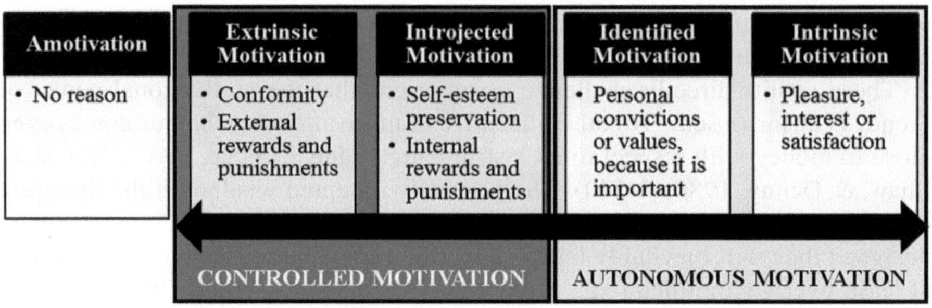

Fig. 12.2 Self-determination continuum and types of motivation according to SDT (Adapted from Deci & Ryan, 2008 with permission)

motivation theories such as goal setting theory (Locke & Latham, 1990, 2002) or empowerment (Thomas & Velhouse, 1990). SDT suggests four motivational types (e.g., Gagné & Deci, 2005) that can be measured (e.g., Gagné et al., 2010), namely intrinsic motivation, identified motivation, introjected motivation and extrinsic motivation. These four types of motivation can be positioned on a self-determination continuum (see Fig. 12.2), that represents the degree to which motivation emanates from the self (i.e., is self-determined; Ryan & Deci, 2000). In other words, we are self-determined when we endorse our actions at the highest level of reflection (Deci & Ryan, 2008).

Intrinsic motivation is usually described as doing an activity for its own sake, for the satisfaction it provides; when intrinsically motivated we find the tasks satisfying in and of themselves. Such motivation is characterized by episodes of "flow", total absorption, concentration and positive emotions. For example, an intrinsically motivated professor may deeply enjoy teaching and having contact with students, and he may see time fly by when in class.

Identified motivation is defined as doing tasks that are in line with one's values, that are important and socially useful and that give meaning to our life, at work or elsewhere. In this case, the tasks can be pleasant to do or not, but we perform them because we perceive them as important. An example could be a nurse who exerts effort to maintain proper elderly patients' hygiene by giving a bath; this task is not necessarily fun to do, but she does it conscientiously since she recognizes it to be important for the patient's health and dignity. On the self-determination continuum, intrinsic and identified motivations can be considered as two autonomous motivation forms.

A less self-determined type of motivation is *introjected motivation.* It can be defined as the search for internal rewards (e.g., boosting one's ego) and the avoidance of internal punishments (e.g., avoiding shame or guilt). This type of motivation is aimed at the protection or enhancement of ego or self-esteem as well as the protection, maintenance or improvement of one's reputation in the workplace. People who display high levels of this type of motivation will work hard to avoid failure, will be disappointed if they do not attain their standards and will oftentimes try to be the best in their field. An example of this type of motivation could be a salesperson who is willing to win at all cost the best ranking in the week's sale, even though it may involve stealing sales from colleagues or selling an inappropriate product only to boost sales.

From a traditional management perspective, *extrinsic motivation* is probably the most salient type of motivation. It involves the search for external rewards (e.g., money) and the avoidance of external punishments (e.g., losing one's job). People with high levels of this motivation avidly search for higher salary or keep a job mainly because of the standard of living it provides, its compensation, pension plan and benefits and because no alternative pays as well in the job market. As these two types of motivation are less self-determined, they can be grouped under the label of controlled motivation.

Finally, *amotivation* represents the relative absence of motivation, the lack of clear direction and the nonexistence of meaning in a job. It is often characterized by learned helplessness and is oftentimes accompanied by experiences of fatigue and exhaustion.

Basic Psychological Needs in the Workplace

SDT posits that the type of motivation adopted, which guides our experience at work (and in life more generally), is mainly influenced by the satisfaction or frustration of our fundamental psychological needs (Ryan, 1995). A psychological need is defined as an essential component that, when satisfied, leads to well-being, self-actualization, adaptation and optimal functioning and that, when dissatisfied, frustrated or thwarted, leads to more ill-being, distress and sub-optimal functioning (e.g., Deci & Ryan, 2000; Sheldon, 2011). In this perspective, a need is a different concept than desire, aspiration, ambition, wish or reason. It is more than desirable, but absolutely necessary to carry out a flourishing life. Furthermore, a need can be proved to be universal and innate, meaning that it is present for all human beings, no matter their geographical location, status or education and is present at birth therefore it does not have to be learned (Deci & Ryan, 2000). Sheldon, Elliot, Kim, and Kasser (2001) carried out a study aimed at determining which psychological needs are really fundamental and important to all human beings. The results demonstrate that the three needs identified by SDT, namely autonomy, competence and relatedness (also called belongingness), are what constitute the "Big Three" of needs to satisfy.

Autonomy refers to yearning to experience ownership of behaviors and act in accordance with our values (deCharms, 1968; Deci, 1975). *Competence* means achieving desired outcomes when putting effort and succeeding when negotiating life's terrains (Skinner, 1995; White, 1959), and *relatedness* implies the need for having mutually satisfying relationships (Baumeister & Leary, 1995; Harlow, 1958).

It appears that autonomy, competence and relatedness are indeed psychological needs since it has been shown on many occasions, and through various spheres of life, types of jobs and cultures, that their satisfaction leads to a multitude of positive consequences (e.g., more positive emotions, energy, performance, and intention to stay; less somatizations, exhaustion, etc.). Complementing this, their partial satisfaction or their frustration leads individuals to experience mitigated or harmful consequences (e.g., more physical problems, absenteeism, exhaustion, and negative emotions; less self-regulation, etc.; see Deci & Ryan, 2000; Ryan, 1995; Ryan & Deci, 2000).

In terms of the universal character of the needs for autonomy, competence and relatedness, many studies conducted in America (e.g., Canada, Brazil, United States), Europe (e.g., France, England, Belgium) and Asia (e.g., Korea, Japan) repeatedly show the same trend: as needs are satisfied, participants report experiencing positive consequences, whereas they report negative outcomes when their needs are dissatisfied or frustrated (Deci & Ryan, 2008). It is thus possible to say that no matter what is the cultural influence conveyed (either by a country or by an organization), these three needs tend to be important to satisfy for optimal functioning.

Finally, regarding the innate aspect of a need, studies conducted with participants of all ages (children, teenagers, adults and elderly) show the importance of satisfying the needs for autonomy, competence and relatedness, and this throughout life (or career) stages (Sheldon et al., 2001). It goes without saying that how these three needs are satisfied varies according to the stage of life or the career the individual is at. For example, the need for competence is not satisfied in the same way for a new employee as it is for an employee with 30 years of experience.

Traditionally, SDT emphasized and studied the importance of *need satisfaction* for optimal functioning. While also stating that *need thwarting* (or frustration) is the explanatory mechanism for sub-optimal functioning, little research has directly tested this assumption. Recent empirical evidence with athletes (Bartholomew, Ntoumanis, Ryan, Bosch, & Thørgesen-Ntoumani, 2011; Bartholomew, Ntoumanis, Ryan, & Thørgesen-Ntoumani, 2011) and workers (Gillet, Fouquereau, Forest, Brunault, & Colombat, 2012) shows that need satisfaction and need thwarting are conceptually different. However, more work is needed to better understand the dynamics between need satisfaction and need thwarting.

Figures 12.3 and 12.4 graphically depict how the satisfaction or frustration of the basic psychological needs at work can have an impact over the types of motivation we will adopt, which in turn has differential behavioral and emotional consequences (e.g., Dagenais-Desmarais, Forest, & Gagné, 2009). The two figures also show the possible levers by which interventions may occur in organizational settings; such interventions are now recognized as effective ways to initiate this “domino effect” postulated by SDT. The next section now turns to a review of those sources of need satisfaction or thwarting in the workplace.

How the Organizational Context Can Promote Self-Determination

SDT posits that the context in which individuals evolve can have an important impact on the extent to which they feel autonomous or controlled (Deci & Ryan, 1985). According to SDT, an environment can be described as autonomy supportive or controlling. Previous research has shown that autonomy-supportive environments will

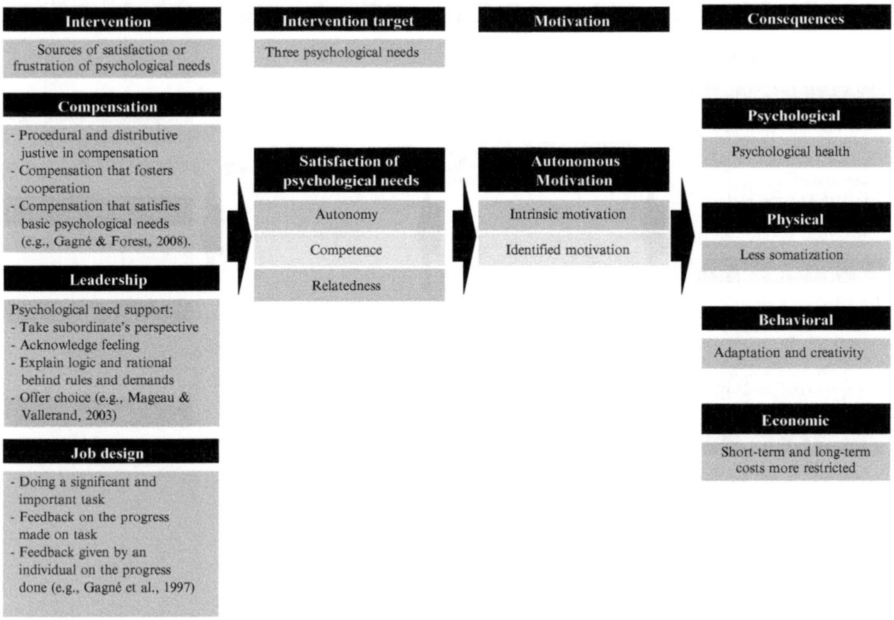

Fig. 12.3 SDT general model of the mediating process by which autonomy-supportive interventions lead to need satisfaction, autonomous motivation, and consequences (From Forest, Crevier-Braud, & Gagné et al. (2009). Copyright 2009 by Ordre des conseillers en ressources humaines agréés. Reprinted with permission)

lead to more positive consequences and controlling environment will lead to less positive consequences and more negative consequences. In this next section, we will describe in further detail these two approaches and their different consequences in the realm of work.

An *autonomy-supportive context* "involves the supervisor understanding and acknowledging the subordinate's perspective, providing meaningful information in a non-manipulative manner, offering opportunities for choice, and encouraging self-initiation" (Baard, Deci, & Ryan, 2004, p. 2048). Although the label refers to the need for autonomy, it should be understood in a larger perspective, and is a means to satisfy all three basic needs (thus it is more accurately a "need-supportive context"). Multiple studies have provided support for the beneficial effect of autonomy support on need satisfaction and autonomous motivation (see Deci & Ryan, 2008, for a review). This interpersonal context has been studied in a wide variety of domains and relationships including education (e.g., Ryan & Grolnick, 1986), parent and child relationship (e.g., Grolnick, Deci, & Ryan, 1997), health (e.g., Williams, Rodin, Ryan, Grolnick, & Deci, 1998), and work (e.g., Baard et al., 2004). Deci, Eghrari, Patrick, and Leone (1994) conducted a laboratory experiment in order to understand the specific factors that form autonomy support. They found three different factors, namely providing a rationale, acknowledging feelings, and conveying choice. These three factors led to greater autonomous motivation.

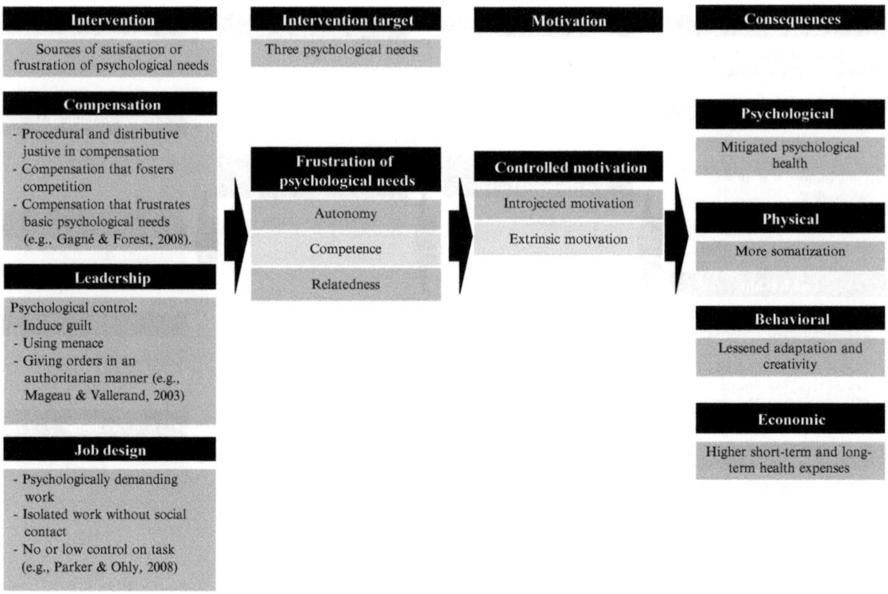

Fig. 12.4 SDT general model of the mediating process by which controlling interventions lead to need frustration, controlled motivation, and consequences (From Forest et al. (2009). Copyright 2009 by Ordre des conseillers en ressources humaines agréés. Reprinted with permission)

Psychologically controlling contexts can be defined as those in which someone or the working context "pressures others to behave in particular ways, either through coercive or seductive techniques that generally include implicit or explicit rewards or punishments" (Black & Deci, 2000, p. 742). Examples of controlling behaviors in a working environment are making an employee feel bad when dissatisfied with his or her work, threatening to take away various privileges in order to pressure the employee into changing his or her behavior, promising rewards as a way to manipulate certain behaviors, and constantly giving orders. A controlling work context undermines employees' autonomous motivation and generates more controlled motivation since it pressures them to think, behave, or feel in certain ways that are detrimental to need satisfaction and increase need thwarting.

It is important to note that psychological control and autonomy support are not the exact opposite of each other (Bartholomew, Ntoumanis, Ryan, Bosch, et al., 2011; Pelletier, Fortier, Vallerand, & Brière, 2001; Silk, Morris, Kanaya, & Steinberg, 2003; Tessier, Sarrazin, & Ntoumanis, 2008). Even though they are to some extent negatively correlated ($r=-.37$; see Bartholomew, Ntoumanis, Ryan, Bosch, et al., 2011), they do not represent the two opposites of a single continuum, but rather two distinct, yet related, approaches. Indeed, a work environment can have some components supporting autonomy (e.g., management's participative leadership style), but at the same time exert some form of psychological control over employees (e.g., pay-for-performance compensation system). Thus, autonomy support and psychological control may coexist in a given organizational context and hence both need to be investigated to obtain a representative portrait of a working environment. The next section will present in more details the different source of support or frustration of psychological needs in the work environment.

Different Sources of Satisfaction and Frustration of the Psychological Needs

According to SDT, both contextual factors and individual factors influence the extent to which one's basic psychological needs are satisfied. In the work context, there are numerous levers on which organizations can take action to meet workers' needs of autonomy, competence and relatedness. According to some recent research, three of the most important levers are (1) the interpersonal relationships that we have at work, especially with our immediate supervisor (Baard et al., 2004), (2) the job design (Gagné, Sénécal, & Koestner, 1997) and (3) the compensation system (Gagné & Forest, 2008). In the following section, each of them will be described and explained with more details.

One Key Player: The Immediate Supervisor

Kelloway and Barling (2010) argue that managers can influence their employees through three main mechanisms: either by serving as a model, by rewarding or punishing them for their attitudes and behaviors at work or by making decisions that can help or stress them. Given the predominance of relations between an employee and his immediate superior, the supervisor is seen as one of the actors most likely to provide a source of autonomy support or psychological control, depending on the interpersonal orientation he uses to interact with his subordinates, or the interpersonal climate he creates through his attitudes and behaviors toward his employees (Baard et al., 2004).

Immediate supervisors can adopt concrete behaviors in order to support the three basic needs of their employees. To support the need for autonomy of their employees, they can encourage an organizational culture of acceptance of honest mistakes and favor initiatives and creative solutions undertaken by the employees. Supervisors can also promote the satisfaction of their employees' need for competence. For instance, they can build on the strengths of their employees when assigning various tasks or projects, or they can give a constructive feedback to enhance employees' awareness of their own competence (Forest, Dagenais-Desmarais, Crevier-Braud, Bergeron, & Girouard, 2010). The immediate supervisor is also known to play an important role in shaping relatedness need satisfaction. A manager that makes it his duty to greet his employees by their name every morning, increases the extent to which those people feel related to him (Forest et al., 2010).

Studies have shown a positive impact of supportive relations between supervisors and subordinates on the need satisfaction they generate, and their positive consequences on work outcomes, including higher employee satisfaction, higher performance, greater effort toward tasks and better acceptance of organizational change (for more details, see Gagné & Deci, 2005). Deci, Connell, and Ryan (1989) also found that supervisors who give a meaningful rationale for completing a task, acknowledge that people might not find an activity interesting, and emphasize choice rather than control have employees who have more trust in the organization, are more satisfied with their job and feel less pressure. Baard and his colleagues (2004) also found that autonomy supportive managerial practices have an indirect positive effect on performance evaluation and psychological adjustment. These results were also found in other cultures (i.e., Bulgaria; Deci et al., 2001). Furthermore, Gagné, Koestner, and Zuckerman (2000) revealed that autonomy support from managers facilitated the acceptance of change in two telecommunication companies.

In contrast, a manager may frustrate employees' needs when he holds controlling attitudes and engages in controlling behaviors towards them. For instance, from a self-determination perspective, management behaviors inducing guilt, using threats, manipulating the employee by the contingency of rewards or giving orders instead of offering choices can be detrimental to employees' psychological need satisfaction (Gillet et al., 2012). In this regard, Richer and Vallerand (1995) have demonstrated that when the interpersonal style of their supervisor is controlling and more specifically, "punitive controlling" (rather than simply non-punitive controlling), employees tend to develop a very low level of intrinsic motivation at work. In contrast, an employee whose supervisor has an "autonomy supportive style" tends to have an intrinsic motivation toward work.

To our knowledge, few studies exist on the specific impact of psychological control in the workplace. In a study, Burstyn, Jonasi, and Wild (2010) were interested in tactics used by health and safety inspectors to ensure compliance with certain health and safety regulations. Their results showed that the inspectors who used more autonomy-supportive tactics were getting more compliance after fewer worksite visits than those who used coercive tactics. In addition, Richer and Vallerand (1995) found that controlling behavior decreased and maintained employee's intrinsic and extrinsic motivation, respectively. Such findings are in line with previous ones and explicitly investigate the dual pathway proposed by SDT. These studies support the idea that controlling behavior has negative workplace outcomes.

As we know that autonomy support and psychological control are embodied in concrete management practices and behaviors, interventions shaping the capacity of training supervisors to engage in autonomy supportive management styles may be especially useful. For example, Deci and colleagues (1989) trained managers to be more autonomy supportive; as a result subordinates reported greater job satisfaction and greater trust toward the organization. Also, Hardré and Reeve (2009) implemented an intervention and showed that 5 weeks after an autonomy-supportive training program, managers were evaluated as being more autonomy supportive than those who did not received this training. Also, their employees were more intrinsically motivated toward their work and more engaged to it. Su and Reeve

(2011) also found in their meta-analysis that autonomy supportive training programs were successful in a variety of settings. These findings are encouraging, since they show that interventions can encourage managers to more effectively foster employees' basic psychological need satisfaction, while reducing need thwarting.

Other Important Players: Colleagues and Human Resources Direction

Apart from the immediate supervisor, it is likely that other individuals play a vital role in supporting employees at work. Coworker relationships are potentially the second most important relations at work, after relationships with one's immediate supervisor. Indeed, Moreau and Mageau (2012) found that colleagues can play a powerful role in well-being at work. Specifically, colleagues' autonomy supportive behaviors showed an incremental contribution to employees' health, subjective well-being and work satisfaction, over the effect of the supervisors' autonomy support. One reason for the effects of colleagues on one another may be their physical and psychological proximity with each other. In fact, coworkers share daily activities, and problems as well as solutions. In this sense, they represent an important source of support for relatedness needs. Moreover, recent research demonstrated that friendship could be beneficial by providing a context where a mutuality of autonomy support is possible (Deci, La Guardia, Moller, Scheiner, & Ryan, 2006). Similarly, in the workplace colleagues can meet one another's autonomy needs. One way in which a colleague may support another's autonomy is, for example, by encouraging him or her to feel free to be who he or she really is rather than feeling pressured to endorse a different image, attitude or behavior (Deci et al., 2006). As for the need for competence, coworkers may impact one another, for instance, by trusting the capacity of their friend to accomplish a task or a part of a common project. In sum, relational climates created by colleagues may support psychological needs in the workplace.

For similar reasons, human resources professionals are likely to be seen as actors who may have a great impact on employees' basic need satisfaction or frustration in many ways. In particular, it seems that the policies and programs implemented by human resources (HR) professionals, especially those that are recognized as best practices, can have a positive influence on employees' needs and motivation at work. Concretely, Sheldon and colleagues (2003, p. 378) propose that "firms that utilize more selective hiring and extensive training should have employees who better fit with the firm and have more organizationally relevant knowledge; such employees are thus more likely to have their competence need satisfied". In another vein, it is possible that the use of work teams or project teams, the implementation of a horizontal structure or the establishment of an open door policy can satisfy employees' need for relatedness. Employees could also feel that their need for autonomy is supported by HR if, for example, HR professionals become ambassadors of a decentralized decision-making policy or a transparency in communication policy (Sheldon et al., 2003). To summarize, because of their role of "employee champion", the human resources management professionals are especially likely to develop supportive relationships to meet the basic psychological needs of autonomy, competence and relatedness of employees. We also acknowledge that human resources professionals can be an important source of need frustration, if they support HR policies leading to increased psychological control within the workplace. In addition, an HR function that is absent from strategic and tactical decision-making and rather confined to operational execution, underrepresented or not consulted for establishing or revising major HR orientations, may run the risk of undermining need satisfaction and autonomous motivation, or arousing employees' need frustration and controlled motivation.

The Impact of Job Characteristics

Among all characteristics of work setting, job design (Gagné et al., 1997) and compensation system (Gagné & Forest, 2008) appear to be the most important features to support the basic needs, because of their relevance in employees' day-to-day experience.

In their model of job characteristics, Hackman and Oldham (1975) suggested that some specific features of job design can engender intrinsic motivation toward work. For instance, in an empirical test of this proposition, Gagné et al. (1997) showed that skill variety, task identity, task significance, autonomy support, job feedback and feedback from different people were all related to intrinsic motivation at work, with the four dimensions of empowerment as mediating variables (e.g., autonomy and meaningfulness). This study demonstrated that interventions shaping various job characteristics are a mean to enhance autonomy satisfaction and increasing intrinsic motivation.

Other characteristics of the work environment may also support or thwart employees' psychological needs. For example, the perception of fit between an employee and his environment (PE fit) can impact the way he or she feels at work (Greguras & Diefendorff, 2009). More particularly, an optimal person-organization fit (PO fit) is related to the autonomy, competence and relatedness needs (Greguras & Diefendorff). A person's congruence within his working group (PG fit) is more specifically related to the relatedness need, whereas a fit between demands and abilities in the work setting (DA fit) is more specifically related to the satisfaction of the competence need (Greguras & Diefendorff). A work environment perceived as fair could also play an important role to support psychological needs (Mayer, Bardes, & Piccolo, 2008), for example, by allowing employees to feel equally important and related to each other, so to satisfy their need of relatedness. This could be illustrated, for instance, in terms of communication systems, where shared information between directors and employees or between departments is viewed as fair.

The Role of Compensation Systems

Although money can be detrimental for employees' self-determination and work motivation, compensation systems can have a positive impact, if used properly. Fairness in the compensation system appears to be crucial for need satisfaction and work motivation. The amount of pay that employees actually receive is important, but the perceptions they have toward distributive justice (i.e., the perception that rewards are distributed fairly among workers) are central. Also, procedural justice (i.e., a fair application of organizational procedures and rules regarding compensation) may be a source of satisfaction or frustration of psychological needs. In their model of compensation effects on work motivation, Gagné and Forest (2008) argue that the amount of pay, distributive justice regarding compensation, ratio of variable versus fixed pay, performance assessment, and level of rewards (individual- or team-based compensation) influence the satisfaction of autonomy, competence and relatedness needs, the development of an autonomous type of motivation and, ultimately, the performance and health of workers.

It is worth noting that, as suggested by equity theory (Adams, 1965), because organizations represent a social context where employees interact with others, they tend to engage in a process of comparison. Doing so, they compare their rewards with same-level workers in other organizations (i.e., external equity) and with colleagues inside of their organization, who have jobs with comparable requirements and level of responsibility and who are perceived as equally competent and successful as them (i.e., internal equity). Finally, employees also assess their rewards in function of their organizational and professional tenure, personal level of competence and their performance at work (i.e., individual equity). If they feel that all these three types of equity are met, their psychological needs would tend to be more satisfied. Up to now, little research supports this theoretical framework, and the relationships between compensation system mode, organizational justice and equity, and self-determination remain to be tested more thoroughly.

Consequences of Self-Determination for Workers' Psychological Health

SDT suggests that employees' need satisfaction or need frustration may have a significant, while different, impact on indicators of employees' psychological health, and empirical evidence supports this claim. More specifically, the psychological processes triggered by need satisfaction or need thwarting appear to lead to differential consequences for employees' mental health.

What Is Psychological Health?

Health has long been considered to be the absence of disease (Seligman, 2008). However, in 1946, the World Health Organization defined health as "a state of complete physical, mental and social well-being, and not merely the absence of disease or infirmity" (p. 100). Nowadays, scholars generally acknowledge that psychological health (also called "mental health" in a medical perspective) has a bidimensional structure (Achille, 2003; Kelloway & Day, 2005; Keyes, 2003), representing both positive and negative dimensions. This conceptualization has been given conclusive empirical support (e.g., see Karademas, 2007; Keyes, 2005; Massé et al., 1998a). The negative component is usually labeled psychological distress, and the positive facet is often labeled psychological well-being (e.g., Keyes, 2006; Massé et al., 1998b, 1998c; Veit & Ware, 1983).

Psychological distress is the component of mental health that has received the most attention in psychology and organizational sciences (Myers & Diener, 1995). Although not strictly limited to specific indicators, it includes in organizational sciences themes such as burnout, depression, anxiety, and stress (Gilbert, Dagenais-Desmarais, & Savoie, 2011).

In comparison to its negative counterpart, *psychological well-being* (PWB) has received only recent interest from the scientific community and understanding of this concept remains heterogeneous (Danna & Griffin, 1999; Harris & Cameron, 2005). Over the last 30 years, a wide variety of PWB conceptualizations have emerged, but are dominated by three main research perspectives (see Dagenais-Desmarais & Savoie, 2012, for a review). The most common themes used to conceptualize psychological well-being are positive affect, life satisfaction, meaning, positive relationships and self-actualization (e.g., Andrews & McKennell, 1980; Berkman, 1971; Bradburn, 1969; Campbell, Converse, & Rodgers, 1976; Diener, 1984; Keyes, 1998; Omodei & Wearing, 1990; Ryan & Deci, 2008; Ryff & Keyes, 1995; Ryff & Singer, 1998). In organizational sciences, psychological well-being is often assimilated to job satisfaction (e.g. Judge & Klinger, 2008), although it is now accepted that well-being at work is not limited to job satisfaction (Wright & Cropanzano, 2004).

As for need satisfaction and need frustration, psychological well-being and distress are two related but distinct phenomena. Indeed, challenging early conceptions of psychological health, studies have demonstrated that the two dimensions appears to be two separate axes rather than two poles of a same continuum (e.g., Karademas, 2007; Massé et al., 1998a; Veit & Ware, 1983). Psychological health can hence be conceptualized as two dimensions that are not simply mirroring each other, and that represent instead two states that may coexist and vary independently of one another. The complete mental health model developed by Keyes and Lopez (2002) offers an interesting representation of the bidimensional conceptualization of psychological health (see Fig.12.5).

In line with this conception of psychological health, practitioners and academics advocate the importance of developing the optimal psychological health of workers rather than merely reducing mental illness. Given the current state of knowledge, promoting optimal psychological functioning should translate into a more complete approach, based both on avoidance of negative mental health and reaching for positive psychological states. Unfortunately, intervention and research efforts are still mainly devoted to preventive approaches, which focus mainly on ill-health at work. In this context, SDT appears to be an insightful framework to inform both research and intervention, and one that offers two paths for shaping the two dimensions of psychological health at work.

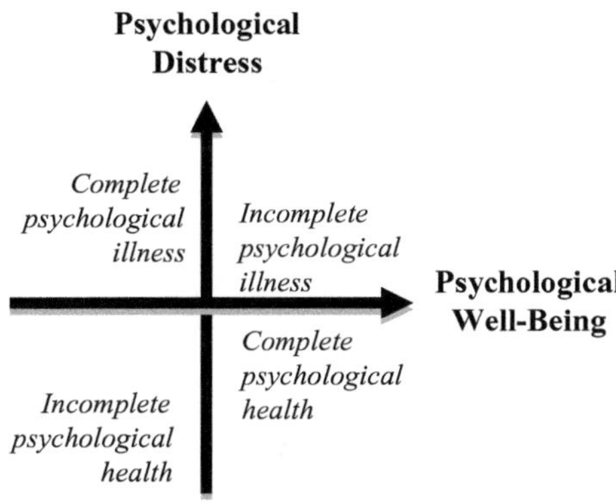

Fig. 12.5 Adaptation of Keyes and Lopez (2002) complete state model (Reprinted with permission)

Empirical findings reveal that need thwarting and need satisfaction may be correlated differentially to psychological health indicators. A recent study among athletes revealed that need thwarting, across all three psychological needs, was a stronger predictor of emotional and physical exhaustion (considered as proxies for distress) and that need satisfaction was a better predictor of vitality (an indicator of well-being; Bartholomew, Ntoumanis, Ryan, et al., 2011). Some studies have also demonstrated that motivation acts as a partial mediator of the path between need satisfaction and well-being (e.g., Milyavskaya & Koestner, 2011). In the workplace, need satisfaction increases work satisfaction, happiness, and self-realization, while need thwarting does the opposite (Gillet et al., 2012).

Beyond need satisfaction or frustration, a few studies have provided support for the direct and indirect effects of autonomy support or control on psychological health. Baard et al. (2004) have found that managers' autonomy support leads to intrinsic need satisfaction, which in return influences psychological health and adjustment. Similarly, testing a SDT model across two cultures, Deci and his colleagues (2001) found that perceived autonomy support is related to the satisfaction of the intrinsic needs for competence, autonomy, and relatedness, and that need satisfaction in turn led to higher work engagement and self-esteem, and lower anxiety. Even in the manufacturing industry where employees had monotonous jobs, workers reporting autonomous motivation also report higher levels of job satisfaction and well-being (Ilardi, Leone, Kasser, & Ryan, 1993). In addition, Shirom, Westman, and Melamed (1999) found that controlling, performance-contingent pay systems, a psychologically controlling practice, had a detrimental impact on blue-collar employees' depression level and somatic complaints. Finally, Niemiec, Ryan, and Deci (2009) have also shown that the pursuit of extrinsically motivated aspirations lead to more ill-being and less well-being and that pursuing intrinsic aspirations leads to more well-being and less distress. These results indicate that not all goal attainment is beneficial to the individual.

In sum, SDT appears to be a conceptual framework particularly useful to better describe, understand and explain both psychological well-being and distress (Gagné & Forest, 2009). Indeed, different autonomy-supportive versus controlling work

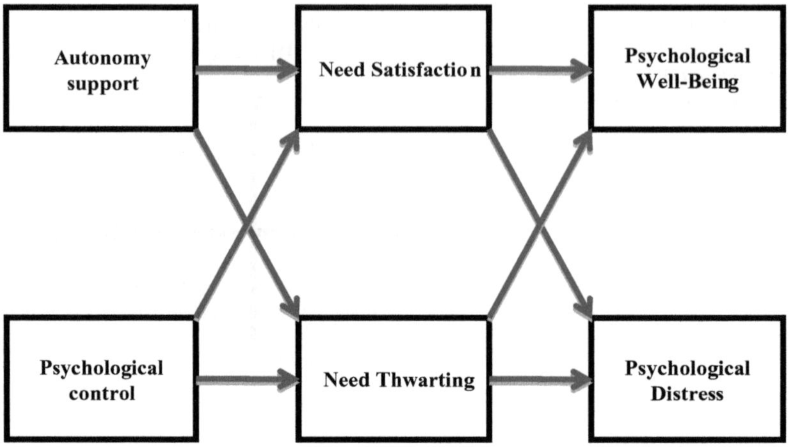

Fig. 12.6 Consequences of self-determination for workers' psychological health

contexts appear to have a domino effect, by influencing need satisfaction and need thwarting, which in turn impact psychological health. Derived from the findings reported here, as well as from other empirical evidences from other life domains, Fig. 12.6 reflects a schematic representation of the relations between autonomy-support/psychological control, employees' need satisfaction/frustration and their well-being/ill-being. This theoretical model argues that, on the one hand, autonomy support leads to more need satisfaction, which leads to more psychological well-being and, on the other hand, psychological control leads to need thwarting, which results in more psychological distress among employees.

How Is SDT Different from What We Already Know

SDT is widely used in various domains such as sport and exercise, education, parenting, psychotherapy, psychopathology, relationships, environment, but has only quite recently been used in the work domain. While SDT has a 35 years history in other domains, the recent popularity in the work domain has created the need for SDT to explicit its added value over previously existing concepts, which are more popular or widely known. Three of those concepts are organizational commitment (Meyer & Allen, 1991), engagement (Bakker, Schaufeli, Leiter, & Taris, 2008) and workaholism (Oates, 1971).

Organizational commitment is defined as the strength of the link that unites an employee to its employer (Klein, Becker, & Meyer, 2009) and can take three different forms, namely affective, normative and continuance commitment. Affective commitment is defined as a positive emotional attachment and a strong identification to the organizational characterized by a desire to stay; employees stay in the organization because they "want to". Normative commitment is defined as a feeling of obligation to stay in the organization characterized by guilt and a sense of reciprocity; this type of commitment implies that employees will want to stay within the organization because they feel they "ought to". Finally, continuance commitment is defined as an evaluation of the high cost of leaving the organization (high sacrifice) and the minimal opportunities for new jobs on the market (low alternatives); people with a high level of this commitment will stay in the organization because they "have to". These definitions share some similarities with the different types of commitment and motivation as outlined by SDT. Affective commitment is relatively similar to intrinsic motivation, normative commitment is similar to introjected motivation and continuance commitment is related to extrinsic motivation. Different theoretical models have hypothesized the link between organizational commitment and work motivation (e.g., Meyer, Becker, & Vandenberghe, 2004; Meyer & Maltin, 2010; Roussel, Dalmas, & Oubrayrie-Roussel, 2009) and usually put commitment as a precursor of work motivation. However, Gagné, Chemolli, Forest, and Koestner (2008) have shown using cross-lagged analyses that work motivation leads to affective and normative commitments and not the other way around. More specifically, they have shown that autonomous motivation leads to affective commitment and that introjected motivation leads to normative commitment. Regarding continuance commitment, results show that the perception of low alternatives for new jobs (the job market is not favorable for the candidate) leads to increase in extrinsic motivation. But does perceiving low alternatives on the job market reflect a form of commitment or just a cognitive analysis of the opportunities one could find elsewhere? We think that perception of the job market can increase extrinsic motivation ("if there are no jobs that pay as much elsewhere, I need to keep this one") but this subcomponent cannot be considered to equal commitment. All in all, SDT share some similarities with organizational commitment with a primary difference being that the concept of work motivation involves the reasons why we put forth effort and behavior, whereas commitment describes the link between individuals and employers. Finally, empirical evidence supports the idea that work motivation is an antecedent to commitment.

The second concept that is somewhat similar to SDT is *engagement* (Schaufeli, Salanova, Gonzalez-Roma, & Bakker, 2002) defined as a positive, fulfilling work-related state of mind that is characterized by vigor, dedication, and absorption. Vigor is defined by having high levels of energy, the capacity to resist to hard work (resilience), and a will to put effort and persist. Dedication can be described as being entirely involved in work, deriving meaning and significance while completing work and experiencing pride, challenge, inspiration, and enthusiasm. Lastly, absorption is defined as being totally absorbed and immersed in time, where time flies by without noticing it. While research has shown that engagement leads to positive consequences such as performance (e.g., Xanthopoulou, Bakker, Demerouti, & Schaufeli, 2009) and that it is theoretically the antithesis of burnout (e.g., González-Roma, Schaufeli, Bakker, & Lloret, 2006), it could be seen as a manifestation of self-determined motivation. SDT-based research has shown that vitality, a concept almost homonymous to vigor, defined as perceived levels of energy – is a consequence of having psychological needs satisfied (e.g., Ryan, Bernstein, & Brown, 2010; Ryan & Deci, 2008) or of having high levels of self-determined motivation (e.g., Niemiec, Ryan, Patrick, Deci, & Williams, 2010; Nix, Ryan, Manly, & Deci, 1999). As of dedication, its definition is clearly in line with the two types of motivation which forms autonomous motivation. Having inspiration, enthusiasm and challenge is closely aligned with what intrinsic motivation is and deriving meaning and significance is similar to identified motivation; this characteristic of engagement would thus be a consequence or a correlate of autonomous motivation. Finally, absorption closely resembles to the concept of flow (Csikszentmihalyi, 1990), which is a transient state characterized by different characteristics such as being immersed and absorbed in what one is doing and not noticing time passing. Our research has shown that self-determined types of motivation are indeed positively related to higher levels of vigor, dedication, and absorption. Research analyzing "engagement" can thus be reinterpreted in that this state is a result of self-determination and need satisfaction.

Workaholism has originally been defined as the "compulsion or the uncontrollable need to work incessantly" (Oates, 1971, p. 11), but recent research has identified two core characteristics of workaholism. The first characteristic is behavioral, working excessively (spending a lot of time at work) and the second is cognitive, working compulsively (the difficultly to control the urge to work and the constant thinking about work; Schaufeli, Bakker, & Salanova, 2006; Schaufeli, Taris, & Van Rhenen, 2008). Van den Broeck et al. (2011) have shown that SDT can shed light on the inconsistent results in line with workaholism. Their research results show that, on the one hand, controlled motivation is related both to compulsive work and excessive work, and that these two components increase exhaustion. On the other hand, autonomous motivation is only linked to excessive work which increases vigor. Thus, it can be said that the negative consequences of what is seen as workaholism may be explained as high levels of controlled motivation.

These three SDT-related concepts – commitment, engagement and workaholism, which have been largely studied (and are known and popular) in the work-related literature, can indeed be understood as similar manifestations to self-determined and controlled types of motivation.

The Example of Canadian Workers

Based on the literature reviewed above, we conducted a cross-sectional study to test an SDT-informed theoretical model according to which autonomy support leads to need satisfaction, which in turn leads to more psychological well-being, while psychological control leads to need thwarting, which results in more psychological distress among employees.

Method

Participants

A sample of 279 Quebec workers from the paramedical sector participated in the study. Participants had a mean age of 37.7 years ($SD = 10.2$ years), and 95 % were women, a number representative of the observed gender distribution in the traditionally female profession composing the sample. Of participants, 77.8 % held a bachelor degree, and 21.9 % completed graduate studies. The vast majority of the sample was working in the public sector (79.2 %), while others were working in the parapublic system (8.2 %), large private companies (4.7 %), small and medium businesses (2.9 %), non-profit organizations or were self-employed (3.2 %). Nearly half of the respondents were living in an urban region (54.1 %). Two-thirds worked full time (35 h/week or more), 19.0 % worked between 25 and 34 h/week, and 14.4 % worked 24 h or less per week. Most respondents were working as professionals (88.5 %), and others had management positions. 20.1 % of them had less than a year of tenure, 34.1 % had 1–5 years of tenure, 24 % had 6–15 years of tenure, and 21.9 % had more than 15 years of tenure.

Measures

The measures used in this study were the Need Satisfaction at Work Scale, the Perceived Autonomy Support Scale for Employees, the Psychological Distress Manifestation Scale and the Psychological Well-Being Manifestation Scale. These questionnaires were chosen because they show adequate psychometrical properties, and their French versions were validated and available. Socio-demographic questions were also included at the end of the questionnaire.

Autonomy Support and Psychological Control

Perceived levels of autonomy support and psychological control were measured with the Perceived Autonomy Support Scale for Employees (PASS-E; Moreau & Mageau, 2012). Based on 21 items and a seven-point scale, employees are asked to assess their supervisor's behaviors. The questionnaire is structured around two higher-order factors (autonomy support – nine items, and psychological control – 12 items), divided into seven subscales. Reliability in this study was adequate, with Cronbach's Alpha coefficients of $\alpha = .92$ and $\alpha = .93$ for the two dimensions.

Need Satisfaction and Need Thwarting

The *Need Satisfaction at Work Scale* was used to measure need satisfaction and thwarting, as perceived by employees themselves (Van den Broeck, Vansteenkiste,

Lens, Soenens, & De Witte, 2010). Composed of 25 items based on a five-point scale, its original dimensional structure comprises one dimension for each basic psychological need, namely autonomy, relatedness, and competence. For each dimension, positive and negative items were interpreted as representing need satisfaction and need thwarting, respectively, leading to a potential 3 × 2 subdimension matrix. In the present study, the Cronbach's Alpha coefficients vary from $\alpha = .81$ for need thwarting to $\alpha = .84$ for need satisfaction.

Psychological Health

To measure the positive dimension of psychological health, the Psychological Well-Being Manifestation Scale (Massé et al., 1998a, 1998b) was used. Comprising 25 items and six factors (Self-Esteem, Social Involvement, Mental Balance, Control of Self and Events, Sociability, and Happiness), the scale showed adequate reliability in this study ($\alpha = .94$ for the total instrument).

To measure the negative component of psychological health, the *Psychological Distress Manifestation Scale* (Massé et al., 1998a, 1998c) was used. Based on 23 items measured on a five-point scale and four dimensions, namely Anxiety/Depression, Irritability, Self-Depreciation, and Social Disengagement, it showed adequate reliability ($\alpha = .95$ for the total instrument).

Results

Correlational Analyses

In order to offer preliminary insight into the hypothesized model, Pearson correlations were analyzed for the SDT components and psychological health (see Table 12.1).

The correlation matrix analysis supported our initial hypothesis. The more managers were perceived as need supportive by their employees, the more workers reported having their psychological needs satisfied and the less they reported having their psychological needs thwarted. To a lesser extent, they also report more well-being and less distress.

The opposite pattern can be observed with psychological control: the more a supervisor is perceived as controlling, the more fundamental needs are thwarted and the less these are satisfied. Its detrimental effect can be observed on psychological health as well, where employees working in such context report less well-being and more distress. A careful observation of the correlation matrix reveals that correlations are stronger for more proximal variables in the SDT sequence we postulated. This suggests a potential mediation effect that was tested in the next set of analyses.

Table 12.1 Correlations and Cronbach's Alpha coefficients (n = 279)

	1	2	3	4	5	6
1. Autonomy support	(.921)					
2. Psychological control	–.680	(.925)				
3. Need satisfaction	.526	–.460	(.842)			
4. Need thwarting	–.535	.537	–.731	(.814)		
5. Psychological well-being	.289	–.227	.526	–.472	(.948)	
6. Psychological distress	–.267	.301	–.422	.468	–.769	(.954)

Note: All coefficients are significant at $p < .01$. Cronbach's Alpha coefficients are presented on the diagonal in parentheses

Path Analysis

In order to test the complete model, in which the mediation processes postulated by SDT lead to psychological health, we performed a path analysis on raw data, with the Maximum Likelihood estimation method using Amos 7.0 (Arbuckle, 2006). In order to assess the fit of the model, different fit indices, residuals and significance of the path coefficients were studied (Kline, 2005). According to generally accepted standards, a model fits the data when the normed chi-square (χ^2/df) does not exceed a value of 3, the Goodness-of-Fit Index (GFI) and Comparative Fit Index (CFI) are higher than .90, the Standardized Root Mean Square Residual (SRMR) is lower than .10 and the Root Mean Square Error of Approximation (RMSEA) is lower than .08, the confidence interval inferior limit being lower than .05 and the higher limit being lower than .10 (Kline).

A first initial model was tested, according to the hypothesized model proposed previously, with the addition of unanalyzed relationships between autonomy support and control, need satisfaction and thwarting, as well as between psychological well-being and distress, as these variables are expected to be conceptually related. Given that most fit indices exceed the recommended values, this model could not be considered to offer a good fit to the data.

We respecified this model to better fit the data by adding two direct effects to the model. The first one included the direct effect of autonomy support on psychological well-being, and the second one represented the direct effect of psychological control on psychological distress. Figure 12.7 illustrates this model. Results indicated that most unstandardized path coefficients were statistically significant and all reflect the expected direction and make sense conceptually. Normed chi-square, GFI, CFI, SRMR and RMSEA were satisfactory.

In order to try to improve the model's fit, we tried to specify different alternative models, by trying to eliminate indirect (mediation) effects and keeping only direct effects. As the models' fit was unsatisfactory, these alternative models were rejected.

This illustration of SDT in the work context reveals that having a supporting supervisor is a determinant of workers' psychological health. Not only does autonomy support have beneficial effect on psychological well-being through the

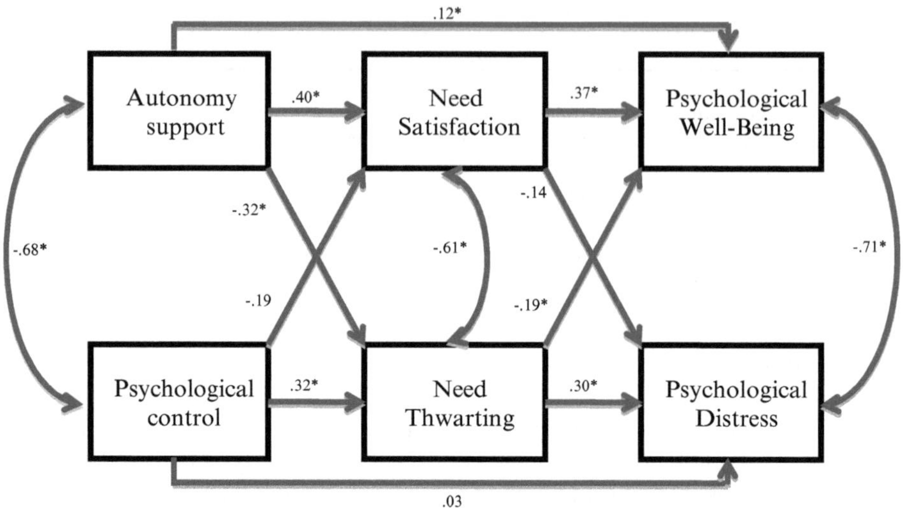

Fig. 12.7 Final explanatory model of psychological health ($n=279$). Standardized coefficients are shown. Significance levels are related to the equivalent unstandardized coefficient. $\chi^2=3{,}457$; $df=2$; $p<.178$; normed $\chi^2=1.728$; GFI=.996; CFI=.998; RMSEA=.051 (low IC=.051, high IC=.140); SRMR=.022

fulfilment of employees' fundamental needs, but it also seems to have, to a lesser extent, a buffer effect on the emergence of distress symptoms, reducing the risk of anxiety, disengagement, and self-depreciation. On the other hand, a psychologically controlling boss, by thwarting employees' basic needs, seems to have a detrimental effect over their mental health. Not only do such management behaviors lead to increased psychological distress, but it also tends, to a lesser extent, to impair workers' well-being. The mediating process by which this occurs is the need satisfaction or thwarting resulting from the supervisory practices. This process can be thought of as the "domino effect" of some managerial practices on psychological health.

This study served as an illustration of a part of the SDT at work model we presented. Some limitations about the study must be raised. First, a cross-sectional design was used and as such the direction of causality is unclear. Also, the sample was representative of a given sector of activity, but the generalizability of the results may have to be limited to a highly educated population working in the healthcare sector. Moreover, the other components of the SDT at work framework (i.e., compensation, job design, as well as physical, behavioral, and economic consequences) would gain to be included in future studies. More research, using longitudinal designs and hard data such as disability records, absenteeism or turnover, would be welcomed in order to better document the process by which the various components identified by SDT interact to affect employees' mental health. However, this study serves as a first example of how SDT can be applied to essential organizational outcomes, in a real-world setting.

Conclusion

SDT is an insightful theory of human motivation that explains various consequences for both the individual and the organization. From a theoretical point of view, it suggests two main paths to human functioning. The positive path provides insights about the inter- and intra-individual processes by which optimal functioning at work is possible, whereas the negative path shed light on the processes leading to detrimental consequences. With regard to psychological health at work more specifically, SDT allows for a better understanding of the dual process by which employees' psychological health can be affected, both positively and negatively. Both paths underline the importance of the organizational and the interpersonal climate in the prediction of work motivation and mental health.

Despite the existence of these two different trajectories to human functioning, most SDT studies focused on the positive path by which autonomy support leads to increased need satisfaction, which in return brings more self-determined motivation. To date, the lack of empirical support for the other half of the SDT model is prominent. Indeed, this "positive-only" approach does not fully portray human functioning, as it is blind to the darker side of motivation and human relationships. As Seligman, Steen, Park, and Peterson (2005) put it about positive psychology:

> Research findings from positive psychology are intended to supplement, not remotely to replace, what is known about human suffering, weakness, and disorder. The intent is to have a more complete and balanced scientific understanding of the human experience (…). We believe that a complete science and a complete practice of psychology should include an understanding of suffering and happiness, as well as their interaction, and validated interventions that both relieve suffering and increase happiness (p. 410).

When applying this perspective to SDT, the need to test the mediation effect of psychological control on need frustration, controlled motivation, and ultimately psychological distress in the workplace is salient. To our knowledge, only one study has tested the complete model, with both positive and negative paths, in a single study in sport (Bartholomew, Ntoumanis, Ryan, et al., 2011), and only one study has done so in the workplace (Gillet et al., 2012). Studying a more exhaustive model leading to optimal mental health would also offer opportunities to investigate more complex relations among variables. Indeed, beyond the two linear trajectories to reach (or not) optimal functioning, the interaction between these two main paths should be further explored.

SDT bridges two trends of research. On the one hand, the prevailing view in psychology and other disciplines focuses on problem solving, limiting dysfunctions and disorders, and healing disease (Bakker & Schaufeli, 2008). On the other hand, emergent approaches, such as positive psychology (Seligman & Csikszentmihalyi, 2000), positive organizational scholarship (Cameron, Dutton, & Quinn, 2003) and positive organizational behavior (Bakker & Schaufeli, 2008; Luthans & Youssef, 2007), study optimal functioning for individuals and organizations. Consistent with these two fields, SDT offers the possibility to address health promotion through two different channels, a positive one and a negative one, yet few empirical studies have used this approach.

We believe it is appropriate to broaden the scope of this discussion to understand how to best optimize psychological health. Traditionally, psychological health has been approached through a biomedical model and a prevention framework that preconize limiting damages, by addressing the risk factors related to diseases (Kimiecik, 2011). To do this, three different intervention levels are proposed, namely *primary prevention* (i.e., eliminating or reducing the causes of mental health problems before they involve the individual, in order to avoid the occurrence of the condition), *secondary prevention* (i.e., reinforcing workers' abilities to cope with risk factors in the workplace), and *tertiary prevention* (i.e., supporting disabled individuals, restoring their previous situation or maximizing the use of their remaining capacities; Randall & Nielsen, 2010; World Health Organization, 2001).

Although necessary for both reaching optimal psychological health and improving mental illness, this approach only focuses on risk factors for illness, including physiological, behavioral, socio-economical, or psychosocial factors (Noblet & Rodwell, 2010). Prevention research within a biopsychosocial framework relies on the assumption that something is wrong and requires fixing (Kimiecik & Lawson, 1996). Hence, prevention does not aim at improving psychological well-being, but rather aims at "returning the body from states of negative functioning back to neutral" (Ryff & Singer, 1998, p. 3). For example, heavy workload is known to be a major risk factor in the workplace (e.g., Ilies, Dimotakis, & De Pater, 2010). By eliminating overload, we reduce the risk of distress among employees, but do we also increase employees' well-being? Acting solely on risk factors is the metaphorical equivalent of removing a thorn in the foot. The pain may be eliminated, but this solution does not by itself elicit optimal health.

More recently, preventionists and researchers in mental health have begun to consider protection factors, or variables that can have a buffering effect to help protect individuals from negative effects of the risk factors (e.g., Reiss & Price, 1996). This approach offers more insight about ways to promote optimal mental health, but once again, interventions aimed at developing protective factors reduce health problems, but do not encourage flourishing and well-being.

Given the strengths and limitations of this widely spread conception of mental health intervention, we suggest a counterpart to factors affecting psychological distress (i.e., risk and protection factors), which received more attention from the scientific community. In order to better understand the individual and organizational variables that can have a positive effect on psychological well-being, we invite the scientific community to dedicate efforts at better understanding what we call *promotion factors*, characteristics of an individual or his environment that have a positive effect on psychological well-being specifically. Up to now, much of the interest of the scientific community focused on risk factors, and to a lesser extent, protection factors. Table 12.2 summarizes this threefold model for a more global intervention framework with regard to complete mental health.

As health prevention typically does not take into consideration the two sides of the medal of psychological health, investigation of the "promotion factors" fostering psychological well-being at work has been left mostly unattended. The literature concerning best promotion factors of optimal mental health is at present unintegrated, and as such it is left to us to explore databases in psychology, organizational behavior, and management in order to extract information on individual and organizational correlates of psychological well-being at work. Given the state of knowledge on what can

Table 12.2 Three levers of intervention for fostering optimal psychological health

Effect over…	Risk factor	Protection factor	Promotion factor
Psychological distress	↗	↘	
Psychological well-being			↗

be called the promotion factors of psychological health at work, we call for a more structured and integrative investigation of these determinants.

Given that psychological distress and well-being are distinct but related dimensions of psychological health (as demonstrated in the study presented above, as well as in previous research), we pose the hypothesis that some variables may have an effect not only over distress, but also on well-being. Some determinants could act as protection factors (i.e., diminishing distress), but also play a role as promotion factors (i.e., increasing well-being). This hypothesis has received some empirical support (e.g., Karademas, 2007). The study we presented is also a good illustration of this, where autonomy support is a both a promotion factor (through its direct and indirect effects over psychological well-being) and a protection factor (because of its mediated effect over psychological distress).

Curiously, many decades after the World Health Organization recognized that health is "not merely the absence of disease" (1946, p. 1), the scientific community continued to investigate psychological health as if it was only a continuum from distress to non-distress. In parallel, positive science scholars began to develop various models of psychological well-being and optimal functioning with little connection to current theoretical models of psychological health (although we acknowledge that some initiatives are now more connected to the field of mental health; e.g., Keyes, 2005). We advocate for building scientific bridges between positive science and health promotion, in order to better understand the various facets of psychological health and to unveil the most efficient levers to optimize it. In such a context, SDT appeared as a theoretical framework capable of reconciling the prevention frame-of-reference and a positive scholarship approach, in order to explain optimal work motivation and employees' mental health. The challenge the scientific community is now facing is to maintain a balance between studying the positive and the negative paths to optimal psychological health.

References

Achille, M. A. (2003). Définir la santé au travail. II. Un modèle multidimensionnel des indicateurs de la santé au travail [Defining health at work. II. A multidimensional model of workplace health indicators]. In R. Foucher, A. Savoie, & L. Brunet (Eds.), *Concilier performance organisationnelle et santé psychologique au travail* (pp. 91–112). Montréal, QC: Éditions nouvelles.

Adams, J. S. (1965). Inequity in social exchange. *Advances in Experimental Social Psychology, 62*, 335–343.

Andrews, F. M., & McKennell, A. C. (1980). Measures of self-reported well-being: Their affective, cognitive and other components. *Social Indicators Research, 8*, 127–155.
Arbuckle, J. L. (2006). *Amos 7.0* [Computer software]. Chicago, IL: Smallwaters Corporation.
Baard, P. P., Deci, E. L., & Ryan, R. M. (2004). Intrinsic need satisfaction: A motivational basis of performance and well-being in two work settings. *Journal of Applied Social Psychology, 34*, 2045–2068.
Bakker, A. B., & Schaufeli, W. B. (2008). Positive organizational behavior: Engaged employees in flourishing organizations. [Ed.]. *Journal of Organizational Behavior, 29*(2), 147–154. doi:10.1002/job.515.
Bakker, A., Schaufeli, W. B., Leiter, M. P., & Taris, T. W. (2008). Work engagement: An emerging concept in occupational health psychology. *Work and Stress, 22*, 187–200.
Bartholomew, K., Ntoumanis, N., Ryan, R., Bosch, J., & Thogersen-Ntoumani, C. (2011). Self-determination theory and diminished functioning: The role of interpersonal control and psychological need thwarting. *Personality and Social Psychology Bulletin, 37*, 1459–1473.
Bartholomew, K., Ntoumanis, N., Ryan, R., & Thøgersen-Ntoumani, C. (2011). Psychological need thwarting in the sport context: Development and initial validation of a psychometric scale. *Journal of Sport & Exercise Psychology, 33*, 75–102.
Baumeister, R. F., & Leary, M. R. (1995). The need to belong: Desire for interpersonal attachment as a fundamental human motivation. *Psychological Bulletin, 117*(3), 497–529.
Berkman, P. L. (1971). Measurement of mental health in a general population survey. *American Journal of Epidemiology, 94*, 105–111.
Black, A. E., & Deci, E. L. (2000). The effects of instructors' autonomy support and students' autonomous motivation on learning organic chemistry: A self-determination theory perspective. *Science Education, 84*, 740–756.
Blais, M., Hess, U., Bourbonnais, J., Saintonge, J., & Riddle, A. (1995). Mens sana ad corpus sanum: Un modèle de motivation-stress-santé appliqué au couple et au travail [A motivation-stress-health model applied to relationships and work]. *Santé mentale au Québec, 2*, 139–162.
Bono, J. E., & Judge, T. A. (2003). Self-concordance at work: Toward understanding the motivational effects of transformational leaders. *The Academy of Management Journal, 46*, 554–571.
Bradburn, N. M. (1969). *The structure of psychological well-being*. Chicago: Aldine.
Brickman, P., Coates, D., & Janoff-Bulman, R. (1978). Lottery winners and accident victims: Is happiness relative? *Journal of Personality and Social Psychology, 36*, 917–927. doi:10.1037/0022-3514.36.8.917.
Brown, K. W., Kasser, T., Ryan, R. M., Linley, P. A., & Orzech, K. (2009). When what one has is enough: Mindfulness, financial desire discrepancy, and subjective well-being. *Journal of Research in Personality, 43*, 727–736.
Burstyn, I., Jonasi, L., & Wild, T. C. (2010). Obtaining compliance with occupational health and safety regulations: A multilevel study using self-determination theory. *International Journal of Environmental Health Research, 20*(4), 271–287.
Cameron, K., Dutton, J., & Quinn, R. (2003). *Positive organizational scholarship: Foundations of a new discipline*. San Francisco: Berrett-Koehler.
Campbell, A., Converse, P. E., & Rodgers, W. L. (1976). *The quality of American life: Perceptions, evaluations, and satisfaction*. New York: Russell.
Csikszentmihalyi, M. (1990). *Flow: The psychology of optimal experience*. New York: Harper & Row.
Csiksznțmihalyi, M. (1999). If we are so rich, why aren't we happy? *The American Psychologist, 54*, 821–827.
Dagenais-Desmarais, V., Forest, J., & Gagné, M. (2009, June). *When your supervisor can influence your psychological health: An empirical verification of autonomy support's Domino effect*. Communication presented at 70th annual convention of Canadian Psychological Association, Montréal, Canada.

Dagenais-Desmarais, V., & Savoie, A. (2012). What is psychological well-being, really? A grass-roots approach from organizational sciences. *Journal of Happiness Studies, 13*(4), 659–668. doi:10.1007/s10902-011-9285-3.
Danna, K., & Griffin, R. W. (1999). Health and well-being in the workplace: A review and synthesis of the literature. *Journal of Management, 25*(3), 357–384.
deCharms, R. (1968). *Personal causation: The internal affective determinants of behavior*. New York: Academic.
Deci, E. L. (1975). *Intrinsic motivation*. New York: Plenum.
Deci, E. L., Connell, J. P., & Ryan, R. M. (1989). Self-determination in a work organization. *The Journal of Applied Psychology, 74*, 580–590.
Deci, E. L., Eghrari, H., Patrick, B. C., & Leone, D. (1994). Facilitating internalization: The self-determination theory perspective. *Journal of Personality, 62*, 119–142.
Deci, E. L., La Guardia, J. G., Moller, A. C., Scheiner, M. J., & Ryan, R. M. (2006). On the benefits of giving as well as receiving autonomy support: Mutuality in close friendships. *Personality and Social Psychology Bulletin, 32*, 313–327.
Deci, E. L., & Ryan, R. M. (1985). *Intrinsic motivation and self-determination in human behavior*. New York: Plenum Publishing Co.
Deci, E. L., & Ryan, R. M. (2000). The 'what' and 'why' of goal pursuits: Human needs and the self-determination of behavior. *Psychological Inquiry, 11*, 227–268.
Deci, E. L., & Ryan, R. M. (2008). Facilitating optimal motivation and psychological well-being across life's domains. *Canadian Psychology, 49*(1), 14–23.
Deci, E. L., Ryan, R. M., Gagné, M., Leone, D. R., Usunov, J., & Kornazheva, B. P. (2001). Need satisfaction, motivation, and well-being in the work organizations of a former eastern bloc country. *Personality and Social Psychology Bulletin, 27*, 930–942.
Diener, E. (1984). Subjective well-being. *Psychological Bulletin, 95*(3), 542–575.
Diener, E., Ng, W., Harter, J., & Arora, R. (2010). Wealth and happiness across the world: Material prosperity predicts life evaluation, whereas psychosocial prosperity predicts positive feeling. *Journal of Personality and Social Psychology, 99*, 52–61.
Easterlin, R. A. (1995). Will raising the incomes of all increase the happiness of all? *Journal of Economic Behavior and Organization, 27*, 35–48.
Easterlin, R. A. (2005). Building a better theory of well-being. In L. Bruni & P. L. Porta (Eds.), *Economics and happiness: Framing the analysis* (pp. 29–64). New York: Oxford University Press.
Easterlin, R. A., Angelescu McVey, L., Switek, M., Sawangfa, O., & Smith Zweig, J. (2010). The happiness-income paradox revisited. *Proceedings of the National Academy of Sciences, 107*(52), 22463–22468. doi:10.1073/pnas.1015962107.
Fernet, C., Gagné, M., & Austin, S. (2010). When does quality of relationships with coworkers predict burnout over time? The moderating role of work motivation. *Journal of Vocational Behavior, 31*, 1163–1180.
Forest, J., Crevier-Braud, L., & Gagné, M. (2009). Mieux comprendre la motivation au travail [For a Better Understanding of Workplace Motivation]. *Effectif, 12*, 23–27.
Forest, J., Dagenais-Desmarais, V., Crevier-Braud, L., Bergeron, E., & Girouard, S. (2010). Le lien entre la santé mentale et la satisfaction des besoins d'autonomie, de compétence et d'affiliation sociale [The relationship between mental health and satisfaction of autonomy, competence, and relatedness needs]. *Gestion, 35*(3), 20–26.
Forest, J., Gagné, M., Girouard, S., Houlfort, N., & Crevier-Braud, L. (2011). *Enquête sur la rémunération: Quelles sont les meilleures pratiques pour vous motiver?* (Rapport Sommaire) [Survey on compensation: What are the best practices to motivate you ? Summary report], Ordre des conseillers en ressources humaines agréés, Montréal, Canada.
Forest, J., Gilbert, M.–H., Beaulieu, G., Le Brock, P., & Gagné, M. (in press). Translating research results in economic terms: An application of economic utility analysis using SDT-based interventions. In M. Gagné (Ed.), *The Oxford handbook of work engagement, motivation, and self-determination theory*. New York: Oxford University Press.

Gagné, M., Chemolli, E., Forest, J., & Koestner, R. (2008). The temporal relations between work motivation and organizational commitment. *Psychologica Belgica, 48*, 219–241.

Gagné, M., & Deci, E. L. (2005). Self-determination theory and work motivation. *Journal of Organizational Behavior, 26*, 331–362.

Gagné, M., & Forest, J. (2008). The study of compensation systems through the lens of self-determination theory: Reconciling 35 years of debate. *Canadian Psychology, 49*, 225–232.

Gagné, M., & Forest, J. (2009). La motivation au travail selon la théorie de l'autodétermination [Workplace motivation according to Self-Determination Theory]. In J. Rojot, P. Roussel, & C. Vandenberghe (Eds.), *Comportement Organisationnel: Vol. 3. Théories des Organisations, Motivation au travail, Engagement Organisationnel* (pp. 215–234). Bruxelles, Belgium: De Boeck.

Gagné, M., Forest, J., Gilbert, M.-H., Aubé, C., Morin, E., & Malorni, A. (2010). The motivation at work scale: Validation evidence in two languages. *Educational and Psychological Measurement, 70*, 628–646.

Gagné, M., Koestner, R., & Zuckerman, M. (2000). Facilitating acceptance of organizational change: The importance of self-determination. *Journal of Applied Social Psychology, 30*, 1843–1852.

Gagné, M., Sénécal, C. B., & Koestner, R. (1997). Proximal job characteristics, feelings of empowerment, and intrinsic motivation: A multidimensional model. *Journal of Applied Social Psychology, 27*, 1222–1240.

Gilbert, M.-H., Dagenais-Desmarais, V., & Savoie, A. (2011). Validation d'une mesure de santé psychologique au travail [Validation of a measure of psychological health at work]. *Revue européenne de psychologie appliquée, 61*(4), 195–203.

Gillet, N., Fouquereau, E., Forest, J., Brunault, P., & Colombat, P. (2012). Organizational factors and psychological needs and their relations with well-being. *Journal of Business and Psychology, 27*, 437–450. doi:10.1007/s10869-011-9253-2.

González-Romá, V., Schaufeli, W. B., Bakker, A. B., & Lloret, S. (2006). Burnout and work engagement: Independent factors or opposite poles? *Journal of Vocational Behavior, 68*, 65–174.

Grant, A. M., & Berry, J. W. (2011). The necessity of others is the mother of invention: Intrinsic and prosocial motivations, perspective-taking, and creativity. *The Academy of Management Journal, 54*, 73–96.

Greguras, G. J., & Diefendorff, J. M. (2009). Different fits satisfy different needs: Linking person-environment fit to employee commitment and performance using Self-Determination Theory. *The Journal of Applied Psychology, 94*, 465–477.

Grolnick, W. S., Deci, E. L., & Ryan, R. M. (1997). Internalization within the family: The self-determination theory perspective. In J. E. Grusec & L. Kuczynski (Eds.), *Parenting and children's internalization of values: A handbook of contemporary theory* (pp. 135–161). New York: Wiley.

Hackman, J. R., & Oldham, G. R. (1975). Development of the job diagnostic survey. *The Journal of Applied Psychology, 60*, 159–170.

Hardré, P., & Reeve, J. (2009). Benefits of training corporate managers to adopt a more autonomy supportive style toward employees: An intervention study. *International Journal of Training and Development, 13*(3), 165–184. doi:10.1111/j.1468-2419.2009.00325.x.

Harlow, H. F. (1958). The nature of love. *The American Psychologist, 13*(12), 673–685.

Harris, G. E., & Cameron, J. E. (2005). Multiple dimensions of organizational identification and commitment as predictors of turnover intentions and psychological well-being. *Canadian Journal of Behavioural Science, 37*(3), 159–169.

Heath, C. (1999). On the social psychology of agency relationship: Lay theories of motivation overemphasize extrinsic incentives. *Organizational Behavior and Human Decision Processes, 78*(1), 25–62.

Howell, R. T., & Howell, C. J. (2008). The relation of economic status to subjective well-being in developing countries: A meta-analysis. *Psychological Bulletin, 13*(4), 536–560.

Ilardi, B. C., Leone, D., Kasser, T., & Ryan, R. M. (1993). Employee and supervisor ratings of motivation: Main effects and discrepancies associated with job satisfaction and adjustment in a factory setting. *Journal of Applied Social Psychology, 23*, 1789–1805.

Ilies, R., Dimotakis, N., & De Pater, I. E. (2010). Psychological and physiological reactions to high workloads: Implications for well-being. *Personnel Psychology, 63*(2), 407–436. doi:10.1111/j.1744-6570.2010.01175.x.

Judge, T. A., & Klinger, R. (2008). Job satisfaction: Subjective well-being at work. In M. Eid & R. J. Larsen (Eds.), *The science of subjective well-being* (pp. 393–413). New York: Guilford Press.

Karademas, E. C. (2007). Positive and negative aspects of well-being: Common and specific predictors. *Personality and Individual Differences, 43*, 277–287.

Kasser, T., & Ryan, R. M. (1993). A dark side of the American dream: Correlates of financial success as a central life aspiration. *Journal of Personality and Social Psychology, 65*, 410–422.

Kasser, T., & Ryan, R. M. (1996). Further examining the American dream: Differential correlates of intrinsic and extrinsic goals. *Personality and Social Psychology Bulletin, 22*, 280–287.

Kasser, T., Ryan, R. M., Zax, M., & Sameroff, A. J. (1995). The relations of maternal and social environments to late adolescents' materialistic and prosocial values. *Developmental Psychology, 31*, 907–914.

Kelloway, E. K., & Barling, J. (2010). Leadership development as an intervention in occupational health psychology. *Work and Stress, 24*(3), 260–279. doi:10.1080/02678373.2010.518441.

Kelloway, E. K., & Day, A. (2005). Building healthy workplaces. What we know so far. *Canadian Journal of Behavioural Science, 37*(4), 223–235.

Keyes, C. L. M. (1998). Social well-being. *Social Psychology Quarterly, 61*(2), 121–140.

Keyes, C. L. M. (2003). Complete mental health: An agenda for the 21st century. In C. L. M. Keyes (Ed.), *Flourishing: Positive psychology and the life well-lived* (pp. 293–312). Washington, DC: American Psychological Association.

Keyes, C. L. M. (2005). Mental illness and/or mental health? Investigating axioms of the complete state model of health. *Journal of Consulting and Clinical Psychology, 73*(3), 539–548.

Keyes, C. L. M. (2006). Subjective well-being in mental health and human development research worldwide: An introduction. *Social Indicators Research, 77*(1), 1–10.

Keyes, C. L. M., & Lopez, S. J. (2002). Toward a science of mental health: Positive directions in diagnosis and interventions. In C. R. Snyder & S. J. Lopez (Eds.), *Handbook of positive psychology* (pp. 45–59). New York: Oxford University Press.

Kimiecik, J. (2011). Exploring the promise of eudaimonic well-being within the practice of health promotion: The "how" is as important as the "what". *Journal of Happiness Studies, 12*, 769–792.

Kimiecik, J., & Lawson, H. (1996). Toward new approaches for exercise behavior change and health promotion. *Quest, 48*, 102–125.

Klein, H. J., Becker, T. E., & Meyer, J. P. (Eds.). (2009). *Commitment in organizations: Accumulated wisdom and new directions*. Florence, KY: Routledge/Taylor & Francis Group.

Kline, R. B. (2005). *Principles and practice of structural equation modeling* (2nd ed.). New York: Guilford Press.

Lawler, E. E. (1971). *Pay and organizational effectiveness*. New York: McGraw-Hill.

Lawler, E. E. (1973). *Motivation in the workplace*. Monterey, CA: Brooks/Cole.

Layard, R. (2005). *Happiness: Lessons from a new science*. London: Penguin.

Lazear, E. P. (2000). Performance pay and productivity. *The American Economic Review, 90*, 1346–1361.

Locke, E. A., Feren, D. B., McCaleb, V. M., Shaw, K. N., & Denny, A. T. (1980). The relative effectiveness of four methods of motivating employee performance. In K. D. Duncan, M. M. Gruneberg, & D. Wallis (Eds.), *Changes in working life* (pp. 363–388). London: Wiley.

Locke, E. A., & Latham, G. P. (1990). *A theory of goal setting and task performance*. Englewood Cliffs, NJ: Prentice-Hall.

Locke, E. A., & Latham, G. P. (2002). Building a practically useful theory of goal setting and task motivation: A 35-year odyssey. *The American Psychologist, 57*, 705–717.

Luthans, F., & Youssef, C. M. (2007). Emerging positive organizational behavior. *Journal of Management, 33*, 321–349.
Manuck, S. B., & Garland, F. N. (1979). Coronary-prone behavior pattern, task incentive, and cardiovascular response. *Psychophysiology, 16*(2), 136–142.
Massé, R., Poulin, C., Dassa, C., Lambert, J., Bélair, S., & Battaglini, A. (1998a). The structure of mental health: Higher-order confirmatory factor analyses of psychological distress and well-being measures. *Social Indicators Research, 45*, 475–504.
Massé, R., Poulin, C., Dassa, C., Lambert, J., Bélair, S., & Battaglini, A. (1998b). Élaboration et validation d'un outil de mesure du bien-etre psychologique: L'ÉMMBEP [Development and validation of a measuring instrument for psychological well-being]. *Revue canadienne de santé publique, 89*(5), 352–357.
Massé, R., Poulin, C., Dassa, C., Lambert, J., Bélair, S., & Battaglini, A. (1998c). Élaboration et validation d'un outil de mesure de la détresse psychologique dans une population non clinique de Québécois francophones [Development and validation of a measuring instrument for psychological distress among a non clinical population of French-speaking Quebec individuals]. *Canadian Journal of Public Health, 89*, 183–187.
Mayer, D. M., Bardes, M., & Piccolo, R. F. (2008). Do servant-leaders help satisfy follower needs? An organizational justice perspective. *European Journal of Work and Organizational Psychology, 17*(2), 180–197.
Meyer, J. P., & Allen, N. J. (1991). A three-component conceptualization of organizational commitment. *Human Resource Management Review, 1*, 64–89.
Meyer, J. P., Becker, T. E., & Vandenberghe, C. (2004). Employee commitment and motivation: A conceptual analysis and integrative model. *The Journal of Applied Psychology, 89*, 991–1007.
Meyer, J. P., & Maltin, E. R. (2010). Employee commitment and well-being: A critical review, theoretical framework and research agenda. *Journal of Vocational Behavior, 77*, 323–337.
Milkovich, G. T., Newman, J. M., & Gerhart, B. (2010). *Compensation* (10th ed.). New York: McGraw-Hill /Irwin.
Milyavskaya, M., & Koestner, R. (2011). Psychological needs, motivation, and well-being: A test of self-determination theory across multiple domains. *Personality and Individual Differences, 50*, 387–391.
Moreau, E., & Mageau, G. A. (2012). The importance of perceived autonomy support for the psychological health and work satisfaction of health professionals: Not only supervisors count, colleagues too! *Motivation and Emotion, 36*(3), 268–286.
Morin, E. M. (2004, August). *The meaning of work in modern times*. Paper presented at the 10th World Congress on Human Resources Management, Rio de Janeiro, Brazil.
Morin, E. M., Savoie, A., & Beaudin, G. (1994). *L'efficacité de l'organisation: Théories, représentations et mesures* [Efficacy of organizations : Theories, representations, and measures]. Montréal, QC, Canada: Gaétan Morin.
Morse, N. C., & Weiss, R. S. (1955). The function and meaning of work and the job. *American Sociological Review, 20*, 191–198.
MOW-International Research Team. (1987). *The meaning of work: An international view*. London: Academic.
Myers, D. G., & Diener, E. (1995). Who is happy? *Psychological Science, 6*, 10–19.
Niemiec, C. P., Ryan, R. M., & Deci, E. L. (2009). The path taken: Consequences of attaining intrinsic and extrinsic aspirations in post-college life. *Journal of Research in Personality, 43*(3), 291–306.
Niemiec, C. P., Ryan, R. M., Patrick, H., Deci, E. L., & Williams, G. C. (2010). The energization of health-behavior change: Examining the associations among autonomous self-regulation, subjective vitality, depressive symptoms, and tobacco abstinence. *The Journal of Positive Psychology, 5*, 122–138.
Nix, G. A., Ryan, R. M., Manly, J. B., & Deci, E. L. (1999). Revitalization through self-regulation: The effects of autonomous and controlled motivation on happiness and vitality. *Journal of Experimental Social Psychology, 35*, 266–284.

Noblet, A. J., & Rodwell, J. J. (2010). Workplace health promotion. In S. Leka & J. Houdmont (Eds.), *Occupational health psychology* (pp. 157–193). Chichester, England: Wiley-Blackwell.

Oates, W. (1971). *Confessions of a workaholic: The facts about work addiction*. New York: World.

Omodei, M. M., & Wearing, A. J. (1990). Need satisfaction and involvement in personal projects: Toward an integrative model of subjective well-being. *Journal of Personality and Social Psychology, 59*(4), 762–769.

Paulsen, R. (2008). Economically forced to work: A critical reconsideration of the lottery question. *Basic Income Studies, 3*(2), Article 3. doi:10.2202/1932-0183.1104.

Pelletier, L. G., Fortier, M. S., Vallerand, R. J., & Brière, N. M. (2001). Associations among perceived autonomy support, forms of self-regulation, and persistence: A prospective study. *Motivation and Emotion, 25*(4), 279–306. doi:10.1023/A:1014805132406.

Pinder, C. C. (1998). *Work motivation: Theory, issues, and applications*. Upper Saddle River, NJ: Prentice Hall.

Randall, R., & Nielsen, K. (2010). Interventions to promote well-being at work. In S. Leka & J. Houdmont (Eds.), *Occupational health psychology* (pp. 88–123). Chichester, England: Wiley-Blackwell.

Reiss, D., & Price, R. H. (1996). National research agenda for prevention research: The National Institute of Mental Health Report. *The American Psychologist, 51*(11), 1109–1115. doi:10.1037/0003-066x.51.11.1109.

Richer, S. F., & Vallerand, R. J. (1995). Supervisors' interactional styles and subordinates' intrinsic and extrinsic motivation. *The Journal of Social Psychology, 135*, 707–722.

Richter, M., & Gendolla, G. H. E. (2007). Incentive value, unclear task difficulty, and cardiovascular reactivity in active coping. *International Journal of Psychophysiology, 63*, 294–301.

Roussel, P., Dalmas, M., & Oubrayrie-Roussel, N. (2009). Les modèles intégrateurs de la motivation au travail [Integrative models of workplace motivation]. In J. Rojot, P. Roussel, & C. Vandenberghe (Eds.), *Comportement Organisationnel: Vol. 3. Théories des Organisations, Motivation au travail, Engagement Organisationnel* (pp. 235–249). Bruxelles, Belgium: De Boeck.

Ryan, R. M. (1995). Psychological needs and the facilitation of integrative processes. *Journal of Personality, 63*, 397–427.

Ryan, R. M., Bernstein, J. H., & Brown, K. W. (2010). Weekends, work, and well-being: Psychological need satisfactions and day of the week effects on mood, vitality, and physical symptoms. *Journal of Social and Clinical Psychology, 29*, 95–122.

Ryan, R. M., Chirkov, V. I., Little, T. D., Sheldon, K. M., Timoshina, E., & Deci, E. L. (1999). The American dream in Russia: Extrinsic aspirations and well-being in two cultures. *Personality and Social Psychology Bulletin, 25*, 1509–1524.

Ryan, R. M., & Deci, E. L. (2000). Self-determination theory and the facilitation of intrinsic motivation, social development, and well-being. *The American Psychologist, 55*(1), 68–78.

Ryan, R. M., & Deci, E. L. (2008). Self-determination theory and the role of basic psychological needs in personality and the organization of behavior. In O. P. John, R. W. Robbins, & L. A. Pervin (Eds.), *Handbook of personality: Theory and research* (pp. 654–678). New York: Guilford Press.

Ryan, R. M., & Grolnick, W. S. (1986). Origins and pawns in the classroom: Self-report and projective assessments of children's perceptions. *Journal of Personality and Social Psychology, 50*, 550–558.

Ryan, R. M., Sheldon, K. M., Kasser, T., & Deci, E. L. (1996). All goals are not created equal: An organismic perspective on the nature of goals and their regulation. In P. M. Gollwitzer & J. A. Bargh (Eds.), *The psychology of action: Linking cognition and motivation to behavior* (pp. 7–26). New York: Guilford Press.

Ryff, C. D., & Keyes, C. L. M. (1995). The structure of psychological well-being revisited. *Journal of Personality and Social Psychology, 69*(4), 719–727.

Ryff, C. D., & Singer, B. (1998). The contours of positive human health. *Psychological Inquiry, 9*(1), 1–28.

Rynes, S. L., & Gerhart, B. (Eds.). (2000). *Compensation in organizations*. San Francisco: Jossey-Bass.

Schaufeli, W. B., Bakker, A. B., & Salanova, M. (2006). The measurement of work engagement with a short questionnaire: A cross-national study. *Educational and Psychological Measurement, 66*, 701–716.

Schaufeli, W. B., Salanova, M., González-Romá, V., & Bakker, A. B. (2002). The measurement of engagement and burnout: A two sample confirmatory factor analytic approach. *Journal of Happiness Studies, 3*, 71–92.

Schaufeli, W. B., Taris, T. W., & Van Rhenen, W. (2008). Workaholism, burnout and engagement: Three of a kind or three different kinds of employee well-being. *Applied Psychology: An International Review, 57*, 173–203.

Schmuck, P., Kasser, T., & Ryan, R. M. (2000). The relationship of well-being to intrinsic and extrinsic goals in Germany and the U.S. *Social Indicators Research, 50*, 225–241.

Seligman, M. E. (2008). Positive health. *Applied Psychology: An International Review, 57*, 3–18.

Seligman, M. E., & Csikszentmihalyi, M. (2000). Positive psychology: An introduction. *The American Psychologist, 55*(1), 5–14.

Seligman, M. E., Steen, T. A., Park, N., & Peterson, C. (2005). Positive psychology progress: Empirical validation of interventions. *The American Psychologist, 60*(5), 410–421.

Shearer, B. (2004). Piece rates, fixed wages and incentives: Evidence from a field experiment. *Review of Economic Studies, 71*, 513–534. doi:10.1111/0034-6527.00294.

Sheldon, K. M. (2011). Integrating behavioral-motive and experiential-requirement perspectives on psychological needs: A two process model. *Psychological Review, 118*(4), 552–569. doi:10.1037/a0024758.

Sheldon, K. M., Elliot, A. J., Kim, Y., & Kasser, T. (2001). What's satisfying about satisfying events? Comparing ten candidate psychological needs. *Journal of Personality and Social Psychology, 80*, 325–339.

Sheldon, K. M., & Kasser, T. (1998). Pursuing personal goals: Skills enable progress, but not all progress is beneficial. *Personality and Social Psychology Bulletin, 24*, 1319–1331.

Sheldon, K. M., Turban, D. B., Brown, K. G., Barrick, M. R., & Judge, T. A. (2003). Applying self-determination theory to organizational research. *Research in Personnel and Human Resources Management, 22*, 357–393.

Shirom, A., Westman, M., & Melamed, S. (1999). The effects of pay systems on blue collar employees emotional distress: The mediating effects of objective monotony and subjective work monotony. *Human Relations, 52*, 1077–1095.

Siegrist, J. (1996). Adverse health effects of high-effort/low-reward conditions. *Journal of Occupational Health Psychology, 1*, 27–41.

Silk, J. S., Morris, A. S., Kanaya, T., & Steinberg, L. (2003). Psychological control and autonomy granting: Opposite ends of a continuum or distinct constructs? *Journal of Research on Adolescence, 13*, 113–128. doi:10.1111/1532-7795.1301004.

Skinner, E. A. (1995). *Perceived control, motivation and coping*. Thousand Oaks, CA: Sage Publications.

Su, Y.-L., & Reeve, J. (2011). A meta-analysis of the effectiveness of intervention programs designed to support autonomy. *Educational Psychology Review, 23*, 159–188.

Tessier, D., Sarrazin, P., & Ntoumanis, N. (2008). The effect of an experimental program to support students' autonomy on the overt behaviours of physical education teachers. *European Journal of Psychology of Education, 23*, 239–253.

Thomas, K. W., & Velhouse, B. A. (1990). Cognitive elements of empowerment: An "interpretive" model of intrinsic task motivation. *Academy of Management Review, 15*(4), 666–681.

Vallerand, R. J., & Houlfort, N. (2003). Passion at work: Toward a new conceptualization. In D. Skarlicki, S. Gilliland, & D. Steiner (Eds.), *Research in social issues in management* (Vol. 3, pp. 175–204). Greenwich, CT: Information Age Publishing Inc.

Van den Broeck, A., Schreurs, B., De Witte, H., Vansteenkiste, M., Germeys, F., & Schaufeli, W. (2011). Understanding workaholics' motivations: A self-determination perspective. *Applied Psychology: An International Review, 60*, 600–621.

Van den Broeck, A., Vansteenkiste, M., De Witte, H., Soenens, B., & Lens, W. (2010). Capturing autonomy, competence, and relatedness at work: Construction and initial validation of the

Work-Related Basic Need Satisfaction Scale. *Journal of Occupational and Organizational Psychology, 83*(4), 981–1002.

Veit, C. T., & Ware, J. E. (1983). The structure of psychological distress and well-being in general populations. *Journal of Consulting and Clinical Psychology, 51*, 730–742.

Vroom, V. H. (1964). *Work and motivation*. New York: Wiley.

White, R. M. (1959). Motivation reconsidered: The concept of competence. *Psychological Review, 66*(5), 297–333.

Williams, G. C., Cox, E. M., Hedberg, V., & Deci, E. L. (2000). Extrinsic life goals and health risk behaviors in adolescents. *Journal of Applied Social Psychology, 30*, 1756–1771.

Williams, G. C., Rodin, G. C., Ryan, R. M., Grolnick, W. S., & Deci, E. L. (1998). Autonomous regulation and adherence to long-term medical regimens in adult outpatients. *Health Psychology, 17*, 269–276.

World Health Organization. (1946). *Constitution of the World Health Organization as adopted by the International Health Conference*, New York 19–22 June, 1946; signed on 22 July 1946 by the representatives of 61 States and entered into force 7 April 1948.Official Records of the World Health Organization (2).

World Health Organization. (2001). *The world health report: 2001: Mental health: New understanding, new hope* (p. 169). Geneva, Suisse: World Health Organization.

Wright, T. A., & Cropanzano, R. (2004). The role of psychological well-being in job performance: A fresh look at an age-old quest. *Organizational Dynamics, 33*(4), 338–351. doi:10.1016/j.orgdyn.2004.09.002.

Wright, T. A., & Cropanzano, R. (2007). The happy/productive worker thesis revisited. In J. J. Martocchio (Ed.), *Research in personnel and human resources management* (Vol. 26, pp. 269–307). Oxford, UK/Greenwich, CT: Elsevier Science/JAI Press.

Xanthopoulou, D., Bakker, A. B., Demerouti, E., & Schaufeli, W. B. (2009). Work engagement and financial returns: A diary study on the role of job and personal resources. *Journal of Organizational and Occupational Psychology, 82*, 183–200.

Zelenski, J. M., Murphy, S. A., & Jenkins, D. A. (2008). The happy-productive worker thesis revisited. *Journal of Happiness Studies, 9*(4), 521–537. doi:10.1007/s10902-008-9087-4.

Chapter 13
The Influence of the Social Environment on Health Behavior

Jennifer G. La Guardia and Heather Patrick

Characteristics of the social environment – at both the macro- and micro-environmental levels – are important for a variety of health outcomes. The social environment directly influences the extent to which people initiate and maintain health behaviors including diet and physical activity, smoking, alcohol consumption, and stress management. Further, the social environment influences how people respond to and manage chronic illnesses and acute health events (e.g., heart attack; cancer diagnosis). Despite the unequivocal importance of the social context, to date most interventions have primarily targeted the individual or macro-level social-environmental variables such as policy rather than addressing the role of more proximal social and relational contexts. The focus of this chapter is to provide a broad overview of the existing literature on the role of relationships in health – both from the perspective of health behavior as primary prevention and from the perspective of navigating health threats and challenges (e.g., an acute health crisis or managing chronic illness) – and to address the importance of understanding and intervening with more proximal players in the social context (e.g., close relationships) for achieving long-term health.

The social context has been construed to include macro-level environmental factors such as laws, public policy and cultural and social norms as well as micro-level environmental factors such as the quality of relationships with health care providers as well as close personal relationships with family, friends, romantic partners, co-workers, and important others. Recently, much attention has been given to the role of public policy in shaping health behavior. This is largely due to the public health success of tobacco policy (e.g., tobacco product taxation; clean indoor acts)

J.G. La Guardia, Ph.D. (✉)
Department of Psychiatry and The Center for Community Health,
University of Rochester Medical Center, Rochester, NY, USA
e-mail: jennifer_laguardia@urmc.rochester.edu

H. Patrick, Ph.D.
Division of Cancer Control and Population Sciences, National Cancer Institute,
National Institutes of Health, Bethesda, MD, USA

N. Weinstein (ed.), *Human Motivation and Interpersonal Relationships: Theory, Research, and Applications*, DOI 10.1007/978-94-017-8542-6_13,

in shaping population-level declines in tobacco use in the US over the past 40 years and the somewhat limited success that individual-level interventions have yielded for population health. More recently, policy changes to affect diet and physical activity behaviors (e.g., increasing availability of parks and recreation space; reducing availability of snack foods and sugar-sweetened beverages in schools) have shown potentially important implications for reducing the incidence of overweight and obesity. However, despite the positive impact that health policy has on shifting cultural and social norms around health behaviors (e.g., acceptability of cigarette smoking), focusing on changes in social policy is not enough. For example, evidence shows that there has been relatively little population-level change in tobacco use in the US over the past 15 years, despite increasingly stringent regulations on when and where people can smoke and steep increases in taxation of tobacco products. Further, evidence regarding the role of the built physical and food environments on exacting broad health behavior change (i.e., physical activity and dietary intake) and health outcomes (i.e., weight status) across the population has been somewhat mixed. Thus, it is important to consider effects of the social context operating at the micro-level.

Micro-level social-environmental factors that affect health include the quality of relationships with various others including health care providers, family, friends, romantic partners, and co-workers. Regarding the health care system, an extensive body of research has focused on patient-provider communication and the ways in which patients' relationships with medical providers influence care received, perceptions of care, and prognosis. Health care practitioners play a critical role in advising patients regarding lifestyle changes around behaviors such as tobacco cessation, diet, physical activity and weight management – all of which are important to primary prevention and effective management of non-communicable diseases that confer the greatest public health burden (e.g., cardiovascular disease, diabetes, cancer). Further, medical care teams are engaged with patients in acute care of major health events (e.g., heart attacks) and ongoing management of chronic conditions (e.g., diabetes, cancer). A large and rich literature suggests that the quality of health care providers' interactions with patients around their health has important implications for initiation and maintenance of health behavior change, as well as treatment adherence in the management of health events and chronic disease (see Williams, this volume). Despite the relatively new emergence of patient-centered care initiatives that attempt to treat the whole person (e.g., medical homes), a critical limitation remains: interventions are still largely focused on the patient only, with little consideration for the complex relationships in which the patient exists outside the care setting.

Understanding how patients function in their ongoing micro-level social contexts is important for several reasons. First, family systems have their own norms around health behaviors (e.g., when, what, and how they eat; the extent to which they are physically active vs. sedentary). Further, family systems differ in their flexibility and willingness to adapt to needed changes for a particular member of that system. Additionally, patients inhabit multiple roles and identities that do not necessarily change as a function of health behavior needs or health status. That is, patients are rarely "just patients." For example, an emerging literature on caregiving during cancer treatment has demonstrated that when women are undergoing treatment, they are often also maintaining their primary caregiving roles in their relationships as wife, mother, sister and friend. Thus, the functional challenge of maintaining these roles and the capacity of the social system to shift responsibilities in response to a patient's health needs is a core factor in whether the patient can reach and maintain health behavior goals for primary prevention and achieve an adequate level of self-care during treatment and management of acute and chronic health conditions. Finally, families are often intimately involved in decisions about lifestyle behavior change as well as treatment decisions for significant illnesses (e.g., cancer), including decisions about what types of treatments are considered, whether treatments are pursued, and when to cease treatment. Culturally competent intervention requires a consideration of how the family and its dynamics play a role in patient's choices around their health behaviors and treatment decisions. Thus, failing to consider the substantial influence of relational partners misses a critical opportunity for improved patient care.

Although a variety of relationships have been shown to influence health – including parents' influence on children and peer influences on each other – in this chapter we focus specifically on romantic relationships, as these relationships represent one of the most significant relationships of adulthood and represent a core arena in which health behavior change and coping with illness is negotiated (Kiecolt-Glaser & Newton, 2001).

The Role of Close Relationships in Initiating & Maintaining Health Behavior Change

The developed world has seen a dramatic shift in major causes of mortality from communicable (i.e., infectious) to non-communicable diseases (e.g., cancer, cardiovascular disease (CVD)). Although a variety of factors in genetics, biology and the physical environment play some role in the development and progression of non-communicable diseases, a convincing body of research has demonstrated the importance of health behaviors – particularly tobacco use, diet, and physical activity – in non-communicable diseases and preventable mortality. Indeed, tobacco use, diet, and physical activity account for 35 % of preventable deaths in the developed world (Mokdad, Marks, Stroup, & Gerberding, 2004). Currently, more than 20 % of US adults smoke and more than two third of US adults are overweight or obese, largely as a result of insufficient physical activity and poor diets characterized by the intake of too many low-nutrient dense foods (e.g., soft drinks, sweet and savory snacks) and intake of too few high-nutrient dense foods (e.g., fruit and vegetables). The obesity epidemic has significant health costs. Twenty-six million U.S. adults have diabetes and 79 million have pre-diabetes, with as many as 1 in 3 expected to have diabetes by 2050 (Centers for Disease Control & Prevention, 2011). Further, 80 million U.S. adults (nearly 1 in 3) have one or more types of CVD (American Heart Association, 2009) and 40.5 % of the population is projected to have some form of

CVD by 2030 (Heidenreich et al., 2011). Cancer is currently the second leading cause of death in the US and is projected to surpass CVD as the leading cause of death in the next few years (NCI, Cancer Facts and the War on Cancer; ACS, Cancer Facts and Figures, 2009), and cancer is strongly tied to health behaviors. Indeed, current estimates suggest that up to 60 % of all cancers could be prevented through primary prevention via lifestyle change (i.e., diet, physical activity, avoiding tobacco use; Policy & Action for Cancer Prevention, 2009). Thus, to improve population health, health behavior change is an important target for interventions.

Many individually-focused approaches to health behavior change have demonstrated efficacy for health behavior change. Indeed, there are many interventions that have been shown to help people to change their dietary and physical activity habits, and cease use of cigarettes and other tobacco products in the short term. However, fewer individually-focused interventions have yielded *maintained* behavior changes over time and in the absence of ongoing intervention. Better engagement of the social environment (i.e., close personal relationships) may be one mechanism by which long-term health behavior change and maintenance may be achieved.

The Impact of Romantic Partners on Health Behaviors

Couples implicitly and explicitly create a relational contract that defines the roles and expectations for each partner as well as the priorities of the couple (La Guardia & Patrick, 2008), including how they approach their lifestyle behaviors. For example, partners influence the extent to which healthy options are available (e.g., what food is available in the house, rules about smoking in the home), how norms are established (e.g., eating meals together at the table or in front of the TV), and how health behaviors fit into the broader goals of the relationship (e.g., to what extent time the couple spends together includes physical activity). Empirical evidence shows convergence of health behaviors (e.g., eating, smoking, exercise) among relationship partners (Ask, Rognmo, Fartein Ask, Røysamb, & Tambs, 2012; Bove, Sobal, & Rauschenbach, 2003; Jurj et al., 2006), such that health behaviors between partners are correlated (Wilson, 2002). Further, not only are health behaviors correlated within couples, but so are risk and development of disease. For example, having an obese spouse increases one's own risk of being obese by 37 % (Smith & Christakis, 2008). Moreover, shared lifestyles of marital partners (e.g., smoking status, frequency of exercise, amount of fat and fiber in the diet) result in greater risk of cardiovascular disease (Macken, Yates, & Blancher, 2000).

On the positive side, the partnership can play an important role in behavioral change, such that health behavior change in one partner may spillover to similar health behavior changes in the other partner (Falba & Sindelar, 2008). For example, those who participate in a weight loss intervention with a partner are more likely to lose weight at 6, 12, and 18 months than those without a partner (Gorin, Phelan, et al., 2005). Further, people who successfully quit smoking are more likely to have smokefree homes (Lee & Kahende, 2007), while having a partner who smokes is one of the most significant risk factors for continued smoking and failure in future quit attempts (e.g., Ferguson, Bauld, Chesterman, & Judge, 2005). Indeed, for more than a decade, scientists have suggested that targeting the relationship as a unit may be more efficacious than targeting individuals (Macken, Yates, & Blancher, 2000). To optimize intervention efficacy, such efforts must be oriented toward the couple – and not merely reflect one-off iterations of individually-based interventions that are now applied to a dyad. To be truly relationship-based, interventions must address not only the specific health behaviors of the individuals that comprise the relationship but also the broader relational context in which these behaviors occur.

Renegotiating the Relational Contract

As noted above, couples create a relational contract that defines the priorities of the couple, including how they approach lifestyle behaviors such as eating, activity levels and tobacco use. Change in health behaviors often requires the couple to make instrumental changes to their daily functioning. For example, to accommodate the addition of a new exercise routine the couple has to negotiate how this change impacts their time together and their shared duties (e.g., changes to childcare). Further, when the behavior is a core element of couple-time (e.g., an after-dinner cigarette is a shared couple experience), the couple must decide how to restructure their activities to accommodate the behavior change while maintaining the feelings of connectedness fostered by the relationship. When inconsistencies arise in lifestyle choices between partners (e.g., one partner is attempting to make dietary changes while the other is not), conflict may arise and can derail desired change (Bove et al., 2003).

Relationship Quality and Health Behaviors

One of the primary areas in which relationship processes have been studied in health behavior change attempts is with regard to social support, broadly defined. Historically, the literature on social support and health has focused more generally on the health benefits of receiving – and to some extent giving – social support, with evidence suggesting that those who perceive greater social support evidence better general health, greater quality of life, and improved prognosis in the context of acute or chronic illness (cf. Kiecolt-Glaser & Newton, 2001; Uchino, 2009). A growing body of research has focused on the role of social support specifically with regard to navigating health behavior change.

Several studies have suggested that behaviors such as expressing confidence in a smokers' ability to quit and acknowledging a partner's success in not smoking – both of which support the smokers' perceived competence and self-efficacy for quitting smoking – are important for facilitating successful cessation (e.g., Cohen et al., 1988; Roski, Schmid, & Lando, 1996). Moreover, when spouses attempt to influence their partners' health behaviors by directly discussing these changes, attempting to work with their partner around changes, and positively reinforcing changes by their partner, partners report that they engage in more health-enhancing behaviors (e.g., improving diet, exercising, reducing/quitting smoking; Lewis & Butterfield, 2007). In contrast, negative forms of support (e.g., criticism) have been found not only to be ineffective for eliciting a desired health behavior change but in fact result in perpetuating the very behavior the partner is attempting to eliminate (e.g., smoking cessation; Rohrbaugh et al., 2001; Shoham, Rohrbaugh, Trost, & Muramoto, 2006). Importantly, the ways in which partners give and experience receipt of social support is not unique to the particular behavioral domain that is being targeted. Indeed, in much the same way that partners have relational contracts regarding various health behaviors and the roles they play in the relationship, partners also have a history of giving and receiving social support to each other. Thus, the specific behaviors that are experienced as supportive, critical, nagging, or encouraging may differ between couples. In this way, how partners support each other is reflective of the broader character of the relationship and highlights one reason why the relationship – and not merely the individuals that comprise the relationship – is an important target for interventions.

Close Relationships in Managing Acute Health Events and Chronic Conditions

When a person's health becomes compromised because of illness, whether it is an acute event (e.g., heart attack) or the insidious onset of illness (e.g., cancer), the whole social system is affected. Although many positive emotions often emerge (e.g., love, care) and the social system shifts its priorities to attend to the patients' health, health events also have the potential to increase the frequency and intensity of many negative emotions for patients and their significant others (e.g., fear, worry, sadness). For example, approximately 20–35 % of cardiac patients have clinically significant depression within 1 year of their cardiac event (Connerney, Shapiro, McLaughlin, Bagiella, & Sloan, 2000; Kaptein, De Jonge, van den Brink, & Korf, 2006; Lane, Carroll, Ring, Beevers, & Lip, 2002; Timberlake et al., 1997), and approximately 35–40 % of patients have significant anxiety symptoms (Andrew, Baker, Kneebone, & Knight, 2000; Lane et al., 2002; Rymaszewska, Kiejna, & Hadrys, 2003). Moreover, spouses have their own intense emotions about their partners' cardiac events, and spouses' distress has been shown to equal or surpass the distress felt by patients across the first year following hospitalization (Artinian, 1991, 1992; Moser & Dracup, 2004). Similarly, across various cancers, clinically significant psychological distress is quite common in the patient (Butler, Koopman, Classen, & Spiegel, 1999; Butler, Koopman, Cordova, Garlan, DiMiceli, & Spiegel, 2003; Massie & Holland, 1990; Northouse et al., 2007; Spiegel, 1996) and the spouse (Couper et al., 2006, 2009; Lavery & Clarke, 1999; Manne et al., 2006; Soloway, Soloway, Kim, & Kava, 2005). The persistence of psychological distress has important implications for both how the couple manages the illness as well as how each partners' health is affected. For example, cardiac patients who continue to experience symptoms of psychological distress during recovery show less adherence to prescribed medications and poorer control of cardiovascular risk-factors (e.g., blood pressure, smoking, cholesterol; Shemesh et al., 2001, 2004), greater risk for new cardiovascular events (Connerney et al., 2000; Doering, Martinez-Maza, Vredevoe, & Cowan, 2008; Kaptein et al., 2006; Pinna Pintor et al., 1992; Saur et al., 2001; Shibeshi, Young-Xu, & Blatt, 2007; Strik, Denollet, Lousberg, & Honig, 2003), and higher rates of early mortality (Barth, Schumacher, & Herrmann-Lingen, 2004; Blumenthal et al., 2003). Further, spouses who have significant levels of stress are more likely to develop their own physical symptoms and risk for illness (Beach, Schulz, Yee, & Jackson, 1997; Schulz & Beach, 1999). Importantly, the relationship can serve as a critical buffer after a health event. Marital quality is a significant predictor of better health outcomes (Robles & Kiecolt-Glaser, 2003). For example, marital quality has been shown to be a potent predictor of length of hospital stay after coronary artery bypass surgery (e.g., Kulik & Mahler, 2006), recurrence of cardiac events after a heart attack (e.g., Orth-Gomer et al., 2000), and rate of survival after congestive heart failure (Rohrbaugh, Shoham, & Coyne, 2006).

Much of the research on the role of close relationships in the context of acute illness has focused primarily on the experience of support provided to the patient by the spouse. For example, after a cancer diagnosis, the more that spouses ask patients about what they feel and need, the more satisfied patients are with their marriage and the better they are able to cope with treatment (Hagedoorn et al., 2000). In contrast, unsupportive behaviors – avoiding health event related discussions, criticizing patients' coping efforts, providing unsolicited advice, and taking over for the patient – have a negative impact on the patient. For example, cancer patients become more distressed when spouses are avoidant or convey discomfort when patients try to talk about their illness (Manne, Ostroff, Winkel, Grana, & Fox, 2005). Further, in cardiac patients, the more wives are hostile toward their husbands after the husbands' cardiac event, the more husbands tend to be psychologically distressed (Fiske, Coyne, & Smith, 1991). When spouses are more hostile or criticize cancer patients for how they are coping with their illness, patients are more distressed (Manne, Ostroff, Sherman, et al., 2004; Manne, Ostroff, Winkel, et al., 2005) and in turn are more likely to avoid coping effectively with their own stress about their illness (e.g., they become less disclosing; Manne, Ostroff, Winkel, et al., 2005). Finally, the more that spouses try to control the patient, the worse off the patient is. For example, in cancer patients, the more spouses are overprotective (Hagedoorn et al., 2000) or try to solve problems *for* patients rather than *with* them (Manne et al., 2004), the more distressed patients are. In congestive heart failure patients, the more spouses are over-involved (e.g., taking over responsibilities or activities the patient can do for himself or herself), the more distressed and the less efficacious patients feel in their daily lives (Benazon, Foster, & Coyne, 2006). Finally, the more spouses are controlling of patients' health related behaviors (e.g., diet, exercise) the less patients engage in these health behaviors and the poorer patients' psychological health over time (Franks et al., 2006).

Emerging evidence has begun to address how acute illness affects the non-ill spouse as well. For example, women with breast cancer who are depressed and have higher levels of distress (and are thus less available to their partners) have been shown to have partners with lower physical health and well-being (Dorros, Card, Segrin, & Badger, 2010). Further, the more spouses of women with metastatic breast cancer found their partner to be unsupportive, the more distressed they felt (Badr, Carmack Taylor, Kashy, Cristofanilli, & Revenson, 2010; Fang, Manne, & Pape, 2001). Similarly, spouses of breast cancer patients who are less satisfied with the support they receive from their partner experience greater negative emotions than those who are satisfied with their partners' support (Hoskins et al., 1996). Thus, although limited data exists, clear evidence suggests that spouses are also affected by how the ill partner copes with and navigates an acute or chronic health condition.

How relational partners collectively cope with illness has been captured in constructs such as dyadic coping (Bodenmann, 1997, 2005), communal coping (Lyons, Mickelson, Sullivan, & Coyne, 1998), and relationship talk (Acitelli & Badr, 2005). Dyadic coping refers to both positive and negative ways that couples work together to manage stress and take care of their relationship amidst the stress (Bodenmann, 1997, 2005). Positive coping is reflected in the extent to which the couple takes time to talk and share their feelings with one another, solves problems jointly, coordinates daily demands, works to maintain the relationship and provides comfort and care for one another. Negative coping is reflected in the extent to which the couple mutually withdraws from contact, either through avoidance or hostile behaviors. Badr and colleagues (2010) found that patients with metastatic breast cancer and their spouses both experienced more cancer-related distress and poorer dyadic adjustment the more they perceived that they withdraw from or avoid each other. In contrast, when patients and spouses are available to be more emotionally and instrumentally supportive of each other, they were better able to collectively take on the challenges of illness (Hagedoorn et al., 2000; Mahrer-Imhof, Hoffmann, & Froelicher, 2007).

Communal coping reflects the extent to which the couple shares their assessment of a threat or stressor, communicates about the situation, and takes collective action in managing the threat (Lyons et al. 1995). In the context of acute health events, the health event becomes something that "we" manage rather than something that any one individual manages. This communal approach (as reflected in "we" talk) has been associated with more positive outcomes in patients with congestive heart failure (Rohrbaugh, Mehl, Shoham, Rielly, & Ewy, 2008).

Relationship talk, a related concept, reflects the extent to which couples discuss the state of their relationship, each partner's needs, and the relational implications of a shared stressor (Acitelli & Badr, 2005), and it has been shown to be particularly important for adjustment in couples coping with chronic illness. For example, when discussing a wife's breast cancer, reciprocal self-disclosure between the patient and her spouse is associated with lower general and cancer-specific distress as well as lower incidence of cancer-related intrusions and avoidance for the patient (Manne et al., 2004). In couples in which one partner has been diagnosed with lung cancer, the more the couple was able to talk about the relationship implications of lung cancer and work to maintain or enhance the relationship, the less distress (Badr, Acitelli, & Carmack Taylor, 2008) and greater adjustment (Badr & Carmack Taylor, 2008) the non-ill partner experienced. Finally, greater mutual constructive communication about cancer related problems is associated with less distress and greater marital satisfaction for both partners in couples coping with cancer (Manne et al., 2006). In contrast, attempts to avoid discussing personal concerns or the cancer itself have been shown to be associated with greater distress in both partners (e.g., Manne et al., 2007).

In sum, partners respond to health crises by calling upon their own coping resources and the collective coping resources of the couple. The relationship serves as an important touch point for support during a health crisis and the responses of partners have important implications for the physical and psychological health outcomes for all involved.

A Note About Physical Intimacy

A key way in which partners maintain intimacy is through their physical connection. However, acute and chronic health conditions can significantly alter this physical connection. Challenges in physical intimacy can occur for a variety of reasons, including physical limitations and disability for the patient created by the health condition itself and/or its treatment; changes in sexual interest or desire, arousal, and performance due to patients' and spouses' emotional response to the health event (e.g., anxiety, depression) or the side effects of drugs (e.g., blood pressure medication and beta blockers for cardiac patients; chemotherapy for cancer patients); and fears about the safety of initiating and engaging each other sexually (Beach et al., 1992; Lindau et al., 2010). The health event can further have a significant impact on patients' pre-health event identity (e.g., loss in their sense of masculinity/femininity) and sense of attractiveness (e.g., physical changes due to scars from surgery; loss of hair due to treatment), which can create additional distress within the couple.

Sexual problems are common after health events, occurring in 50–75 % of those who have a cardiac event (e.g., heart attack, bypass surgery) and 50–80 % of those with cancer [e.g., 60–80 % prostate cancer, Stanford et al., 2000; 50 % ovarian cancer, Carmack Taylor, Basen-Engquist, Shinn, & Bodurka, 2004], and become a key issue for improving quality of life after such events. Indeed, sexuality is viewed as important to life and health, particularly among those with chronic or life threatening illnesses (Hill et al., 2011; Lindau & Gavrilova, 2010; Lindau, Gavrilova, & Anderson, 2007; Lindau et al., 2007; Lindau, Surawska, Paice, & Baron, 2011). Yet, despite the well-known impact of health events on sexuality and the importance of it for quality of life, patients and their spouses report that is one of the areas that is most difficult to navigate with one's partner in the context of acute or chronic health conditions (Badr & Taylor, 2009; Boehmer & Clark, 2001; Lindau et al., 2011). Moreover, it is a topic that receives very little attention in treatment. Lindau and colleagues (2012) reported that 1/3 of women and less than 1/2 of men received discharge instructions about sex following treatment for a cardiac event. Further, failure to receive counseling at discharge predicts loss of sexual activity for both men and women at 1 year post-event (Lindau et al., 2012). Thus, health events are clearly *relational*. That is, acute and chronic health conditions influence not only the person who has the illness but also their proximal social network, particularly their romantic partner. Importantly, health conditions also influence the relationship in ways that can create emotional and psychological distance in the relationship at a time when connection is needed most.

The Relationship as an Intervention Target

Across the health care continuum – from primary prevention to management of acute and chronic illnesses – relationships are an important social context in which individuals navigate the challenges inherent in these health issues. Relationships are more than the sum of the individuals of which they are comprised. Relationships have their own character, history, norms and culture and thus reflect a direct target for intervention.

In the context of health behavior interventions, relationships may be a particularly important target. To date, many individually-based interventions have failed to achieve long-term maintenance, which may be, in part, because individuals live not in clinical trials but rather in ongoing family and relational contexts that may support or impede behavior change efforts. Further, although policies operating at a macro-level can do much to address social norms around health behaviors (e.g., smoking), close relationships represent a more proximal target that may be particularly important to leverage in the context of diminishing returns that increasing public policies have yielded (e.g., unchanged population-level smoking rates over the past 20 years). Several recent efforts have aimed to engage relationship partners in lifestyle behavior interventions, though these studies vary in the degree to which the relationship – and not merely the individuals that comprise relationships – are engaged. For example, in a trial aimed at improving adherence to cholesterol-lowering regiments, including lifestyle behavior change, patients were randomly assigned to receive usual care or an enhanced intervention in which patients received telephone calls regarding information about hypercholesterolemia and strategies for managing this indicator of CVD. Spouses received separate calls that provided this same information about the patient's condition as well as tips for how to best support the patient in achieving treatment and management goals around topics such as diet, physical activity, doctor-patient communication, and medication adherence. Although there were no differences between usual care and enhanced intervention participants on biological indicators of changes in cholesterol profile, patients in the intervention group evidenced improved diet (i.e., lower intake of total calories, fat, and saturated fat) and greater moderate-intensity physical activity (Voils, Coffman, Yancy, et al., 2013). Matsuo and colleagues (Matsuo, Kim, Murotake, et al., 2010) randomly assigned abdominally obese men to no intervention, direct lifestyle intervention, or indirect lifestyle intervention in which patient's wives were provided with the lifestyle intervention treatment but men (patients) were not. Men in both the direct and indirect intervention groups evidenced significant weight loss and improvements in other metabolic syndrome symptoms. Notably, in the indirect intervention group, both men and their non-patient wives lost weight and had decreased incidence of metabolic syndrome, suggesting that indirect lifestyle intervention by engaging a spouse in treatment may be effective for improving health status in patients with metabolic syndrome. Still other research has focused on the role of communal coping (i.e., "we" talk) by health compromised smokers and their spouses. This research found that pre-treatment we-talk in which partners described smoking as "our" problem rather than "your" problem or "my" problem was associated with greater smoking cessation rates at 12 months, as was residualized change in we-talk throughout the course of intervention (Rohrbaugh, Shoham, Skoyen, Jensen, & Mehl, 2012).

In a recent systematic review of partner support for smoking cessation among pregnant and postpartum women, Hemsing and colleagues (Hemsing, Greaves, O'Leary, Chan, & Okoli, 2012) found that there were very few effective smoking cessation interventions for pregnant and postpartum women that include or target male partners. As evidenced by this brief review, there have been increasing efforts to target multiple members of families and relationships across a range of health behaviors that have been implicated as major causes of preventable morbidity and mortality. However, very few of these interventions have truly targeted the couple or the ongoing relationship dynamics that may facilitate or impede health behavior change efforts.

Research in the context of coping with acute and chronic health conditions has shown tremendous promise for the utility and efficacy of intervening with couples rather than just the patient. A significant body of this work has occurred in the treatment of various cancers. For example, research by Manne et al. (2005) demonstrated that a couples-focused group intervention aimed at enhancing support exchanges and coping skills in couples reduced depression and anxiety, increased behavioral and emotional control, and increased well-being in patients with early stage breast cancer. The benefit of using this couples' intervention over typical psychosocial care was particularly important for women who rated their partners as more unsupportive pre-intervention or for those who reported greater physical impairment at baseline. Research by Scott, Halford, and Ward (2004) has also demonstrated benefits of a couples coping training intervention (CanCOPE) over medical information education training and patient-only coping training for couples in which the woman has early stage breast or gynecologic cancer. The intervention focused on improving couples' communication about cancer, including learning how to more effectively self-disclose and empathically listen and validate each other. Results showed that couples who received the intervention increased observable supportive communications, and both partners receiving the intervention reported reductions in required effort for effective coping. Further, for patients, the intervention decreased psychological distress, reduced their need to avoid intrusive negative thoughts about cancer, improved self-perceptions about their sexuality, and fostered greater intimacy in their relationship. In a recent study using a brief intervention with couples in which a partner was diagnosed with localized prostate cancer, Manne and colleagues (2011) showed that couples who began an Intimacy-Enhancing Therapy intervention with higher cancer-specific distress, lower marital satisfaction, lower intimacy, and poorer communication, showed significant improvement in these outcomes versus usual care. Finally, Mc Lean and colleagues (2008) used Emotion-Focused Couples Therapy with advanced cancer patients and their spouses and showed that couples showed relational growth and improved marital functioning, even during the end stages of cancer. Taken together, the findings from this emerging body of research suggests that treating the couple, including elements of the relationship that are crucial for improved experience of social support, is beneficial for patient and spouse, and for physical and relational health.

Conclusions

The transition of major causes of morbidity and mortality from communicable to non-communicable diseases has created a number of challenges for individuals, researchers, and policy makers. Lifestyle behaviors – maintaining a healthy diet, engaging in regular physical activity and avoiding tobacco use and exposure – are critical to preventing and managing the diseases that contribute the most to the public health burden. However, long-term maintenance of these behaviors has remained elusive. This may be due, in part, to the fact that most interventions have focused either on individuals or broader aspects of the social system such as healthcare delivery and public health policy. As described here, a burgeoning area of research has used the context of acute health events and chronic disease management as test-beds for understanding how close relationships can be leveraged to improve health behavior change, medication adherence, patient prognosis, and the emotional and psychological well-being of relationship partners. Thus, close relationships represent an important, proximal target for study and intervention. Interventions that address the dynamics of the social context as a core element of their interventions provide benefit not just to the patient, but also to the partner and the relationship as a whole.

References

Acitelli, L. K., & Badr, H. J. (2005). My illness or our illness? Attending to the relationship when one partner is ill. In T. A. Revenson, K. Kayser, & G. Bodenmann (Eds.), *Emerging perspectives on couples' coping with stress* (pp. 137–156). Washington, DC: American Psychological Association.

American Cancer Society. (2009). *Cancer facts and figures 2009*. Atlanta: American Cancer Society; 2010.

American Heart Association. (2009). *Heart disease and stroke statistics update*. Dallas, TX: American Heart Association.

Andrew, M. J., Baker, R. A., Kneebone, A. C., & Knight, J. C. (2000). Mood state as a predictor of neuropsychological deficits following cardiac surgery. *Journal of Psychosomatic Research, 48*, 537–546.

Artinian, N. T. (1991). The stress experience of spouses of coronary artery bypass patients during hospitalization and six weeks post discharge. *Heart and Lung, 20*(1), 52–59.

Artinian, N. T. (1992). Spouse adaptation to mate's CABG surgery: 1-year follow-up. *American Journal of Critical Care, 1*, 36–42.

Ask, H., Rognmo, K., Fartein Ask, T., Røysamb, E., & Tambs, K. (2012). Non-random mating and convergence over time for alcohol consumption, smoking, and exercise: The Nord-Trøndelag Health Study. *Behavior Genetics, 42*, 354–365.

Badr, H., Acitelli, L. K., & Carmack Taylor, C. L. (2008). Does talking about their relationship affect couples' martial and psychological adjustment to lung cancer? *Journal of Cancer Survivorship, 2*, 53–64.

Badr, H., & Carmack Taylor, C. L. (2008). Effects of relational maintenance on psychological distress and dyadic adjustment among couples coping with lung cancer. *Health Psychology, 27*, 616–627. PubMed: 18823188.

Badr, H., & Carmack Taylor, C. L. (2009). Sexual dysfunction and spousal communication in couples coping with prostate cancer. *Psychooncology, 18*(7), 735–746.

Badr, H., Carmack Taylor, C. L., Kashy, D. A., Cristofanilli, M., & Revenson, T. A. (2010). Dyadic coping in metastatic breast cancer. *Health Psychology, 29*(2), 169–180. doi:10.1037/a0018165.

Barth, J., Schumacher, M., & Herrmann-Lingen, C. (2004). Depression as a risk factor for mortality in patients with coronary heart disease: A meta-analysis. *Psychosomatic Medicine, 66*, 802–813.

Beach, E. K., Maloney, B. H., Plocica, A. R., Sherry, S. E., Weaver, M., Luthringer, L., et al. (1992). The spouse: A factor in recovery after acute myocardial infarction. *Heart and Lung, 21*(1), 30–38.

Beach, S. R., Schulz, R., Yee, J. L., & Jackson, S. (1997). Negative and positive health effects of caring for a disabled spouse: Longitudinal findings from the Caregiver Health Effects study. *Psychology & Aging, 15*, 259–271.

Benazon, N. R., Foster, M. D., & Coyne, J. C. (2006). Expressed emotion, adaptation and patient survival among couples coping with chronic heart failure. *Journal of Family Psychology, 20*, 328–334.

Blumenthal, J. A., Lett, H. S., Babyak, M. A., White, W., Smith, P. K., Mark, D. B., et al. (2003). Depression as a risk factor for mortality after coronary artery bypass surgery. *Lancet, 362*, 604–609.

Bodenmann, G. (1997). Dyadic coping-a systemic-transactional view of stress and coping among couples: Theory and empirical findings. *European Review of Applied Psychology, 47*, 137–140.

Bodenmann, G. (2005). Dyadic coping and its significance for marital functioning. In T. A. Revenson, K. Kayser, & G. Bodenmann (Eds.), *Couples coping with stress: Emerging perspectives on dyadic coping* (pp. 33–50). Washington, DC: American Psychological Association.

Boehmer, U., & Clark, J. A. (2001). Communication about prostate cancer between men and their wives. *The Journal of Family Practice, 50*(3), 226–231.

Bove, C. F., Sobal, J., & Rauschenbach, B. S. (2003). Food choices among newly married couples: Convergence, conflict, individualism, and projects. *Appetite, 40*, 25–41.

Butler, L. D., Koopman, C., Classen, C., & Spiegel, D. (1999). Traumatic stress, life events, and emotional support in women with metastatic breast cancer: Cancer-related traumatic stress symptoms associated with past and current stressors. *Health Psychology, 18*(6), 555–560.

Butler, L. D., Koopman, C., Cordova, M. J., Garlan, R. W., DiMiceli, S., & Spiegel, D. (2003). Psychological distress and pain significantly increase before death in metastatic breast cancer patients. *Psychsomatic Medicine, 65*(3), 416–426.

Cancer Facts & The War on Cancer. National Cancer Institute. http://training.seer.cancer.gov/disease/war/
Carmack Taylor, C. L., Basen-Engquist, K., Shinn, E. H., & Bodurka, D. C. (2004). Predictors of sexual functioning in ovarian cancer patients. *Journal of Clinical Oncology, 22*(5), 881–889.
Centers for Disease Control and Prevention. (2011). *National diabetes fact sheet: National estimates and general information on diabetes and prediabetes in the United States.* Washington, DC: Centers for Disease Control and Prevention.
Cohen, S., Lichtenstein, E., Mermelstein, R., Kingsolver, K., Baer, J., & Karmarck, T. (1988). Social support interventions for smoking cessation. In B. H. Gottleib (Ed.), *Marshalling social support: Formats, processes and effects*. New York: Sage.
Connerney, I., Shapiro, P. A., McLaughlin, J. S., Bagiella, E., & Sloan, R. P. (2000). In-hospital depression after CABG surgery predicts 12-month outcome. *Lancet, 358*, 1766–1771.
Couper, J. W., Bloch, S., Love, A., Duchesne, G., Macvean, M., & Kissane, D. W. (2006). The psychosocial impact of prostate cancer on patients and their partners. *MJA, 185*, 428–432.
Couper, J. W., Bloch, S., Love, A., Duchesne, G., Macvean, M., & Kissane, D. W. (2009). Coping patterns and psychosocial distress in female partners of prostate cancer patients. *Psychosomatics, 50*, 375–382.
Doering, L. V., Martinez-Maza, O., Vredevoe, D. L., & Cowan, M. J. (2008). Relation of depression, natural killer cell function, and infections after coronary artery bypass in women. *European Journal of Cardiovascular Nursing, 7*(1), 52–58.
Dorros, S. M., Card, N. A., Segrin, C., & Badger, T. A. (2010). Interdependence in women with breast cancer and their partners: An interindividual model of distress. *Journal of Consulting and Clinical Psychology, 78*(1), 121–125.
Falba, T. A., & Sindelar, J. L. (2008). Spousal concordance in health behavior change. *Health Services Research, 43*(1 Pt 1), 96–116. doi:10.1111/j.1475-6773.2007.00754.x.
Fang, C. Y., Manne, S. L., & Pape, S. J. (2001). Functional impairment, marital quality, and patient psychological distress as predictors of psychological distress among cancer patients' spouses. *Health Psychology, 20*, 452–457.
Ferguson, J., Bauld, L., Chesterman, J., & Judge, K. (2005). The English smoking treatment services:One-yearoutcomes.*Addiction,100*(Suppl2),59–69.doi:10.1111/j.1360-0443.2005.01028.
Fiske, V., Coyne, J. C., & Smith, D. A. (1991). Couples coping with myocardial infarction: An empirical reconsideration of the role of overprotectiveness. *Journal of Family Psychology, 5*, 4–20.
Franks, M. M., Stephens, M. A. P., Rook, K. S., Franklin, B. A., Keteyian, S. J., & Artinian, N. T. (2006). Partners' provision of health-related support and control to patients participating in cardiac rehabilitation. *Journal of Family Psychology, 20*(2), 311–318.
Gorin, A., Phelan, S., Tate, D., Sherwood, N., Jeffery, R., & Wing, R. (2005). Involving support partners in obesity treatment. *Journal of Consulting and Clinical Psychology, 73*(2), 341–343.
Hagedoorn, M., Kuijer, R. G., Buunk, B. P., DeJong, G. M., Wobbes, T., & Sanderman, R. (2000). Marital satisfaction in patients with cancer: Does support from intimate partners particularly affect those who need it most? *Health Psychology, 19*, 274–282.
Heidenreich, P. A., Trogdon, J. G., Khavjou, O. A., Butler, J., et al. (2011). Forecasting the future of cardiovascular disease in the United States: A policy statement from the American Heart Association. *Circulation, 123*, 933–944.
Hemsing, N., Greaves, L., O'Leary, R., Chan, K., & Okoli, C. (2012). Partner support for smoking cessation during pregnancy: A systematic review. *Nicotine and Tobacco Research, 14*, 767–776.
Hill, E. K., Sandbo, S., Abramsohn, E., Makelarski, J., Wroblewski, K., Wenrich, E. R., et al. (2011). Assessing gynecologic and breast cancer survivors' sexual health care needs. *Cancer, 117*, 2643–2651.
Hoskins, C. N., Badker, S., Budin, W., Ekstrom, D., Maislin, G., Sherman, D., et al. (1996). Adjustment among husbands of women with breast cancer. *Journal of Psychosocial Oncology, 14*, 41–69.
Jurj, A. L., Wen, W., Li, H. L., Zheng, W., Yang, G., Xiang, Y. B., et al. (2006). Spousal correlations for lifestyle factors and selected diseases in Chinese couples. *Annals of Epidemiology, 16*(4), 285–291.

Kaptein, K. I., De Jonge, P., van den Brink, R. H. S., & Korf, J. (2006). Course of depressive symptoms after myocardial infarction and cardiac prognosis: A latent class analysis. *Psychosomatic Medicine, 68*, 662–668.

Kiecolt-Glaser, J. K., & Newton, T. L. (2001). Marriage and health: His and hers. *Psychological Bulletin, 127*, 472–503.

Kulik, J. A., & Mahler, H. I. M. (2006). Marital quality predicts hospital stay following coronary artery bypass surgery for women but not men. *Social Science & Medicine, 63*, 2031–2040.

La Guardia, J. G., & Patrick, H. (2008). Self-determination theory as a fundamental theory of close relationships. *Canadian Psychology, 49*, 201–209.

Lane, D., Carroll, D., Ring, C., Beevers, D. G., & Lip, G. Y. H. (2002). The prevalence and persistence of depression and anxiety following myocardial infarction. *British Journal of Health Psychology, 7*(1), 11–21.

Lavery, J. F., & Clarke, V. A. (1999). Prostate cancer: Patients' and spouses' coping and marital adjustment. *Psychology, Health & Medicine, 4*, 289–302.

Lee, C. W., & Kahende, J. (2007). Factors associated with successful smoking cessation in the United States, 2000. *American Journal of Public Health, 97*, 1503–1509.

Lewis, M. A., & Butterfield, R. M. (2007). Social control in marital relationships: Effect of one's partner on health behavior. *Journal of Applied Social Psychology, 37*(2), 298–319.

Lindau, S. T., Abramsohn, E., Gosch, K., Wroblewski, K., Spatz, E. S., Chan, P. S., et al. (2012). Patterns and loss of sexual activity in the year following hospitalization for acute myocardial infarction (a United States National Multisite Observational Study). *The American Journal of Cardiology, 109*, 1439–1444.

Lindau, S. T., & Gavrilova, N. (2010). Sex, health, and years of sexually active life gained due to good health: Evidence from two US population based cross sectional surveys of ageing. *BMJ, 340*, 1–11.

Lindau, S. T., Gavrilova, N., & Anderson, D. (2007). Sexual morbidity in very long term survivors of vaginal and cervical cancer: A comparison to national norms. *Gynecologic Oncology, 106*, 413–418.

Lindau, S. T., Gosch, K., Abramsohn, E., Chan, P., Krumholz, H., Spatz, E., Wroblewski, K., et al. (2010). *Gender differences in loss of sexual activity 1-year after an acute myocardial infarction (AMI)*. Presentation at American Heart Association's Forum on Quality of Care and Outcomes Research in Cardiovascular Disease and Stroke, Washington, DC.

Lindau, S. T., Schumm, P., Laumann, E. O., Levinson, W., O'Muircheartaigh, C. A., & Waite, L. J. (2007). A study of sexuality and health among older adults in the United States. *The New England Journal of Medicine, 357*(8), 762–774.

Lindau, S. T., Surawska, H., Paice, J., & Baron, S. R. (2011). Communication about sexuality and intimacy in couples affected by lung cancer and their clinical-care providers. *Psychooncology, 20*, 179–185.

Lyons, R. F., Mickelson, K. D., Sullivan, M. J. L., & Coyne, J. C. (1998). Coping as a communal process. *Journal of Social and Personal Relationships, 15*, 579–605.

Macken, L. C., Yates, B., & Blancher, S. (2000). Concordance of risk factors in female spouses of male patients with coronary heart disease. *JCRP, 20*(6), 361–368.

Mahrer-Imhof, R., Hoffmann, A., & Froelicher, E. S. (2007). Impact of cardiac disease on couples' relationships. *Journal of Advanced Nursing, 57*(5), 513–521.

Manne, S. L., Norton, T., Ostroff, J., Winkel, G., Fox, K., & Grana, G. (2007). Protective buffering and psychological distress among couples coping with breast cancer: The moderating role of relationship satisfaction. *Journal of Family Psychology, 21*, 380–388.

Manne, S. L., Ostroff, J. S., Norton, T., Fox, K., Goldstein, L., & Grana, G. (2006). Cancer-related relationship communication in couples coping with early stage breast cancer. *Psycho-oncology, 15*, 234–247.

Manne, S. L., Ostroff, J. S., Sherman, M., Heyman, R. E., Ross, S., & Fox, K. (2004). Couples' support-related communication, psychological distress, and relationship satisfaction among women with early stage breast cancer. *Journal of Consulting and Clinical Psychology, 74*(4), 660–670.

Manne, S. L., Ostroff, J. S., Winkel, G., Fox, K., Grana, G., Miller, E., et al. (2005). Couple-focused group intervention for women with early stage breast cancer. *Journal of Consulting and Clinical Psychology, 73*, 634–646. doi:10.1037/0022-006X.73.4.634.

Manne, S. L., Ostroff, J. S., Winkel, G., Grana, G., & Fox, K. (2005). Partner unsupportive responses, avoidant coping, and distress among women with early stage breast cancer: Patient and partner perspectives. *Health Psychology, 24*(6), 635–641.

Massie, M. J., & Holland, J. (1990). Depression and the cancer patient. *Journal of Clinical Psychiatry, 51*, 12–17. PubMed: 2195008.

Matsuo, T., Kim, M. K., Murotake, Y., Numao, S., et al. (2010). Indirect lifestyle intervention through wives improves metabolic syndrome components in men. *International Journal of Obesity, 34*(1), 136–145.

McLean, L. M., Jones, J. M., Rydall, A. C., Walsh, A., Esplen, M. J., Zimmermann, C., et al. (2008). A couples intervention for patients facing advanced cancer and their spouse caregivers: outcomes of a pilot study. *Psychooncology, 11*, 1152–1156.

Mokdad, A. H., Marks, J. S., Stroup, D. F., & Gerberding, J. L. (2004). Actual causes of death in the United States, 2000. *JAMA, 291*(10), 1238–1245.

Moser, D. K., & Dracup, K. (2004). Role of spousal anxiety and depression in patients' psychosocial recovery after a cardiac event. *Psychosomatic Medicine, 66*, 527–532.

Northouse, L. L., Mood, D. W., Montie, J. E., Sandler, H. M., Forman, J. D., Hussain, M., et al. (2007). Living with prostate cancer: Patients' and spouses' psychosocial status and quality of life. *Journal of Clinical Oncology, 25*, 4171–4177.

Orth-Gomer, K., Wamala, S. P., Horsten, M., Schenck-Gustafsson, K., Schneiderman, N., & Mittleman, M. A. (2000). Marital stress worsens prognosis in women with coronary heart disease: The Stockholm Female Coronary Risk Study. *JAMA, 284*, 3008–3014.

Pinna Pintor, P., Torta, R., Bartolozzi, S., Borio, R., Caruzzo, E., Cicolin, A., et al. (1992). Clinical outcomes and emotional-behavioural status after isolated coronary surgery. *Quality of Life Research, 1*, 177–185.

Policy and action for Cancer Prevention: Food, nutrition, and physical activity. (2009). Washington, DC: World Cancer Research Fund/American Institute for Cancer Research.

Robles, T. F., & Kiecolt-Glaser, J. K. (2003). The physiology of marriage: Pathways to health. *Physiology & Behavior, 79*(3), 409–416.

Rohrbaugh, M. J., Mehl, M. R., Shoham, V., Reilly, E. S., & Ewy, G. (2008). Prognostic significance of spouse "we-talk" in couples coping with heart failure. *Journal of Consulting and Clinical Psychology, 76*, 781–789.

Rohrbaugh, M. J., Shoham, V., & Coyne, J. C. (2006). Effect of marital quality on eight-year survival of patients with heart failure. *American Journal of Cardiology, 98*, 1069–1072.

Rohrbaugh, M. J., Shoham, V., Skoyen, J. A., Jensen, M., & Mehl, M. R. (2012). *We*-talk, communal coping, and cessation success in a couple-focused intervention for health-compromised smokers. *Family Process, 51*, 107–121.

Rohrbaugh, M. J., Shoham, V., Trost, S., Muramoto, M., Cate, R., & Leischow, S. (2001). Couple-dynamics of change resistant smoking: Toward a family-consultation model. *Family Process, 40*, 15–31.

Roski, J., Schmid, L. A., & Lando, H. A. (1996). Long-term associations of helpful and harmful spousal behaviors with smoking cessation. *Addictive Behaviors, 21*(2), 173–185.

Rymaszewska, J., Kiejna, A., & Hadrys, T. (2003). Depression and anxiety in coronary artery bypass grafting patients. *European Psychiatry, 18*, 155–160.

Saur, C. D., Granger, B. B., Muhlbaier, L. H., Forman, L. M., McKenzie, R. J., Taylor, M. C., et al. (2001). Depressive symptoms and outcome of coronary artery bypass grafting. *American Journal of Critical Care, 10*(1), 4–10.

Schulz, R., & Beach, S. R. (1999). Caregiving as a risk factor for mortality. *JAMA, 282*(23), 215–2219.

Scott, J. L., Halford, W. K., & Ward, B. G. (2004). United we stand? The effects of a couple-coping intervention on adjustment to early stage breast or gynaecological cancer. *Journal of Consulting and Clinical Psychology, 72*(6), 1122–1135.

Shemesh, E., Rudnick, A., Kaluski, E., Milovanov, O., Salah, A., Alon, D., et al. (2001). A prospective study of posttraumatic stress symptoms and non-adherence in survivors of a myocardial infarction (MI). *General Hospital Psychiatry, 23*, 215–222.

Shemesh, E., Yehuda, R., Milo, O., Dinur, I., Rudnick, A., Vered, Z., et al. (2004). Posttraumatic stress, nonadherence, and adverse outcome in survivors of a myocadial infarction. *Psychosomatic Medicine, 66*, 521–526.

Shibeshi, W. A., Young-Xu, Y., & Blatt, C. M. (2007). Anxiety worsens prognosis in patients with coronary artery disease. *Journal of the American College of Cardiology, 49*, 2021–2027.

Shoham, V., Rohrbaugh, M. J., Trost, S., & Muramoto, M. (2006). A family consultation intervention for health-compromised smokers. *Journal of Substance Abuse Treatment, 31*, 395–402.

Smith, K. P., & Christakis, N. A. (2008). Social networks and health. *Annual Review of Sociology, 34*, 405–429.

Soloway, C. T., Soloway, M. S., Kim, S. S., & Kava, B. R. (2005). Sexual, psychological and dyadic qualities of the prostate cancer 'couple'. *BJU International, 95*, 780–785.

Spiegel, D. (1996). Cancer and depression. *British Journal of Psychiatry, 168*(Suppl. 30), 109–116.

Stanford, J. L., Feng, Z., Hamilton, A. S., Gilliland, F. D., Stephenson, R. A., Eley, J. W., et al. (2000). Urinary and sexual function after radical prostatectomy for clinically localized prostate cancer: The Prostate Cancer Outcomes Study. *JAMA, 283*(3), 354–360.

Strik, J., Denollet, J., Lousberg, R., & Honig, A. (2003). Comparing symptoms of depression and anxiety as predictors of cardiac events and increased health care consumption after myocardial infarction. *Journal of the American College of Cardiology, 42*(10), 1801–1807.

Timberlake, N., Klinger, L., Smith, P., Venn, G., Treasure, T., Harrison, M., et al. (1997). Incidence and patterns of depression following coronary artery bypass graft surgery. *Journal of Psychosomatic Research, 43*, 197–207.

Voils, C. I., Coffman, C. J., Yancy, W. S., Jr., Weinberger, M., Jeffreys, A. S., Datta, S., et al. (2013). A randomized controlled trial to evaluate the effectiveness of CouPLES: A spouse-assisted lifestyle change intervention to improve low-density lipoprotein cholesterol. *Preventive Medicine, 56*(1), 46–52. PMID 23146744.

Wilson, S. E. (2002). The health capital of families: An investigation of the inter-spousal correlation in health status. *Social Science Medicine, 55*(7), 1157–1172.

[illegible]

Chapter 14
Motivation in the Client-Counselor Relationship

Martin F. Lynch

The role of motivation in the client-counselor relationship was recently given attention in a special section of the journal, *The Counseling Psychologist*, which included an invited target article (Ryan, Lynch, Vansteenkiste, & Deci, 2011), several responses to the target article (Carter, 2011; Kim, 2011; Scheel, 2011), and a reply (Lynch, Vansteenkiste, Deci, & Ryan, 2011). Across these articles, there was broad agreement that client motivation plays a central role in the therapeutic endeavor, and special consideration was given to the role of the therapist in fostering client motivation for change in the context of the client-counselor relationship. After briefly summarizing some of the key points in that discussion, the present chapter seeks to extend the conversation by addressing how an understanding of client motivation might inform a recently proposed model for the therapeutic relationship, a model that builds on current thinking about the common and specific factors in therapy (Wampold & Budge, 2012).

Describing Client Motivation Along a Continuum, from Controlled to Autonomous

In their target article, Ryan and colleagues (2011) observed that motivation can be described along a continuum. At one end of the continuum lies external or controlled motivation, and at the other end lies internal or autonomous motivation. Describing motivation along a continuum essentially captures the fact that a person's actions in a particular domain of behavior or for a particular action can be experienced by the person as more or less volitional. In other words,

M.F. Lynch (✉)
Warner School of Education, University of Rochester, Rochester, NY, USA
e-mail: mlynch@warner.rochester.edu

N. Weinstein (ed.), *Human Motivation and Interpersonal Relationships: Theory, Research, and Applications*, DOI 10.1007/978-94-017-8542-6_14,

motivation can be described in terms of the *perceived locus of causality* (Ryan & Connell, 1989), which refers to the extent to which a person experiences the causes of his or her actions as coming from outside or from inside the self. When motivated by rewards, pressures, threats, or other forms of control, people experience less volition in their actions; they feel as though their behavior is under the contingency of some anticipated consequence, whether reward or punishment, that is separable from the behavior itself, and to that extent they have an external perceived locus of causality. On the other hand, when people engage in actions for reasons that are more internal, such as seeing the importance of the action for oneself, experiencing the action as consistent with one's other values, or finding it enjoyable, their motivation is experienced as less under the control of external contingencies and as more internally motivated, that is, as more volitional or autonomous; accordingly, their perceived locus of causality is more internal. Although motivation is viewed as a continuum, that is, as a continuous metric ranging from external at one end to internal at the other end, by convention points along the axis are demarcated with the labels *introjection*, *identification*, and *integration*, reflecting increasingly more autonomous motivation.

As applied to counseling, the continuum of motivation suggests that clients can come with a motivation for change that is more external and controlled, or with a motivation for change that is more internal and autonomous. An example of external motivation for counseling might be the client who feels pressured by an employer or a spouse to seek therapy, or, in a more extreme case, who has been mandated for treatment by the court. More internally motivated would be the client who perceives the value of counseling for him- or herself, and who feels volitional about making the choice to seek counseling. These differences in the quality of motivation have implications for counseling, as research suggests that clients whose motivation is more internal tend to stay in counseling longer (that is, they are less likely to drop out or terminate early), obtain better counseling outcomes, and maintain counseling-related change longer than do those whose motivation is more external (Lynch et al., 2011; Ryan et al., 2011).

Importantly, based on their review of the literature Ryan and colleagues (2011) made the argument that internal or autonomous motivation in the client is preferred by therapists from virtually every theoretical approach, even those approaches with which the concept of autonomy is not theoretically consistent. That is, most therapists prefer that their clients come to counseling and engage in the therapeutic process because they *want* to. The following section draws on Ryan and colleagues to summarize how client motivation is treated in the behavioral, cognitive-behavioral, psychodynamic, and existential-humanistic traditions, before returning to the self-determination theory perspective. Specific focus is given to the role of the client-therapist relationship within each of these traditions in fostering client motivation, in particular autonomous motivation, for counseling.

Motivation and the Relationship in Major Approaches to Counseling

Although in practice most therapists prefer it when clients are in counseling because they themselves want to be there, there are important differences in how therapists approach their own role with respect to client motivation, from screening out those whose motivation is deemed to be 'too low,' to actively prompting and shaping a client's motivation through rewards and other contingencies, to supporting and facilitating the client's own motivation for change from within. In other words, there are important differences in how counselors view their role in the client-counselor relationship with respect to motivation. To a large extent, these differences can be traced to the underlying theoretical orientation of the counselor, with some approaches being more *outcome-oriented* and others being more *process-oriented.* As Ryan and colleagues (2011) noted, outcome-oriented therapies "often have well-defined ideas about what the clients should do and aim for," while process-oriented therapies "often explicitly avoid any quick focus on specified outcomes, engaging instead in a more open-ended exploration and search" (p. 198). Another way of saying this is that outcome-focused therapists control the agenda for therapy, often from the start of the relationship, while process-oriented therapists allow the agenda to emerge in the context of the relationship, in the course of working with the client. The following sections briefly describe how these theoretical differences influence the way counselors view both their role and the nature of the client-counselor relationship.

Behavioral Approaches

Among the outcome-oriented perspectives are behavioral approaches, the most influential of which can be traced back to Skinner's (1974) operant conditioning. In operant conditioning, behavior is held to be under the control of external contingencies, or reinforcers. A *reinforcer* can be anything in the environment, separable from the behavior itself, that increases the likelihood that a behavior will be repeated in the future. As such, this would be considered external motivation, in its purest form, in the taxonomy provided by the continuum of motivation discussed earlier. In behavior therapy, the objective is to identify a target behavior to be changed – whether to increase or decrease its frequency of occurrence – and by means of a *functional analysis* to locate the reinforcer or reinforcers in the environment that control its occurrence. Once that has been done, reinforcement contingencies can be set in place or removed, to increase or decrease the frequency of occurrence of the target behavior. Behavior change thus is prompted by the management of reinforcement contingencies in the environment. Motivationally speaking, it is about the external control of client behavior and the promotion of change from without, such that clients would, presumably, ordinarily experience an external perceived locus of causality with respect to any changes they undergo.[1]

In its purest form, behavior therapy would not be interested in client autonomy or with promoting internal motivation for change; indeed, autonomy and internal motivation would be considered to be unobservable 'epiphenomena' (Watson, 1913) or 'fictional inner causes' (Skinner, 1953) which, as such, could not possibly be the target of behavioral intervention. In actual practice, however, behavior therapists show considerable interest in eliciting volitional engagement from clients. This can be noted in the way that behavioral therapists discuss therapist attitudes and obligations in the context of the therapy relationship. For example, behavior therapists typically emphasize transparency, explicitness, and consensus with their clients about the goals of treatment, viewing the therapy relationship as collaborative (Antony & Roemer, 2003). This emphasis can be seen especially at the very beginning of the relationship in terms of the collaborative formulation of the treatment plan (Meichenbaum, 1986). It could be argued that this emphasis on establishing a collaborative relationship with the client, with the implicit acknowledgment of the importance of clients' "volition, voice, and input in the context of therapy" (Ryan et al., 2011, p. 208), is not consistent with the basic tenets of operant conditioning specifically or of behaviorism more generally. Whether consistent with the underlying theory or not, it indicates a recognition on the part of many behavior therapists that clients' volitional engagement in the tasks of therapy seems to matter, and moreover that the therapist has a role in fostering that volitional engagement. Indeed, one noted behavior therapist has stated that applied behavior analysis, a form of behavioral intervention often used in the treatment of autism and autistic spectrum disorders, can be and is ideally administered in an autonomy supportive manner.[2]

Cognitive and Cognitive-Behavioral Approaches

Cognitive behavior therapy (CBT), like behavior therapy, is an outcome-focused approach. A key feature distinguishing cognitive-behavioral from behavioral approaches is that the former specifically acknowledges the important role played by cognitions in mediating between the environment and behavior; cognitions, in other words, are not mere epiphenomena. Beliefs and expectations are examples of

[1] Technically speaking, because radical behaviorism does not acknowledge the relevance of psychological mediators, it is difficult to refer to this as a model of *motivation*, per se (see Ryan et al., 2011). To the extent that behavioral approaches rely on external reinforcers to shape behavior, it still seems meaningful however to refer to the client's phenomenal experience in terms of the perceived locus of causality for their behavior.

[2] Dr. David R. Donnelly, behavior therapist and author, personal communication, April 18, 2012.

the kind of cognitions that transform an environmental input into a behavioral output. Specifically, self-efficacy beliefs (Bandura, 1989, 1996) reflect one's twin convictions that a certain behavior leads reliably to a particular outcome, and that one is capable of performing that behavior, oneself. Thus, in CBT, motivation is conceptualized in terms of the client's beliefs about self-efficacy: does the client believe that treatment, or a certain therapeutic task assigned within treatment, will be beneficial, and does the client further believe he or she is capable of undertaking the treatment or performing the task? A client for whom one or both of these beliefs is not sufficiently strong is not likely to be motivated to enter or to continue in counseling. Indeed, research supports the importance of the client's efficacy beliefs (Caprara & Cervone, 2000; Westra, Dozois, & Marcus, 2007). In terms of the continuum of motivation discussed earlier, it is important to point out that a client might feel self-efficacious with respect to counseling, but her motivation might be either self-efficacious and controlled (that is, believing actions lead to outcomes and that one is capable of performing those actions, but feeling pressured about doing so) or self-efficacious and autonomous (holding the twin self-efficacy beliefs, while feeling volitional about acting on them). That is, self-efficacy and autonomy are orthogonal constructs or dimensions of client motivation.

As in behavioral therapy, the client-therapist relationship in CBT is characterized by transparency. In the context of CBT, transparency means describing the treatment to the client upfront and in detail. This serves a twofold purpose: on the one hand, it allows the therapist to gauge the client's motivation or "willingness to proceed" (Steketee, 1993, p. 96), and on the other hand, by obtaining the client's consent to treatment (viewed as an ethical mandate) the therapist enlists the client's volitional engagement in therapy. The client who is not willing to proceed may be screened out from treatment *a priori* (e.g., Bieling, McCabe, & Antony, 2006; Linehan, 1993), which underscores the fact that willingness or volition may be viewed as a prerequisite for treatment in some outcome-focused approaches. The basic point, as with behavior therapy, is that in practice many cognitive-behavioral therapists value volitional engagement, that is to say, autonomous motivation, in their clients.

Beyond an emphasis on transparency, which typically plays its most important role at the beginning of the therapy relationship, in the CBT tradition the client-counselor relationship can be used to support client motivation in ways that are more controlling or more autonomy supportive. Dialectical behavior therapy (DBT) is an adaptation of CBT that draws on other traditions and has been used primarily in the treatment of borderline personality disorder. Linehan (1993) has suggested that DBT therapists develop a warm relationship with the client so that the relationship can be used to provide leverage in motivating clients to undertake change; the threat of withdrawing a valued relationship can be enough to get the uncooperative or unwilling client to re-engage in therapy. In this respect, the relationship can thus be used in a controlling way, as a reward or external motivator, in terms of the continuum of motivation.

Potentially at the more autonomy supportive end of the continuum would be the kind of *collaborative empiricism* recommended in cognitive therapy (Beck &

Weishaar, 2008), a distinct approach to therapy that shares much in common with CBT. Here, client and therapist work collaboratively to identify examples of the client's distorted thinking that presumably are contributing to the client's current problems; client and therapist then work together to replace the distorted cognitions with more adaptive alternatives, trying them out in the laboratory of the client's daily life. Successes and failures can be discussed at the next session, and the process can be repeated as necessary. The collaborative nature of the relationship is intended to promote client identification with the goals and process of treatment, and through the process of joint "exploration and discovery" (Beck, Rush, Shaw, & Emery, 1979, p. 32) to promote what in the continuum of motivation would be considered more internal or autonomous motivation in the client. The relationship, in other words, serves an autonomy supportive role. Indeed, within the cognitive therapy tradition therapists are encouraged to emphasize empowering clients to make their own choices, in the context of a relationship characterized by the more 'humanistic' qualities of empathy and warmth (e.g., Beck, Freeman, & Associates, 1990). Notably, efforts have been made in recent work to explicitly integrate the concept of autonomy within cognitive behavioral interventions (Britton, Patrick, Wenzel, & Williams, 2011; Dwyer, Hornsey, Smith, Oei, & Dingle, 2011).

Psychodynamic Approaches

Contemporary psychodynamic approaches, which have evolved from Freud's psychoanalytic perspective, tend to be more process-oriented than outcome-oriented. Psychodynamic approaches include, for example, ego psychology, self-psychology, interpersonal psychoanalysis, and object-relations approaches. Although there are important differences, all appreciate that human behavior is motivated by conscious and unconscious forces, and that these different sources of motivation can lead to conflict that at times manifests itself as symptoms. Psychodynamic approaches place great emphasis on the role of the relationship in understanding and working with client motivation. Key concepts in this regard include transference, resistance, and transparency.

Before turning to these concepts, an initial distinction needs to be made. Psychodynamic psychotherapy can be either *supportive* or *insight-oriented* (Dewald, 1969; Wolitzky, 2003). Supportive therapy is considered appropriate for clients with fewer intellectual or interpersonal resources who therefore require more direct support for their ego in the form of guidance or directives, while insight-oriented therapy allows for deeper exploration of past experiences and unconscious motivations. In terms of client motivation and the relationship, supportive therapy tends to provide more structure in the therapeutic work; this in itself does not necessarily detract from client autonomy, but to the extent that it makes use of the therapist's role as an authority who provides guidance and directives, supportive therapy would typically be engaging clients at the more external end of the motivational continuum, likely focusing on a form of external motivation called *introjection*, in which one's motivation is only partially internalized and is based on gaining another's approval or avoiding shame. On the other hand, when providing insight-oriented therapy psychodynamically oriented psychotherapists explicitly value promoting greater self-regulation in the client as "one of the basic goals of insight-oriented therapy" (Dewald, 1969, p. 109). In other words, dynamic therapists adjust the level of support for client autonomy to the degree of the client's ego strength.

Within psychodynamic approaches, *transference* refers to a relationship process that has important implications for working with client motivation (Gill, 1982). Transference reflects the understanding that feelings from early relationships, typically with caregivers or other influential figures, carry over to future relationships. These feelings become activated in the context of a relationship with someone who resembles the early caregiver in some important respect; typically this process happens unconsciously. When transference takes place in the context of the therapeutic relationship, the therapist's task is to help the client to separate past experiences from present reality, thereby freeing the client from past determinisms. In a sense, then, working with transference is about enhancing clients' autonomy, specifically, their ability to engage their present experiences in relationships at a more reflective level, disentangling them from past experiences, and to integrate them into their sense of self. For Freud, especially when transference with the therapist was positive it could contribute to client motivation for therapy. This is because, in addition to attributing competence and authority to the therapist, a positive transference also implied positive feelings toward the therapist. In motivational terms, such idealization of the therapist could help to move client motivation along the continuum from external regulation to introjection and, possibly, identification. We tend to value those to whom we attribute competence, especially when we like and feel connected to them, and this valuing tends to promote internalization.

On the other hand, clients often demonstrate *resistance*. That is, they can experience a lack of willingness, or even opposition, to moving forward in therapy. Such resistances can be related to transference, to the extent that strong, negative feelings toward a past relationship figure may be activated (again, typically unconsciously) in the presence of the therapist. They can also, however, reflect other defensive processes at work in the client (Gill, 1982). Importantly, for the psychodynamic therapist resistance does not represent a failure in motivation on the client's part; rather, resistance is something to be explored with the client, with interest and curiosity, in order to understand the purpose it is serving in the moment. Indeed, exploration of resistance in an open, respectful, nonjudgmental atmosphere can go a long way toward deepening the client's interest, curiosity, and therefore motivation for participating in the therapeutic process (Gabbard, 2005; Schafer, 1983). Motivation that is characterized by interest and curiosity is by definition internal. Importantly, the dynamic approach to working with resistance underscores the point that, within the psychodynamic tradition, motivation is generally viewed as a *process* that is embedded within the therapeutic relationship, rather than as a *prerequisite* before therapy can even begin. Indeed, since the time of Freud dynamic therapists have increasingly emphasized the importance of relationships in human motivation, including motivation for change (see for example Basch, 1995; Bowlby, 1988; Winnicott, 1965).

In contrast to the way it is treated in more outcome-focused approaches such as those represented by behavioral and cognitive-behavioral therapy, *transparency* about the procedures and goals of therapy may not be as explicit in psychodynamic approaches. In part, this reflects the psychodynamic principle that important aspects of motivation, including the possibility of various defensive processes, remain unconscious within the client, especially at the beginning of therapy. Within this framework, transparency does not carry the same meaning as it does from the behavioral and cognitive behavioral perspectives. Client assent remains of critical importance, but it is more about assent to a process than assent to a set of goals, where the process reflects a willingness to engage in self-exploration within the context of the therapeutic relationship.

Existential-Humanistic Traditions

Often grouped together are the existential and humanistic perspectives; both are process-oriented and begin with the assumption that growth is an inherent propensity of living things and that the therapist's job, when working with the client, is to remove the obstacles to growth. A corollary of this assumption is that the therapist cannot instill motivation into the client from outside, but can only foster and promote the client's own motivation for change and growth.

Drawing upon existentialist philosophy, with its emphasis on freedom and responsibility, existentially oriented therapists focus on client autonomy from the start of the therapeutic relationship. Autonomy is an explicit value within the existential approach, but beyond this, existential therapists call attention to the tension between freedom and responsibility that most clients experience, a tension that leads to anxiety. At its heart, the kind of existential anxiety that clients face is about choice, that is, about the engagement of their autonomy: not just choice about whether to pursue this relationship over that relationship, or this career opportunity over that career opportunity. Rather, the key choice with which clients are faced is the choice about whether or not to live *authentically*, that is, "to be aware of what is real and genuine (without distortion or defense) as well as to be the author of one's existence, taking responsibility and engaging one's freedom" (Ryan et al., 2011, p. 225). Thus the choice to live authentically includes within itself the choice to engage one's autonomy. Transparency is valued as a quality of the relationship, rather than as an upfront obligation to spell out the goals and methods to be used, although in the interest of authenticity therapists are encouraged to remove the shroud of mystery that often surrounds these, as well (Yalom, 2002). A major task of the therapist is to promote client autonomy, beginning with the client's motivation for being in therapy (or choosing to leave it) and including the client's responsibility for the problems he or she is experiencing in life. Yalom described the therapist's role in this process in this way:

> My task was to remove obstacles blocking my patient's path. I did not have to do the entire job; I did not have to inspirit the patient with the desire to grow, with curiosity, will, zest for life, caring, loyalty, or any of the myriad characteristics that make us fully human. No, what I had to do was to identify and remove obstacles. The rest would follow automatically, fueled by the self-actualizing forces within the patient. (p. 1)

Humanistic perspectives begin with the organismic principle noted above, perhaps best represented by what in Rogers' (1951) person-centered approach is called the self-actualizing tendency. A key assumption in these approaches is that human nature is "inherently trustworthy, growth-oriented, and guided by choice" (Elliot, Greenberg, & Lietaer, 2004, p. 493). Regarding client motivation and the therapeutic relationship, Rogers (1957) believed that the therapist who provided genuineness, empathy, and unconditional positive regard could create the necessary and sufficient conditions for supporting the client's own motivation in the direction of self-actualization. Typically, this is accomplished through *reflection*, the process of clarifying the client's motivation for change as well as the barriers to change that exist for the client.

Also relevant for understanding client motivation are Rogers' views on the self-concept. Basically, Rogers argued that because we are capable of thinking about ourselves both as we actually, currently are and as we would ideally like to see ourselves, the possibility exists for us to experience ourselves as falling short of our personal ideal (Rogers, 1961). When this happens, we experience a decrement to self-esteem that plays an important role in motivating many people to seek counseling. Rogers believed that clients could come closer to their ideal view of self in the context of a therapeutic relationship characterized by genuineness, empathy, and unconditional positive regard (Rogers & Dymond, 1954). Importantly, recent empirical work has shown that people feel closer to their ideal view of self in relationships they experience as autonomy supportive (Lynch, La Guardia, & Ryan, 2009).

Thus, client autonomy is valued by therapists within each of these theoretical traditions, behavioral, cognitive-behavioral, psychodynamic, and existential-humanistic. Although it is not in every case self-evident that autonomy as a construct is consistent with the theoretical framework underlying each of these traditions (Ryan et al., 2011), in practice therapists across traditions prefer to work with clients whose motivation for being in counseling is autonomous rather than pressured or controlled. Further, they see themselves and the therapeutic relationship as playing a role, whether in screening out clients *a priori* whose motivation is not adequate or in fostering client autonomy through therapist attitudes and practices such a transparency, providing structure, working collaboratively, showing interest and curiosity, being nonjudgmental and accepting, and taking the client's perspective. At this point I would like to turn to another theoretical perspective, self-determination theory (SDT), that explicitly acknowledges the importance of autonomy, not only as an aspect of motivation, but as an essential factor in human development and relationships.

Self-Determination Theory and Client Motivation

Early empirical work within the self-determination theory tradition established the importance of the distinction between intrinsic motivation and extrinsic motivation, and from this early work emerged the continuum of motivation described earlier in this chapter (see Deci & Ryan, 1985). As noted, the continuum fundamentally suggests that motivation for activity in any domain of behavior can be described in terms of its relative autonomy, or, in attributional terms, in terms of the perceived locus of causality.

Self-determination theory (SDT) introduces another important set of constructs that have relevance for understanding client motivation and the role of the client-therapist relationship in promoting client motivation. Specifically, SDT argues that all humans have a set of three basic psychological needs, the satisfaction of which is essential for growth and well-being. These are the needs for relatedness, for competence, and for autonomy. SDT suggests these basic needs are an inherent aspect of human nature and thus play a critical role in human development. In brief, relatedness refers to the need to experience meaningful and reciprocal closeness in relationships with others; competence has to do with the need to feel effective and optimally challenged in one's environment; and autonomy, which is drawn from the existential tradition, pertains to the need to feel oneself to be the author of one's actions, to be able to make choices and to be, authentically, oneself. Relationships and contexts which support the satisfaction of these needs tend to promote more internal motivation and well-being, whereas relationships and contexts that inhibit or thwart satisfaction of the needs tend to be associated with external motivation or even avoidance, and with ill-being.

Although relatedness and competence undoubtedly play an important role, thus far much of the research that has explored the application of SDT to psychotherapy has focused on the need for autonomy (Britton, Williams, & Connor, 2008; Pelletier, Tuson, & Haddad, 1997; Zuroff et al., 2007). In a recent study that touches on both relatedness and autonomy, Lynch (2013) found evidence that people were more willing to turn to partners for emotional support in relationships in which they felt both secure attachment and autonomy support from the relationship partner. Although this study looked at everyday relationships rather than the client-therapist relationship, it underscores the relevance of the *quality* of the relationship for people's willingness to seek emotional support. Prior research has, in fact, identified important benefits for clients when their motivation for counseling is autonomous: they tend to stay in therapy longer, to derive more benefit from therapy, and to maintain therapy-related change longer than clients whose motivation for therapy is pressured or controlled (Lynch et al., 2011; Ryan et al., 2011). Further, the research suggests that counselors' way of being with the client can have a direct impact on the quality of the client's motivation for counseling. Specifically, when clients experience their therapist as being autonomy supportive (rather than controlling), their motivation for participating in their own therapy tends to become more internal and self-regulated, that is, more autonomous, even if it started out at the external end of the continuum of motivation. Within the SDT framework, motivation is dynamic and responsive to cues and affordances in the interpersonal environment, underscoring the crucial role played by the therapeutic relationship in promoting client motivation.

At this point I wish to turn to a model for the therapeutic relationship recently proposed by Wampold and Budge (2012), after which I will return to clarify the role I believe that client motivation should occupy in that model.

The Relationship in Psychotherapy: Common and Specific Factors

Addressing the debate in the literature over the relative contributions of specific versus common factors in psychotherapy, Wampold and Budge (2012) proposed a model that involves three relationship pathways that bridge the gap between the basic, initial alliance between client and therapist and therapeutic outcomes. The three pathways include: (1) the real relationship between therapist and client, (2) the creation of expectation through explanation and treatment, and (3) using the specific ingredients of treatment to induce the client to participate in healthy actions. In the model, outcomes are divided into quality of life outcomes and symptom reduction outcomes. Pathways (1) and (2) mediate between the client-therapist alliance and the outcome of quality of life, while pathways (2) and (3) mediate between the alliance and symptom reduction.

The model calls for the establishment of an initial therapeutic bond or alliance between client and therapist. Among other things, the establishment of this alliance is based on the client's assessment (often rapid, involving both conscious and unconscious processes) of the therapist's trustworthiness. Wampold and Budge (2012) address client motivation at this initial phase of therapy, arguing that the ability to form an alliance "will be augmented when the patient affirmatively seeks the treatment for felt distress" (p. 606). In other words, in line with the major approaches to psychotherapy discussed earlier in this chapter, the model acknowledges the benefits of client willingness (autonomy, volition) in seeking professional assistance. Citing the paper by Ryan and colleagues (2011), the authors further acknowledged that the client's "motivation for change can impact the patient's engagement while in therapy" (p. 606) even after the formation of the alliance; they do not, however, further address the role of motivation with respect to the three relationship pathways, to which I now turn.

The model proposed by Wampold and Budge (2012) suggests that, once an alliance has been successfully established, there are "three pathways through which the relationship acts to produce therapeutic benefit" (p. 607). The first pathway, called the *real relationship*, refers to a "transference-free genuine relationship based on realistic perceptions" (p. 607). The real relationship, also referred to in the model as 'belongingness' and 'social connection,' is beneficial, that is, therapeutic, because it is a "relationship with an important and significant other who is invested in the patient's well being" (Wampold & Budge, p. 611). As the existential and humanistic traditions argue, the relationship itself is healing. Ultimately, the therapeutic virtue of the relationship stems, as the authors argue, from the fact that connectedness is essential for survival among human beings. In other words, Wampold and Budge are here invoking what in SDT are referred to as basic psychological needs, the social-emotional nutriments considered essential for well-being, growth, and development that serve as fundamental human motives. In essence, they are making a motivational argument: what is therapeutic about this first relationship pathway, called the *real relationship* in the model, is that it provides an opportunity for clients to satisfy the basic psychological need for relatedness. As noted, in the Wampold-Budge model, the *real relationship* pathway produces benefits for quality of life rather than symptom reduction, *per se*.

The second relationship pathway is called *creation of expectations*. Here, the idea is that the relationship with the therapist engenders hope in the client, hope that 'things can get better.' On the one hand, the very act of seeking services can engender hope, even before any relationship with the therapist has been established. But the relationship provides a critical component. Specifically, partly because the therapist has been imbued, within the culture, with a certain authority and recognized expertise, leading the client to attribute to the therapist a certain power to help, and partly because the therapist provides words and actions that tap into the purportedly universal power of ritual, the client accepts the therapist's *adaptive explanation* of the problems the client is experiencing. Further, embedded within the therapist's adaptive explanation is the implicit promise that there is a means of action that, when followed, will lead to positive change. Both the adaptive explanation and relevant therapeutic tasks are essential elements in this relationship pathway. Thus, once the client has accepted the adaptive explanation, the client develops the expectation that participating in the therapeutic actions (also described as therapeutic rituals) will allow the client to gain control or mastery over his or her problems. Wampold and Budge (2012) explain this process in terms of the development of self-efficacy beliefs. That is, as with the first relationship pathway – the *real relationship* – this second pathway, too, derives its therapeutic impact from what is fundamentally a motivational process. In their model, *creation of expectations* has a direct beneficial impact on both therapeutic outcomes, that is, on both quality of life and symptom reduction.

The third relationship pathway is called *participation in healthy actions*. With this third pathway, Wampold and Budge (2012) emphasize that the engagement in therapeutic tasks noted in the second pathway does more than create positive expectations of change. Successful therapy leads the client to participate in activities that are in themselves helpful – for example, by replacing maladaptive behavior patterns with more adaptive ones. Such would be activities and tasks that lead to greater integration into the wider community of family, work and society. Because therapeutic activities and tasks address a specific deficit or provide a specific coping skill, the benefits that accrue from this third relationship pathway have an impact on symptom reduction. Note that, because the authors speak of *inducing* the client to engage in these helpful tasks, there is a motivational aspect to this third pathway, as well. Although they do not elaborate on what it means for the therapist to 'induce' client behavior, the image created is one of the therapist acting on the client from the outside. I will return to this point, below.

In sum, the model proposed by Wampold and Budge (2012) prescinds from the debate between common versus specific factors and views the "effectiveness of therapy as a holistic process" (p. 618). In this model, "the characteristics of attachment/belongingness, empathy, and expectations provide a neurological and social context for establishing a real relationship, therapeutically creating expectations, and participating in healthy actions that all contribute to positive outcomes with the psychotherapy process" (p. 618).

Conclusion: A Motivational Modification of the Model

Wampold and Budge (2012) have proposed a model that purports to explain the beneficial effects of psychotherapy in terms of the therapeutic relationship. I would like to conclude by suggesting that the model of the therapeutic relationship that they have proposed is substantially a motivational model. First, the model explicitly acknowledges the importance of client motivation upon entering therapy, in terms of its potential to affect the working alliance. Although Wampold and Budge did not state it, implicit was a recognition that it is not just the quantity but the *quality* of client motivation that matters (indeed, as noted, they cited the Ryan et al. 2011 paper when addressing the relation between client motivation and the alliance). In other words, their model implicitly acknowledges the relevance of *autonomous* motivation for counseling. I suggest, in line with Ryan and colleagues (2011), that the role of autonomous motivation be made explicit in the model.

Furthermore, the therapeutic impact of the first two relationship pathways in the Wampold-Budge model can be attributed to processes that are essentially motivational in nature: the *real relationship* yields therapeutic benefits precisely because it taps into a basic psychological need for relatedness shared species-wide by all human beings, and the *creation of expectations* depends for its impact on the relevance of efficacy beliefs, discussed earlier in the chapter in the context of cognitive-behavioral approaches to motivation. In self-determination theory terms, self-efficacy can be reframed in terms of the basic psychological need for competence, although, as noted earlier, SDT would emphasize that self-efficacy and autonomy are orthogonal constructs. The third pathway, inducing client participation in healthy actions, implies a motivational role for the therapist; in light of Ryan and colleagues (2011), I would suggest this role would best be accomplished through the adoption of an autonomy supportive stance on the part of the therapist: as empirical evidence in the SDT tradition indicates, the quality of the motivation with which one engages in therapeutic activities – whether more autonomous, or more controlled – has important implications for the degree to which the client will internalize his or her experience, persist in change, and experience benefit.

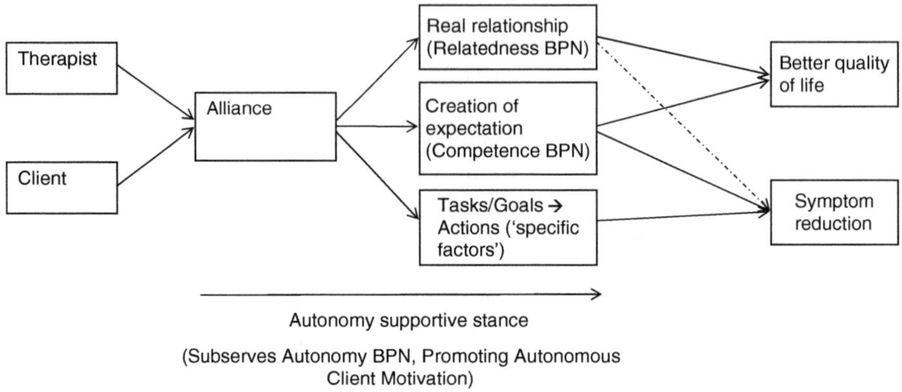

Fig. 14.1 Motivational modification of the relationship in psychotherapy model (Adapted from Wampold and Budge 2012). *BPN* basic psychological need

On this basis, I would like to propose a modification of the Wampold and Budge (2012) model of the therapeutic relationship that specifically incorporates the role of motivation. The model is depicted in Fig. 14.1. As underscored by Ryan and colleagues (2011, Lynch et al. 2011), the client's autonomous motivation is facilitated through an autonomy supportive stance on the part of the therapist. This stance operates at the very start of the relationship and facilitates the development of the alliance. Because client motivation remains important throughout, and is responsive to aspects of the interpersonal situation, the client-therapist relationship is ideally characterized as autonomy supportive in an ongoing way, permeating the three relationship processes specified in the model.

The first pathway, called the *real relationship* by Wampold and Budge (2012), can be understood in terms of the basic psychological need for relatedness. This motivational principle describes both process and content, that is, it pertains both to the quality of the relationship and the nature of the interactions between client and therapist and to the fact that the relationship itself is healing. In line with SDT, along with warmth and dependability, an autonomy supportive stance on the therapist's part is expected to foster the kind of relationship that satisfies the need for relatedness. This is because autonomy support involves taking interest in the other's point of view, and is closely linked with authenticity in the existential tradition. An authentic relationship is a real relationship, in the sense proposed by Wampold and Budge. As noted in Fig. 14.1, I believe it is possible that this relationship pathway may also have an impact on symptom reduction, to the extent that many client problems are linked to relationship difficulties; the therapeutic relationship, as noted by Yalom (2002), is, after all, a dress rehearsal for life.

The second pathway, *creation of expectations*, can be conceptualized in terms of the basic psychological need for competence. The cognitive expectations, as derived from self-efficacy theory and described in terms of self-efficacy beliefs, are critical for motivation: believing that action leads to outcome and that I am capable of the action are both essential components or perhaps prerequisites of motivation. But the reason why this second relationship pathway is both motivating and *healing* is because it, too, taps into a basic, human psychological need, the need for competence, the satisfaction of which leads to well-being. Trying out new, adaptive behaviors that are optimally challenging provides opportunities for experiencing competence. Again, because self-efficacy and autonomy are orthogonal, the therapist's autonomy supportive stance in facilitating the client's self-efficacy beliefs (and self-efficacy efforts, in relation to the tasks of therapy) remains important.

The third relationship pathway involves what Wampold and Budge refer to as *inducing* the client to participate in healthy behaviors. In line with SDT (Lynch et al., 2011; Ryan et al., 2011), I suggest that this therapeutic relationship pathway is best served if therapists facilitate their clients' internal, autonomous motivation for engaging in the relevant therapeutic tasks by adopting an autonomy supportive stance. (The term 'induce' carries the unfortunate connotation of applying pressure from outside to bring about an outcome, perhaps artificially or even prematurely, as when a medical professional induces labor. *Evoking* – literally, 'calling forth' – might be a motivationally more appropriate term.) The motivational continuum suggests that clients can engage in therapeutic activities for reasons that are either more external or more internal, and therapists can motivate their clients in ways that are more controlling or more autonomy supportive; the research, however, suggests that the results will be better internalized and more beneficial when the client's motivation is further toward the internal, that is, autonomous, end of the continuum. Toward this end, tasks and goals can be decided on collaboratively, in line with the cognitive therapy tradition.

This leads me to return to a point with which the chapter began: that client motivation, specifically autonomous motivation, is a central aspect of the therapeutic process (Lynch et al., 2011; Ryan et al., 2011). It plays a critical role in whether clients will seek to initiate a counseling relationship, and, as underscored in my revised version of Wampold and Budge's (2012) model, is an essential element in what it is that makes the therapy relationship effective, beneficial, and healing.

References

Antony, M. M., & Roemer, L. (2003). Behavior therapy. In A. S. Gurman & S. Messer (Eds.), *Essential psychotherapies* (pp. 182–223). New York: Guilford.

Bandura, A. (1989). Human agency in social cognitive theory. *The American Psychologist, 44*, 1175–1184.

Bandura, A. (1996). *Self-efficacy: The exercise of control*. New York: Freeman.

Basch, M. F. (1995). *Doing brief psychotherapy*. New York: Basic Books.

Beck, A. T., Freeman, A., & Associates. (1990). *Cognitive therapy of personality disorders*. New York: Guilford.

Beck, A. T., Rush, A. J., Shaw, B. F., & Emery, G. (1979). *Cognitive therapy of depression*. New York: Guilford.

Beck, A. T., & Weishaar, M. E. (2008). Cognitive therapy. In R. J. Corsini & D. Wedding (Eds.), *Current psychotherapies* (8th ed., pp. 263–294). Belmont, CA: Thomson Brooks/Cole.

Bieling, P. J., McCabe, R. E., & Antony, M. M. (2006). *Cognitive-behavior therapy in groups*. New York: Guilford Press.

Bowlby, J. (1988). *A secure base: Clinical applications of attachment theory*. New York: International Universities Press.

Britton, P. C., Patrick, H., Wenzel, A., & Williams, G. C. (2011). Integrating motivational interviewing and self-determination theory with cognitive behavioral therapy to prevent suicide. *Cognitive and Behavioral Practice, 18*, 16–27.

Britton, P. C., Williams, G. C., & Conner, K. R. (2008). Self-determination theory, motivational interviewing, and the treatment of clients with acute suicidal ideation. *Journal of Clinical Psychology, 64*, 52–66.

Caprara, G. V., & Cervone, D. (2000). *Personality: Determinants, dynamics and potentials*. Cambridge, UK: Cambridge University Press.

Carter, J. A. (2011). Changing light bulbs: Practice, motivation, and autonomy. *The Counseling Psychologist, 39*, 261–266.

Deci, E. L., & Ryan, R. M. (1985). *Intrinsic motivation and self-determination in human behavior*. New York: Plenum.

Dewald, P. A. (1969). *Psychotherapy: A dynamic approach*. New York: Basic Books.

Dwyer, L. A., Hornsey, M. J., Smith, L. G., Oei, T. P., & Dingle, G. A. (2011). Participant autonomy in cognitive behavioral group therapy: An integration of self-determination and cognitive behavioral theories. *Journal of Social and Clinical Psychology, 30*, 24–46.

Elliot, R., Greenberg, L. S., & Lietaer, G. (2004). Research on experiential psychotherapies. In M. J. Lambert (Ed.), *Bergin and Garfield's handbook of psychotherapy and behavior change* (5th ed., pp. 493–539). New York: Wiley.

Gabbard, G. O. (2005). *Psychodynamic psychiatry in clinical practice* (4th ed.). Washington, DC: American Psychiatric Publishing.

Gill, M. M. (1982). *The analysis of transference: Vol. I. Theory and technique*. Madison: International Universities Press.

Kim, B. S. K. (2011). Client motivation and multicultural counseling. *The Counseling Psychologist, 39*, 267–275.

Linehan, M. M. (1993). *Cognitive-behavioral treatment of borderline personality disorder*. New York: Guilford.

Lynch, M. F. (2013). Attachment, autonomy, and emotional reliance: A multilevel model. *Journal of Counseling and Development, 91*(3), 301–312.

Lynch, M. F., La Guardia, J. G., & Ryan, R. M. (2009). On being yourself in different cultures: Ideal and actual self-concept, autonomy support, and well-being in China, Russia, and the United States. *The Journal of Positive Psychology, 4*, 290–304.

Lynch, M. F., Vansteenkiste, M., Deci, E. L., & Ryan, R. M. (2011). Autonomy as process and outcome: Revisiting cultural and practical issues in motivation for counseling. *The Counseling Psychologist, 39*, 286–302.

Meichenbaum, D. (1986). Cognitive-behavior modification. In F. H. Kanfer & A. P. Goldstein (Eds.), *Helping people change* (3rd ed., pp. 346–380). New York: Pergamon.

Pelletier, L. G., Tuson, K. M., & Haddad, N. K. (1997). Client motivation for therapy scale: A measure of intrinsic motivation, extrinsic motivation, and amotivation for therapy. *Journal of Personality Assessment, 68*, 414–435.

Rogers, C. R. (1951). *Client-centered therapy*. Boston: Houghton-Mifflin.

Rogers, C. R. (1957). The necessary and sufficient conditions of therapeutic change. *Journal of Consulting and Clinical Psychology, 21*, 95–100.

Rogers, C. R. (1961). *On becoming a person: A therapist's view of psychotherapy*. Boston: Houghton Mifflin.

Rogers, C. R., & Dymond, R. F. (Eds.). (1954). *Psychotherapy and personality change*. Chicago: University of Chicago Press.

Ryan, R. M., & Connell, J. P. (1989). Perceived locus of causality and internalization: Examining reasons for acting in two domains. *Journal of Personality and Social Psychology, 57*, 749–761.

Ryan, R. M., Lynch, M. F., Vansteenkiste, M., & Deci, E. L. (2011). Motivation and autonomy in counseling, psychotherapy, and behavior change: A look at theory and practice. *The Counseling Psychologist, 39*, 193–260.

Schafer, R. (1983). *The analytic attitude*. New York: Basic Books.

Scheel, M. J. (2011). Client common factors represented by client motivation and autonomy. *The Counseling Psychologist, 39*, 276–285.

Skinner, B. F. (1953). *Science and human behavior*. New York: The Free Press.

Skinner, B. F. (1974). *About behaviorism*. New York: Knopf.

Steketee, G. S. (1993). *Treatment of obsessive compulsive disorder*. New York: Guilford.

Wampold, B. E., & Budge, S. L. (2012). The 2011 Leona Tyler award address: The relationship – And its relationship to the common and specific factors of psychotherapy. *The Counseling Psychologist, 40*, 601–623.

Watson, J. B. (1913). Psychology as the behaviorist views it. *Psychological Review, 20*, 158–177.

Westra, H. A., Dozois, D. J. A., & Marcus, M. (2007). Expectancy, homework compliance, and initial change in cognitive behavioral therapy for anxiety. *Journal of Consulting and Clinical Psychology, 75*, 363–373.

Winnicott, D. W. (1965). *Maturational processes and the facilitating environment*. Madison, CT: International Universities Press.

Wolitzky, D. L. (2003). The theory and practice of traditional psychoanalytic treatment. In A. S. Gurman & S. Messer (Eds.), *Essential psychotherapies* (pp. 24–68). New York: Guilford.

Yalom, I. D. (2002). *The gift of therapy*. New York: Harper Collins.

Zuroff, D. C., Koestner, R., Moskowitz, D. S., McBride, C., Bagby, M., & Marshall, M. (2007). Autonomous motivation for therapy: A new non-specific predictor of outcome in brief treatments of depression. *Psychotherapy Research, 17*, 137–148.

Chapter 15
Self-Determination and the Patient-Health Practitioner Relationship

Geoffrey C. Williams

Introduction

Self-Determination Theory (SDT; Deci & Ryan, 2000; Ryan & Deci, 2000) is a general theory of human motivation and has been successfully applied in many life domains, including the health domain (Ryan, Patrick, Deci, & Williams, 2008). It is our thesis that SDT is uniquely suited among theories to research the doctor patient relationship, as well as to use its principles of supporting human needs for autonomy, competence and relatedness to guide health care practitioners, medical educators, medical ethicists, policy makers, and insurers to improve patient mental health, physical health, quality of life, and the cost-effective delivery of care. Interestingly, biomedical ethics (Beauchamp & Childress, 2001, 2009) and medical professionalism (American Board of Internal Medicine [ABIM], 2002) have elevated enhancing patient autonomy to a primary outcome of health care, equivalent to that of improving length and quality of life. These changes are mandated for health practitioners and create the context of the practitioner-patient relationship. With these changes, no further empirical verification is needed to justify whether or not practitioners should support patient autonomy. Interventions that do not respect patient autonomy (e.g., interventions that thwart or undermine patient autonomy) need to be excluded from practice because they fail to meet standards of ethical care and medical professionalism (see Table 15.1 for the top goals of medicine).

SDT is uniquely positioned among motivation theories to inform health care because it provides measures for patient perceptions of need supportiveness (including autonomy support), patient autonomy, and perceived competence. The SDT model for health behavior provides a framework on how interventions designed to support patient psychological needs also result in enhanced physical and mental health

G.C. Williams, MD, PhD (✉)
Departments of Medicine and Clinical and Social Sciences in Psychology, University of Rochester, Rochester, NY, USA
e-mail: Geoffrey_Williams@URMC.Rochester.edu

N. Weinstein (ed.), *Human Motivation and Interpersonal Relationships: Theory, Research, and Applications*, DOI 10.1007/978-94-017-8542-6_15,

Table 15.1 Fundamental principles of MEDICAL PROFESSIONALISM IN THE NEW MILLENNIUM: A PHYSICIAN CHARTER

Principle of primacy of patient welfare. The principle is based on a dedication to serving the interest of the patient. Altruism contributes to the trust that is central to the physician-patient relationship. Market forces, societal pressures, and administrative exigencies must not compromise this principle
Principle of patient autonomy. Physicians must have respect for patient autonomy. Physicians must be honest with their patients and empower them to make informed decisions about their treatment. Patients' decisions about their care must be paramount, as long as those decisions are in keeping with ethical practice and do not lead to demands for inappropriate care
Principle of social justice. The medical profession must promote justice in the health care system, including the fair distribution of health care resources. Physicians should work actively to eliminate discrimination in health care, whether based on race, gender, socioeconomic status, ethnicity, religion, or any other social category

outcomes based on a meta-analysis of 184 health-related studies (Ng et al., 2012). Finally, building on SDT and medical ethics we will discuss the importance of practitioner-patient relationships in the prevention and treatment of cardiovascular diseases, diabetes, cancer, and somatization. Please proceed if you are willing.

The Goals of Health Care, Our Code of Biomedical Ethics, and Self-Determination Theory

In order to understand the practitioner-patient relationship and the explanatory role that SDT plays in that relationship, it is important to first understand the context, or social surround, in which the relationship exists. The context of the practitioner-patient relationship is represented by medicine's code of ethics with patients and society (Beauchamp & Childress, 2009). As of 2002, health care professionals from around the world have a parallel Charter of Medical Professionalism (ABIM, 2002) that also supports this code of ethics. The ethics are intended to ensure that patients who enter relationships with practitioners will find them *competent* and *trustworthy* to provide expert advice to the patient and society on matters of health and wellbeing. Expert advice is intended to close a perceived competence gap for patients. The code of medical ethics is an implied contract for practitioners to follow in working with their patients.

To further understand this contract, consider what motivates people to go to health care practitioners and what motivates practitioners to see patients. Patients want to improve or maintain their health based on the recommendations and treatments provided by those who they perceive can improve the likelihood they can reach their health goals as well as their other life goals that depend on being healthy. Patients' aspiration for good health is intrinsic (Grouzet et al., 2005; Williams, 2002), but many health-related behaviors they are asked to engage in are extrinsically motivated (e.g., getting a colonoscopy, or taking a medication to lower cholesterol). Practitioners care for patients in part for extrinsic reasons (payment).

At the same time, they can derive intrinsic motivation through interest and curiosity about their work as well as satisfaction of their needs for perceived competence, relatedness to their patients and colleagues, and autonomy afforded by their work (American College of Physicians, 2005). Thus, patients and practitioners have a complex mix of intrinsic and extrinsic motives regarding their relationship and behaviors, making SDT relevant to the practitioner-patient relationship. The recent addition of respecting and enhancing patient autonomy to this code of ethics (Beauchamp & Childress, 2001, 2009) makes SDT even more important in understanding the practitioner relationship and how ethical and professional health care is delivered.

Around 12 years ago, biomedical ethics and medical professionalism identified three equally valued and highest goals of medicine. The first goal, or ethic, is primacy of patient welfare, which involves working to improve the welfare of patients and society. This combines the principles of 'do no harm' from Hippocrates (circa 400 BC; The Hippocratic Oath, 1943), and 'beneficence', which means to intervene actively when patient health can be improved, and to inform patients of potential outcomes of treatment and costs of care. This means practitioners cannot meet professional standards of care if they do not provide an opinion or recommendation regarding a treatment known to improve or preserve health. The second goal is that practitioners must respect (i.e., support) patient autonomy. Practitioners must be honest with their patients and empower them to make informed decisions about their treatment. The elevation of the respect for patient autonomy in these recent updates means that practitioner autonomy support and patient autonomy have become mandated medical outcomes in and of themselves which need no empirical support to justify measuring them or to train all practitioners and health care systems how to provide care that supports patient autonomy. The third goal is for practitioners to support equal access to care for all patients and to avoid discrimination. These ethics and goals of professionalism form the social surround in which the practitioner-patient relationship exists.

It may be surprising to some that professionalism already mandates practitioners act to support autonomy in all interventions. It may also be unexpected to many patients that they need to take responsibility for their own treatment. Until autonomy was elevated to primary outcome of care in 2000 AD, clinicians, researchers, and many patients assumed that patients were simply supposed to do what the doctor said to do. This bias is most evident in the controlling definitions of compliance and adherence to treatment outcomes that are used pervasively in the health care field by clinicians, public health policy makers, and researchers alike. Compliance and adherence are expressed as percentages of the amount of patient behavior divided by what is recommended by the health authority, and interventions are interpreted in the health outcomes research to be successful or not based on whether patients behave as the authority prescribes they do. Medical studies categorize all noncompliant patients as 'negative outcomes', thus possibly diminishing and obscuring the positive effects of interventions that respect patient autonomy have on both quality and length of life. Studies that report adherence and compliance outcomes are likely to underestimate the health effects and cost effectiveness of interventions that enhance patient autonomy.

With the new ethic's mandate for autonomy, interventions that increase compliance through coercion or pressure are likely to be unethical and unprofessional because they intend to control patient behavior, rather than enhance patient autonomy in order to show an increase in compliant behaviors. Further, research about interventions that work by controlling patients are at risk of being irrelevant to delivery of health care because patients can choose freely whether they accept recommended treatments or not. This makes the control paradigm that underlies compliance research largely irrelevant to the practice of twenty-first century medicine, and quite possibly implies such research conduct is unethical and unprofessional.

The new code of biomedical ethics and professionalism mandates that an autonomy paradigm, rather than a control paradigm, be used to research and deliver health care interventions. Interventions need to enhance autonomy, or at least be *intended* to enhance autonomy, and therefore should be tested in a manner that promotes the development of autonomy. SDT is relevant to this new paradigm in several ways. Outcomes in SDT studies are tested under free choice conditions, which are the same conditions in which medicine is practiced. In addition, SDT is the only theory that provides guidance on the role of autonomy in human experience. This includes providing a mechanism of how autonomy changes (internalization), how to measure it directly, and which interventions enhance autonomy. SDT also measures the satisfaction of the two other aspects that a professional relationship intends to provide for patients: a perception of being able to competently improve or maintain patient health (perceived patient and practitioner competence) and a trusting relationship (relatedness). Therefore, all three of SDT's psychological needs appear in the new autonomy paradigm of biomedical ethics and professionalism. This implies that health interventions not only need to be tested for effectiveness in enhancing patient length of life, but also need to be tested for their effects on patient perceptions of autonomy, competence, and relatedness before they are deemed ready for translation into everyday practice.

The autonomy paradigm calls for researchers, clinicians, policy makers, and educators to redefine the concept of compliance or adherence to that of patient autonomy itself. The relevant outcome of the intervention is to support patients to be as autonomous (i.e., volitional) as much as possible with regard to their health behaviors. This autonomous outcome would broadly categorize health care interventions as successful if patient autonomy was supported, even if patients choose not to follow recommended treatments. Thus, after a consultation, patients who willingly choose not to accept treatment would be considered as a positive outcome. The target of the intervention for the practitioner is now shifted to focus on facilitating the patient making an informed and volitional decision to pursue treatment (e.g., make a lifestyle change, take a medication, or to have an operation), rather than trying to control the patient into behaving by providing different levels of copays for treatments to reduce insurers' costs or by exerting interpersonal pressure to comply. The current control paradigm outcome categorizes these patients who volitionally decline treatment as failures of the intervention. According to an autonomy paradigm, these patients are coded as successes; for example in the case of a patient with terminal cancer or on dialysis who decides not to continue chemotherapy or dialysis treatments, given it is a fully autonomous decision. A few studies have begun to document the benefits of supporting autonomy and relatedness in health care. One recent study in the ICU with terminally ill patients showed that an intervention designed to elicit and support patient wishes regarding continuing intensive care treatments or not resulted in better quality of life, was more cost-effective, and that patients who received this intervention lived longer (Temel et al., 2010). This extends findings from an earlier SDT based study of patients in a long-term care facility (Kasser & Ryan, 1999) showing that patient reports of autonomy were predictive of living longer.

Studies of medication use and adoption and maintenance of healthy lifestyles do not distinguish whether patients are volitionally noncompliant or not when they do not adhere to recommended treatments (Osterberg & Blaschke, 2005). Current adherence rates are approximately 50 % for both prescribed medications and recommendations to make lifestyle changes. This is true even for patients with coronary heart disease where uses of several types of medications (aspirin, beta-blockers, LDL-cholesterol lowering medications) or being regularly physically active are known to prolong life. This does not account for the 30 % of prescriptions given to patients that are never started. An autonomy paradigm would determine those that do not want to take the medication when fully aware of the possible benefits in addition to determining those who had benefit from taking the treatment. Future care would focus on determining whether patients change their minds about accepting treatment willingly (i.e., have become autonomously oriented to the treatment), rather than expending clinician time to get them to behave, or trying to teach them how to comply. Importantly, practitioners would no longer be punished with lower income or losing their job in current 'pay for performance' schemes when their patients chose not to accept a certain treatment. These pay for performance schemes have not been shown to improve health outcomes (Kaplan, Kessler, & Greenfield, 2012) for patients, and are likely unethical because practitioners may no longer respect patient autonomy as a result of being rewarded to control patients to comply with their recommendations. SDT research, among other health care studies, indicates that patient health outcomes (e.g., length and quality of life), medication use, healthier behaviors, and particularly behavior maintenance is worse in pay for performance schemes.

The history of autonomy's evolution as a part of biomedical ethics parallels the study of the doctor-patient relationship (i.e., health psychology) and we review that briefly here. For a more in depth discussion of these issues, see Williams and Deci (2012) and Beauchamp and Childress (2001, 2009). The absence of patient autonomy from the practitioner-patient relationship and medical ethics can be traced back to the nineteenth century when Thomas Percival (1803) wrote the first modern version of biomedical ethics that included only 'do no harm' (The Hippocratic Oath, circa 400 BC, 1943) and 'beneficence'. The ethic of beneficence required practitioners to actively intervene when patient welfare could be improved, as well as to inform patients of both the side effects and costs of those treatments. Percival and most health practitioners assumed that patients would do what was recommended because the patient would always act to close the competence gap by following directions. The American Medical Association adapted Percival's ethics in the mid-1800s (Konold, 1962) and these remained unchanged until the year 2000.

Even though medical ethics did not change until the new millennium, astute researchers and clinicians noted that as medical treatments became more effective, patient motivation became increasingly important for success. The assumption that all patients would simply behave as doctors recommended began to be actively challenged starting in the 1950s and 1960s, when clinicians and health researchers noted that patients had better outcomes when they became actively involved in their care (Engel, 1961; Korsch, Gozzi, & Francis, 1968). Engel hypothesized that there were significant psychosocial aspects of disease and illness; specifically asserting that the manner in which practitioners related to their patients could affect patient outcomes (e.g., the blood sugar levels of diabetics; Engel, 1977). This association has been confirmed in several studies by employing SDT's empirical measures of practitioner need supportiveness, patient autonomy, and perceived competence (Senecal, Nouwen, & White, 2000; Williams, Freedman, & Deci, 1998; Williams, McGregor, Zeldman, Freedman, & Deci, 2004).

There are several important aspects of how these ethics and needs are relevant to health care. We turn to a brief theoretical discussion of some of these considerations before we examine the rich and growing empirical base that demonstrates when practitioners support patient psychological needs, the quality of patient motivation is enhanced and their welfare improves.

Consideration 1: Most health related behaviors are adopted for extrinsic reasons, and thus are explained in part by organismic integration theory – one of five sub-theories of SDT. Organismic integration theory states that internalization is the process in SDT by which people take on new behaviors that tend to feel external to the self and transforms the regulation of that behavior to autonomous self-regulation. The internalization process occurs naturally over time and it is facilitated when health authorities and important others (e.g., friends and family members) support patients' psychological needs. Most health professionals are paid for their consultations. In the past, these consultations were paid directly to the professional by the patient, but in recent decades, they have been shifted to third party payers. This shift has complicated the practitioner-patient relationship by introducing the possibility that practitioners might act in the interest of the payer rather than that of their patients. Pay for performance schemes are intended to do just this, and SDT theorists predict that pay for performance may undermine practitioner autonomy supportiveness because practitioner pay is withheld if their patients fail to comply with their treatments. Pay for performance is expected to forestall internalization of autonomy, to lower perceived competence, and to worsen health outcomes. This is likely to occur until patient autonomy is accepted as a primary outcome of care, practitioners are trained in how to support autonomy, and compliance outcomes are replaced by outcomes that code volitional non-adherence positively. In short, practitioners need to be responsible for their own behavior (e.g., making clear recommendations and enhancing patient autonomy regarding treatment), but practitioners should not be penalized or rewarded for making patients comply with treatment.

Instead of penalizing practitioners whose patients willing choose not to accept treatment, the health care system needs to teach and support practitioner facilitation of patient autonomous self-regulations, rather than forcing patient compliance. To optimally facilitate internalization, the practitioner-patient relationship needs to support all three SDT needs. This process of need support starts with gathering accurate information about patient concerns, health risks, behaviors, and general aspirations, while developing rapport. Need support also requires practitioners to elicit patient perspectives about their current behaviors, understanding of their diseases, and their perspectives about possible treatments. Need support also involves providing direct recommendations on how to improve or maintain health as well as acknowledging patient perspectives on the recommendations made. Information regarding diagnosis, prognosis, and effective treatment options are necessary parts of promoting autonomous self-regulation, but this information is insufficient to be motivating by itself. Eliciting patient perspectives and providing information needs to be followed by checking to see if patients are willing to accept the recommended treatments or lifestyle change. In order to facilitate internalization of autonomous self-regulation, practitioners need to acknowledge that patients can decide not to pursue recommended treatment or changes. Supporting patient initiatives for change also facilitates internalization. Unconditional positive regard and a non-judgmental relationship need to be maintained throughout care to promote internalization (please see Table 15.2 that lists current understanding of practitioner behaviors that are need supportive). These same approaches to patient care appear in Motivational Interviewing's (Resnicow & McMaster, 2012), elicit-provide-elicit model, in principles of medical interviewing (Lipkin, Putnam, & Lazare, 1995), and in informed decision-making (Woolf et al., 2005). The 5A's model for practitioners brief counseling for health behavior change recommended by the US Preventive Services Task Force (Whitlock, Orleans, Pender, & Allan, 2002) also follows this pattern: Assess risk, Advise on treatment, Agree on treatment, Assist treatment with skills building, problem solving and medications, and Arrange follow up. All of these approaches identify that respecting patient autonomy explicitly is important for facilitating change. SDT proposes that each of these approaches that respect autonomy in the context of a positive relationship will facilitate change by enhancing the process of internalization along the extrinsic continuum of autonomous motivation.

Consideration 2: Patient autonomy is to be supported in most, but not all, circumstances according to biomedical ethics and professionalism. Practitioners and policy makers are obligated to act in the interest of society in general, as well as in the interest of the individual. Patients can be denied treatments in the setting of scarce resources. A treatment can be denied if providing it would harm society in general, or if the treatment would provide no benefit to patients while using expensive resources that are needed for the care of others. In order to determine which treatments are the most beneficial, interventions that are efficacious are compared on cost-effectiveness using a standardized outcome of cost per quality adjusted life year saved (Maciosek et al., 2006). Because supporting patient autonomy motivates

Table 15.2 A list of need-supportive behaviors derived from self-determination theory

Autonomy support
1. Elicit and acknowledge the patient's perspectives and feelings
2. Explore the patient's values and how they relate to the behavior being addressed
3. Provide a clear rationale for advice given
4. Provide effective options for change and acknowledge the option of not changing
5. Support the patient's self-initiation for change
6. Minimize pressure and control
Competence support
1. Be positive that the patient can succeed
2. Provide accurate, effectance-relevant feedback
3. Identify barriers to change
4. Engage the patient in skills-building and problem-solving
5. Develop a plan that is appropriate for the patient's abilities
6. Reframe failures as short successes
Relatedness support
1. Develop empathy
2. Develop a warm, positive interpersonal relationship
3. Remain non-judgmental and provide unconditional positive regard

health behavior change (e.g., abstinence from tobacco) and is associated with improved quality of life, interventions that work by enhancing personal autonomy, relatedness, and perceived competence are likely to be more cost effective than interventions designed to work by controlling them.

Treatments that are desired by patients can be withheld if practitioners feel they are harmful to patients. Examples include providing increased doses of narcotics for someone with chronic pain or ordering prostatic specific antigen (PSA) to screen for prostate cancer. Patients can become addicted to narcotics or sell the medications to others for profit. At the same time, patients' need for pain control must be addressed as reasonably as possible. In the case of PSA, when this test is used for men without symptoms, the false positive rate is so high that more patients are harmed by the subsequent workup than benefit from treatment for the cancer. The US Preventive Services Task Force deemed PSA as harmful to patients when used to screen for new cases of the disease (Moyer, 2012). PSA can still be effectively used as a marker of disease once a diagnosis has been made, just not when initially screening for the disease.

Consideration 3: Autonomy is now a health outcome in its own right. Health care practitioners can provide effective and professional care even if their patients choose not to follow their treatments, if patients' autonomy is respected. Research is called for to determine what interventions are more effective in enhancing autonomy, relatedness, and perceived competence, and to determine the active components of these interventions.

Consideration 4: Many patients are unaware that practitioners are mandated to support/respect their autonomy. More than 50 % of patients want doctors to make the final specific recommendation regarding the treatment options for their conditions (Levinson, Kao, Kuby, & Thisted, 2005). It is autonomy-supportive to provide specific recommendations when patients ask for them, so long as it is done in a manner that does not leave patients feeling controlled by the practitioner. To force patients to make their own decision without a recommendation would be unethical (as a form of abandonment) and unprofessional, if there is evidence that one treatment would be expected to be better than another. Patients would likely experience not receiving advice to start a treatment if it is known to be effective as controlling when informed later on of the treatment. Further, forcing them to make a choice without practitioner guidance may elicit feelings of anxiety and helplessness if patients do not feel competent to make decisions. At the same time, to be autonomy supportive, practitioners need to encourage patients to actively participate in decision making whenever possible. Over time, in the context of a positive and supportive relationship, patients are expected to naturally internalize autonomous self-regulation around medical decision making, particularly once they have experience with the disease and its management. Consider the case of an adult patient with a new diagnosis of type 2 diabetes. At first, patients are scared and unfamiliar with how foods will affect their blood sugar, how to check their blood glucose, and what medications would be best for initial treatment. They are likely to have no experience with the disease or its treatment. With a supportive and caring patient-provider relationship, patients learn what raises and lowers their blood sugars often better than their doctors and they are likely to begin autonomously regulating their treatment.

In spite of the extrinsic nature of practitioner motivation for treating patients as well as the extrinsic regulations patients have for healthy behaviors, the practitioner-patient relationship can satisfy all three of SDT's psychological needs. Positive, caring interpersonal relationships between practitioners and patients are energizing for both parties (American College of Physicians, 2005). Practitioners and patients can experience increases in perceived competence and autonomy as they learn to manage their symptoms, adapt to new diagnoses, establish effective treatment plans, and participate in end of life care. Thus, the models for understanding the complexities of motivation in health care today would be best approached assessing both intrinsic and extrinsic motivation pathways over time for practitioners and patients.

Motivation and the CDC's Million Hearts Initiative

Motivation is defined within SDT as psychological energy directed at a particular goal. This definition is well suited for understanding practitioner-patient relationships because once a diagnosis is made or a health risk is identified, treatments are directed at particular health goals (e.g., having an LDL cholesterol less than 100 mg/dl) associated with longer life and better quality of life. The problem many practitioners have is that they are only taught to recommend specific health behaviors (e.g., losing weight, being physically active or taking a medication on a daily basis) to reach those goals, but do not attend to creating the kind of interpersonal climate that brings out patients' higher quality psychological energies needed by many patients to adopt and sustain the recommended health behaviors. Patients experience higher quality motivation when their practitioners support their psychological needs of autonomy, competence, and relatedness.

In order to illustrate how these needs and their support result in improved mental and physical health, consider a Centers for Disease Control (CDC) initiative called Million Hearts (Centers for Disease Control, 2012; Frieden & Berwick, 2011) that is intended to prevent one million heart attacks and strokes over 5 years. To accomplish this, the CDC calls for practitioners to deliver interventions for 4 health goals represented by the ABC's: A-appropriate use of **A**spirin; B-**B**lood pressure control; C-**C**holesterol management; and, S-**S**moking cessation. By attaining these 4 health goals, there would be 80 % fewer cardiovascular events. The challenge is how to implement the intervention in a manner that supports practitioner motivation to deliver the recommendations, and patient motivation to adopt the healthy lifestyles and use of the medications when needed. This requires practitioners and patients to know what the risks are, what the healthy targets are, and most importantly what energizes people to reach their health-related goals. The CDC and the Public Health Service have been informing health care practitioners about these goals for decades (Institute of Medicine [IOM], 2010; McGinnis & Foege, 1993; Mokdad, Marks, Stroup, & Gerberding, 2004) in a number of clinical guidelines; including those for nutrition (Dietary Guidelines for Americans, 2010), physical activity (U.S. Department of Health and Human Services, 2008), hypertension (Chobanian, Bakris, & Black, 2003), cholesterol (Expert Panel on Detection, Evaluation, and Treatment of High Blood Cholesterol in Adults, 2001), appropriate aspirin use (United States Preventive Services Task Force [USPSTF], 2009), and tobacco use and dependence (Fiore et al., 2008). The treatment goals have been evolving as new evidence is compiled. For example, the cholesterol goals are expected to change again soon based on an updated guideline from the National Cholesterol Education Program (NCEP). This update is likely to emphasize that maintaining even lower levels of low density lipoprotein cholesterol (LDL-C) over our lifetime is important to prevent cardiovascular events and lengthen life. SDT may be useful for guiding health care systems in creating need supportive work climates for health care practitioners so that they internalize a value for delivering the treatment, and providing training in how to facilitate patient internalization of autonomous self-regulation and perceived competence for these healthy behaviors. According to SDT, if the quality of the self-regulation with respect to the ABC's is autonomous, patients will live longer, and the years they live will be of better quality. Before returning to the different qualities of motivation that can underlie these health behaviors, here is a brief description of heart health related behaviors in the US.

About half of the US population has at least 1 major risk factor for cardiovascular disease that can be changed to improve heart health. Over 40 % of US citizens are inactive (less than 30 min of walking 5 days a week), one third are obese (obesity triples risk for CVD), 30 % have uncontrolled high blood pressure (CVD risk doubles for every 20 mmHg of systolic blood pressure above 115 mmHg), 21 % smoke cigarettes regularly (smoking more than triples risk for CVD), 16 % have high cholesterol (1 % increase in CVD risk for every 1 % increase LDL Cholesterol), and 10 % have diabetes (Centers for Disease Control, 2012). Diabetes is, in part, caused by too little physical activity and overeating. Once people have diabetes, their CVD risk rises so much that they have the equivalent risk of people who have already had a heart attack. High cholesterol, smoking, high blood pressure, and diabetes risks are synergistic in causing CVD (Yusuf, Hawken, & Ounpuu, 2004). Only 50 % of people who would benefit from aspirin take it daily or every other day (Maciosek et al., 2006). In 1993, The CDC clearly identified (McGinnis & Foege, 1993; Mokdad et al., 2004) that three behaviors account for about 40 % of early deaths in the US and about 70 % of health care costs. These behaviors are tobacco use, physical inactivity, and over eating. These three behaviors underlie the excess CVD risk that Million Hearts seeks to reduce and require self-regulation to change. These behaviors also cause other diseases including cancer, emphysema, and diabetes (Chiuve, McCullough, Sacks, & Rimm, 2006; Kushi, et al., 2006; Schroeder, 2007; Woolf, 2008). The fourth motivated behavior that underlies whether the American people can reach the Million Heart goals is that of medication use. A full 1/3 of initial medication prescriptions are never filled, and only 50 % of those that are filled once are continued by patients after 6 months (Osterberg & Blaschke, 2005). In order to reduce cardiovascular disease events, patients will likely need to take aspirin when appropriate, statin medications to lower LDL-cholesterol, and medications to lower blood pressure. It is the combination of healthy lifestyle and use of medications that can lower risk by 80 %. Promoting either health option alone will likely fall short of preventing CVD risks. SDT based interventions have been shown to increase autonomous self-regulation (ASR) for healthier nutrition, physical activity, smoking cessation, and taking medication and perceived competence (PC) in several randomized trials. In turn, ASR and PC predicted the health outcome, and mediated the relationships between the interventions and the health outcomes. Before examining those trials, the various qualities of motivation patients have around these behaviors will be reviewed briefly.

SDT may offer clues on how health risk information is provided by policy makers and how individual practitioners can effectively deliver these health messages so that their patients internalize a value for these goals in a manner that leaves them feeling more willing and able to attain them. At the treatment level, autonomy is reflected in a continuum of regulations that patients experience around initiating and maintaining behaviors that are known to result in improved cardiovascular health. By focusing on a need supportive approach, the Million Hearts program will also result in better quality of life because autonomous self-regulation and perceived competence are predictive of better mental health (wellbeing) in multiple studies, while simultaneously predicting initiation and maintenance of healthier behavior (Ng et al., 2012).

Organismic Integration Theory (Self-Determination Theory, 2012) proposes that people will naturally internalize a value for new challenges when they are presented to us. Our changing world has left us sedentary, stressed from overwork, and overeating, which results in weight gain. This weight gain causes high cholesterol, high blood pressure, cancer, and high blood sugar (e.g., resistance to insulin) leading to diabetes. Health interventions are intended to increase the speed with which people internalize the regulation of inactivity and overeating by checking cholesterol and blood pressure, and then acting to reduce risk. However, SDT proposes (and studies support) the quality of the regulation (e.g., energization) that results from the intervention varies along a continuum of autonomy as a function of the need supportiveness of the authority presenting the intervention. Amotivation is the lowest quality and quantity of motivation. People who are amotivated are not even willing to try to reach a particular goal, and they may also feel unable to reach it if they tried to. When people are unaware of their health risk or the benefit of a particular treatment, they are amotivated. The process of informed decision-making can result in extrinsic forms of self-regulations along the autonomy continuum if done in a need supportive manner. When we are naïve to the goal, we have no autonomous self-regulation or perception of competence that we can reach the goal. For example, many men aged 45 and older simply do not know that taking a baby aspirin each day would lower their risk of having a heart attack by 20 % and that this benefit now outweighs the possibility of experiencing serious gastrointestinal bleeding from taking the aspirin and other factors. Similarly, many women over age 55 do not know that taking a baby aspirin each day reduces their risk for an important type of stroke (ischemic stroke) by 20 % and that this offsets adverse risks. About half the people who would benefit from taking aspirin remain amotivated, or are unwilling, to take the aspirin for these benefits in part because they are unaware of whether the aspirin would benefit them. Interestingly, men do not get the stroke benefit, and women do not get the heart attack benefit from taking aspirin. So, for the over 45 year old men and the over 55 year old women with average or below risk for gastrointestinal bleeding, providing the information that aspirin use is of benefit is necessary, but not sufficient, to reduce or eliminate amotivation. Clarifying the goal and highlighting why it is important allows people to decide if they want to take aspirin or not, although they may still not believe the evidence, reject the goal behavior, and remain with high levels of amotivation. Other people begin the process of internalization after this discussion and develop extrinsic regulations for taking the aspirin. It is unlikely that patients enjoy taking an aspirin, so this behavior is not likely to be intrinsically motivated. Practitioners meet with people that reject the medical benefits of treatment everyday and because support of autonomy is mandated, learning to support patients around these decisions is important. Yet, studies of medical interviewing indicate that practitioners fail to do this in more than 80 % of encounters (Braddock, Edwards, Hasenberg, Laidley, & Levinson, 1999).

Further comments about amotivation are needed before turning to the remainder of the autonomy continuum. When behaviors are more complex than taking a pill each day, such as learning to eat in a way that maintains healthy body weight (Body Mass Index, or BMI, is between 18 and 25 kg/m^2) and to eat a diet low in saturated fats in order to lower LDL-cholesterol and reduce risk for heart attacks and strokes, perceived competence is an important part of amotivation. Repeated failures to achieve a healthy body weight, to stop smoking or lower cholesterol, coupled with the threat of a heart attack or stroke, can lead to amotivation. In this case, the amotivation results from not feeling able to achieve the desired outcome, and is comparable to learned helplessness. This is particularly so when one is at risk for cancer or heart disease from the unregulated behavior. When patients are found to be amotivated to adopt a behavior, the appropriate response from practitioners is to explore why patients have no energy to try to change. Is it because the person simply does not know about the benefit? Or is it that they do not want to do the behavior or do not feel competent to achieve the outcome? Practitioners would act differently with patients based on the whether the cause of the amotivation was unwillingness or a feeling of incompetence. Typical practitioner responses in this situation are to simply provide the information or to tell them to change. If patients are unwilling to change, listening and acknowledging patient perspectives and fully acknowledging that they do not have to change are important elements of facilitating autonomy and relatedness. In addition, practitioners can consider exploring what patients feel would need to happen before they would want to change. If patients feel unable (incompetent) to change, offer skills building, problem solving and supporting early initiatives for change, and being positive that the patients can succeed are important areas for the practitioner to cover. Merely providing the risk and benefit information again is not sufficient to motivate people to change.

Once patients accept that taking an aspirin will decrease risk, and assuming that they feel able (competent) to take a pill on a daily basis, people can experience different qualities of regulations around taking the aspirin. The next level on the continuum is that of external control. People may feel forced to take an aspirin each day because their doctor or spouse says they have to take it or because they fear that they will become sick or die if they do not. Often when people first hear of a new diagnosis such as hypertension (high blood pressure) and are asked to restrict sodium intake to less than one teaspoon per day (<1,500 mg/day), they feel externally controlled by the doctor, nutritionist, or the government who make the recommendation. For people feeling high levels of external control, they take aspirin or consume less sodium only to avoid the threat of punishment, heart attack, stroke, or death. Over time, the natural process of internalization may reduce the experience of external control and if the practitioner or authority supports psychological needs while delivering the message it may reduce the patient experience of being controlled. People who behave only because of external control are likely to stop the behavior if the contingency is removed. This happens in several ways if they no longer believe that the behavior reduces the risk. For example, if a family member, friend, or voice on the Internet questions whether there is a benefit, individuals may no longer value the outcome. Similarly, if people no longer fear death or do not want to live as a function of depression or having a life-ending disease, the contingency is removed and the behavior is expected to stop. Practitioners need to be aware that highly externally controlled people may lose their motivation suddenly and need to be ready to find out why this has happened, while still respecting patient decisions to stop (i.e., supporting autonomy and relatedness). If practitioners simply expect patients to do what they are told and their perspective is never explored, practitioners will be unaware that some patients are feeling highly controlled with respect to their prescriptions. These practitioners miss an opportunity to facilitate their patients' internalization of more autonomous regulations for taking the medication. Exploring patient reasons for taking a medication at the time of prescription and afterward may be one way to increase long-term medication use.

Introjection is the next level of regulation experienced by people on the autonomy continuum and is characterized by doing the behavior in order to avoid feeling negative emotions such as guilt or shame. An example of introjected regulation would be taking an aspirin daily to lower risk of CVD because patients feel guilty or ashamed if they do not take it. In the very common experience of introjection, the entity controlling patients are the patients themselves. The experience of introjection as a motivator is a poor quality of experience over the long term with higher levels of depression, anxiety, and somatic symptoms resulting from the internal pressure. People high in introjection are often ambivalent about the behavior – that is they feel "damned if they do it, and damned if they don't." Practitioners are likely to hear (if they listen closely) that patients feel guilty for not taking their medication or if they have relapsed to smoking after a period of abstinence. Patients often feel as though their practitioners will be mad at them for not doing as told, even if the practitioner has never expressed any such feelings.

Together, external control and introjection are frequently combined in a higher order subscale called controlled regulation. which is distinct from controlled self-regulation because the locus of causality is outside of the self. Both types of autonomous self-regulation (identified and integrate) come from within the self. Also, no clinical intervention has been shown to decrease perceptions of external control or introjections. Gains in health behaviors to date come from variations in autonomous forms of self-regulation.

Identification is the first form of autonomous self-regulation on the continuum, and is characterized by patients' perceptions that they are engaged in the behavior because it is personally valued. This is exemplified when patients take aspirin regularly or follow healthy diets because these actions are important for their health. When patients engage in identification, they feel positively about their behavior and have been shown to persist longer in health behaviors motivated by this level of autonomy for dental flossing and brushing, stopping smoking, losing weight and being physically active (Ng et al., 2012). Practitioners can support and enhance this quality of motivation by supporting their psychological needs for autonomy, competence, and relatedness.

Integrated self-regulation is experienced when patients value the behavior itself (eating a healthy diet) and feel that by engaging in the behavior it will lead to other valued outcomes (e.g., taking aspirin to prevent heart attacks); it also allows them to spend more quality years with their family and friends. There is one SDT intervention that shows that smokers' aspirations for health was increased when practitioners asked smokers about their life aspirations and how smoking helped them or hindered them from achieving their goals. After 18 months, aspirations for health and abstinence for tobacco were both increased in the intervention group compared to controls (Niemiec, Ryan, Deci, & Williams, 2009). It has not been established if the aspiration for health changed first or if the abstinence occurred first, and a replication of this effect is needed for confirmation.

Finally, intrinsic motivation occurs when a behavior is enjoyable or interesting in its own right. It is positively energizing simply by engaging in it. Exercising is enjoyable for some people (perhaps 30 %). Intrinsic motivation is not on the extrinsic continuum. It is a higher quality of energy more like what people feel with identified and integration regulations than what people experience from introjection or external control. Unfortunately, there are few intrinsically motivating behaviors related to health care. Most health behaviors are engaged for extrinsic reasons (to live longer, with a better quality of life), and thus the highest quality motivation most patients have is extrinsic autonomous self-regulation. Practitioners will most likely have to introduce patients to many health related goals, rather than relying on patients to find these goals themselves.

Humans can feel multiple levels of these regulations at the same time. For example, feeling both introjected and identified at the same time may be a source of ambivalence and can be a barrier for change. A patient with both these levels of regulation may respond best with a double-sided reflection from the practitioner once mixed feelings are elicited. With both sides of the ambivalence acknowledged in the setting of a positive relationship, this patient may be better able to make a choice about what to do that is most consistent with his or her values. Internalization is the natural process by which a person begins to regulate a new behavior or to change the regulation of a current behavior to a more autonomous form or self-regulation. Learning to deal with patients experiencing multiple levels of regulation at the same time is challenging, and determining which ones are most amenable to change in a manner that leaves them with improved welfare and autonomy will require careful research.

In order to facilitate internalization of autonomous self-regulation, SDT proposes that the health care climate (the need supportiveness of the practitioner-patient relationship) needs to be supportive of autonomy. If patients experience the relationship as controlling, it is likely to undermine patient autonomy and welfare. The features of an autonomy supportive relationship that have been part of clinical interventions shown to enhance autonomy and subsequent behavior include eliciting and acknowledging patient perspectives, providing a menu of effective treatment options, supporting patient initiatives (as long as they are not felt to be directly harmful – for example, taking antibiotics for viral infections), providing a rationale for direct advice given, exploring how relevant health behaviors relate to patients' values or aspirations in life, and minimizing control. More research is needed to confirm the active components of autonomy support and to identify new ways to support autonomy with less cost.

SDT posits that perceived competence increases only when the need for autonomy has been satisfied. Stated in another way, when patients want to make a change, teaching them how to do so will unlikely be perceived as controlling, but teaching them how to change when they do not want to change is much more likely to be experienced as controlling. Features of the practitioner-patient relationship that are competence enhancing are being positive that patients can be successful, reframing past failures as short successes, providing accurate feedback in a non-judgmental manner, identifying barriers, skills building and problem solving, and developing a plan that is appropriately challenging to patients' skill and experience level. Practitioners also are expected to be more successful in enhancing patient competence if they identify an optimal level of challenge from patients before trying to skills build. Training below patient levels of optimal challenge are often experienced as boring (de-energizing), while training above patient level of optimal challenge may lead to amotivation if patients do not experience improvement or success.

Relatedness is the third need in SDT. Features of practitioner-patient relationships that satisfy this need include providing unconditional positive regard (particularly in the face of failure to achieve desired goals), being empathic, and providing a consistently warm interpersonal relationship. Relatedness also means being available for patients over time. The long-term relationships with patients in primary care are important in building trust and understanding patient values, resulting in relationships that are frequently satisfying for both practitioner and patient. This led the American Board of Internal Medicine to emphasize the importance of maintaining this relationship as a featured aspect of professionalism (American College of Physicians, 2005; the features of autonomy, competence, and relatedness supportive relationships are listed in Table 15.2).

Empirical Studies of SDT in Health Care – On the Promotion of Physical and Psychological Health

SDT has examined the relations of need support, need satisfaction, and internalization to physical and psychological health over the past two decades and 184 data sets have been published that formed the basis of a meta-analysis (Ng et al., 2012). Rather than discuss each of these studies with respect to their positive associations of patients' perceptions of a need supportive relationship with their practitioners, the results will be described in aggregate. Need supportiveness was significantly positively correlated with increased physical activity in 30 studies with tobacco abstinence for smokers in 4 studies and improved dental hygiene in 3 studies. In addition to predicting important physical health outcomes, need supportiveness also predicted greater perceived competence for physical activity, tobacco abstinence, and dental outcomes. Autonomous self-regulation for those same outcomes was also positively related to needs support. A similar pattern was found for the meta-analyzed correlations in the studies which assessed mental health outcomes. When patients reported higher needs support they had fewer symptoms of depression and anxiety, as well as a better quality of life. In contrast, controlled regulations (introjects and external control) related negatively to psychological and physical health outcomes and positively to ill-being.

In a subsequent path analysis that included over 13,000 patients from these studies, Ng et al. found confirmation for the Self-Determination Model for Health Behavior (Ryan et al., 2008; Williams et al., 2002) in which (1) need support related positively to autonomous self-regulation and perceived competence; (2) autonomous

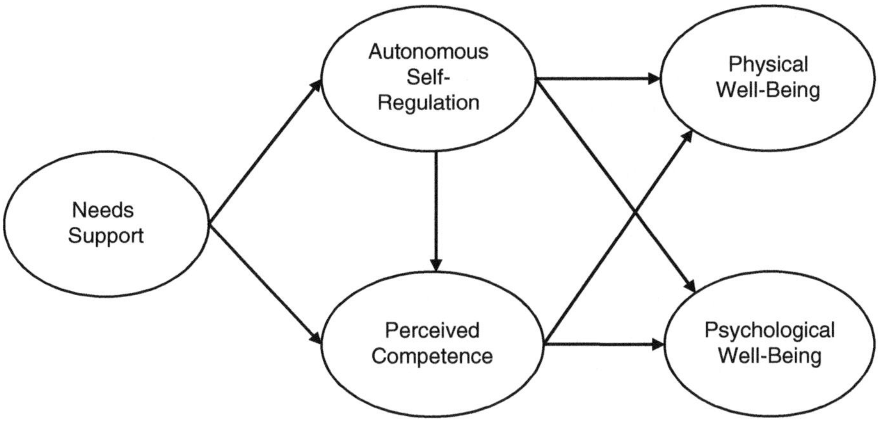

Fig. 15.1 SDT model for health behavior change in the clinical setting (Over 13,000 study participants included in this analysis (Ng et al., 2012))

self-regulation related positively to perceived competence, physical health, and psychological health; and (3) perceived competence related positively to physical and psychological health. This is represented in Fig. 15.1.

Overall, the results of SDT health care studies represented by Ng et al. (2012) meta-analysis underscore the importance of need support, need satisfaction, and internalization for physical and psychological health; especially given that data were obtained from a large number of studies, with different investigators, in different health domains, and from several cultures. Yet a critical limitation is the correlational nature of the data used in the analysis, which precludes a conclusion of causality for these associations. Fortunately, several randomized clinical trials have been conducted using SDT to assess whether physical and psychological health is improved when interventions provide support for basic psychological need satisfaction in the context of treatment. This research has demonstrated the efficacy of SDT-based interventions for behaviors such as tobacco dependence (Williams et al., 2006a), cholesterol (Williams et al., 2006b), weight loss maintenance (Silva et al., 2011; West et al., 2011), physical activity (Fortier, Sweet, O'Sullivan, & Williams, 2007), dental hygiene (Münster Halvari & Halvari, 2006; Münster Halvari, Halvari, Bjørnebekk, & Deci, 2012), and diabetes care (Williams, Lynch, & Glasgow, 2007). Together, the randomized controlled trials have shown that autonomous self-regulation and perceived competence are facilitated in health care climates that provide support for basic psychological needs and that autonomous self-regulation and perceived competence are the psychological mechanisms by which maintenance of health-behavior change occurs (Ryan et al., 2008).

Taken together, these results show that need support, need satisfaction, and internalization relate consistently and positively to physical and psychological health. Moreover, these data suggest that interventions that enhance patient autonomy result in more life years lived and, in better quality life years. When practitioners support patient psychological needs both patient welfare and autonomy are enhanced, thus meeting our highest ethical standards. One of these studies found the SDT intervention for tobacco dependence to be quite cost effective compared to other intensive interventions for tobacco dependence and to other health interventions in general (Pesis-Katz, Williams, Niemiec, & Fiscella, 2011).

When SDT-based interventions have been applied to achieving the clinical targets of the Million Hearts Initiative, they have resulted in important improvements in markers of cardiovascular health. These studies resulted in increased 12-month prolonged abstinence from tobacco, which reduces heart attacks by 50 % (U.S. Department of Health and Human Services, 2004), and lower LDL cholesterol, which also reduces heart attack and stroke rates (1 % reduction in LDL-Cholesterol results in a 1 % reduction in heart attacks). SDT based interventions have been shown to increase physical activity that is known to reduce heart attacks by 20 %. The SDT mediators of autonomy and perceived competence are negatively associated with depressive symptoms and anxiety that are predictive of CVD events. While there are no SDT studies on hypertension management or aspirin use, the SDT based interventions resulted in greater medication use for smoking cessation (Williams et al., 2006a) and are associated with greater medication use for management of a variety of conditions (Williams, Rodin, Ryan, Grolnick, & Deci, 1998b), including diabetes and being HIV positive (Kennedy, Goggin, & Nollen, 2004; Williams et al., 2009).

The practical implications from SDT based research for practitioners are that when they provide support for patient autonomy, competence, and relatedness, patient mental and physical health outcomes are likely to improve and that these interventions are consistent with medical professionalism and biomedical ethics. Initial evidence suggests these SDT guided interventions will reduce heart attacks and strokes by increasing patient motivation for taking medications (e.g., aspirin, and medications to lower cholesterol and blood pressure to their goal levels), improving nutrition, and being physically active. To accomplish this, the principles of SDT and biomedical ethics need to be integrated with the CDC's Million Hearts targets. Successful implementation of Million Hearts would need to include training for practitioners on how to support patient autonomy and perceived competence, and possibly a method to assess these as process indicators, and to provide those markers as feedback for practitioners in the electronic medical record (EMR). While this may seem premature on the basis of the empirical evidence, recall that biomedical ethics mandates that autonomy be supported while interventions are delivered. Thus, the rationale behind training practitioners to support psychological needs, assess patient need satisfaction, and provide patient level of motivation as feedback is not empirical. Instead the justification is a mandate from biomedical ethics and professionalism.

Practitioner-Patient Communication, the Medical Interview, and Self-Determination Theory

Principles of motivation may also be helpful in informing other aspects of how practitioners interact with patients that go beyond motivating patients to engage in healthy behavior. SDT based interventions are by nature 'patient-centered' because they start from patients' perspectives and seek to enhance patient autonomy, rather than to control them with punishments or rewards in order to achieve compliance with treatment recommendations. These patient centered styles of relating to patients have been identified and taught since the 1950s and 1960s, when researchers and clinicians began to examine the practitioner-patient relationship in earnest. The field of Health Psychology emerged at that time. Patient-centeredness evolved from Carl Roger's work on Client Centered Therapy (1951), from George Engel's challenges for medicine to adopt a new medical model based on a biopsychosocial approach (1961, 1977), and from Barbara Korsch and colleagues videotaping medical encounters in emergency rooms to identify why some patients did not benefit from the treatments prescribed (Korsch, Gozzi, & Francis, 1968). Engel challenged medicine to consider psychological and social explanations for illnesses that he referred to as 'dis-ease'. He coined the term 'biospsychosocial model' as a way for medicine to expand to from its more limited biomedical paradigm (1977). He suggested that how practitioners interacted with patients could affect patient medical outcomes (page 132, 1977). For example, he suggested that what a practitioner said to a patient with diabetes may well affect that patient's blood sugar.

> Even with the application of rational therapies, the behavior of the physician and the relationship between patient and physician powerfully influence therapeutic outcome for better or worse. These constitute psychological effects which may directly modify the illness experience or indirectly affect underlying biochemical processes implicated in the disease (11). Thus, insulin requirements of a diabetic patient may fluctuate significantly depending on how the patient perceives his relationship with his doctor.

Research from several SDT studies on diabetes has supported his hypothesis that the extent to which patients experience their practitioners as need supportive correlates with patients' level of glycemic control (Senecal et al., 2000; Williams, Freedman, et al., 1998; Williams, Lynch, et al., 2007; Williams, McGregor et al., 2004; Williams, Patrick, et al., 2009). Engel continued in that same article:

> Furthermore, the successful application of rational therapies is limited by the physician's ability to influence and modify the patient's behavior in directions concordant with health needs. Contrary to what the exclusionists would have us believe, the physicians role is, and always has been, very much of educator and psychotherapist. To know how to induce peace of mind in the patient and enhance his faith in the healing powers of his physician requires psychological knowledge and skills, not merely charisma. These too are outside of the biomedical framework.

Much of this work in the second half of the 1900s focused on the importance of practitioner-patient relatedness, which was named "therapeutic alliance" by DiMatteo & DiNicola (1982), and offered as an alternative term for 'compliance.' Patient-centered approaches were called for to place patients' symptoms and biomedical diseases in the psychosocial context of their lives (Engel, 1977; Lipkin et al., 1995; Stewart et al., 1995). Kaplan, Greenfield, and Ware (1989), Miller and Rollnick (2002; Rollnick, Miller, & Butler, 2008), among others, contributed to an evidence base that called for recognizing and supporting patients as active agents in their treatment; suggesting that patients' outcomes were likely related to the quality of the practitioner-patient relationship, specific aspects of the communication style used by the practitioner, and the motivation of the patient. Efforts of some Motivational

Interviewing and SDT researchers have explored possible overlap and differences of these two approaches that were recently published in a special issue of the International Journal of Behavioral Nutrition and Physical Activity (ISBNPA, 2012).

Engel himself trained hundreds of practitioners in a 'biopsychosocial' fellowship at the University of Rochester over the course of his career. Many of these individuals have gone on to become leaders in the field of health care communication. Engel frequently conducted interviews with patients and observed learners' interviews on 'interview rounds' as a way to teach the biopsychosocial approach within the doctor-patient relationship. He commented that the medical interview was the procedure that practitioners used the most in their careers to care for patients. For example, a primary care practitioner working full time might have over 300,000 interviews with patients in their career, most of which last 10–15 min each. These relationships can last for over 30 years! Expert observation with feedback and systematic study of the doctor patient interaction grew into its own field that is now overseen by the American Academy on Communication in Healthcare (AACH). By 1995, when an important summary of work related to the medical interview was published (Lipkin et al., 1995), over 7,000 articles had been published on the topic, and recently the American Academy on Communication in Healthcare [AACH] (2012) formed, which is devoted to improving health through better communication and relationships with patients. The AACH embraces practitioners of all types and includes patients to be sure both sides of the relationship are represented. A recent summary of the physician patient communication effect on healing was published in 2009 (Street, Makoul, Arora, & Epstein, 2009) and underscores the importance of positive relationships in health.

This literature highlights that patients are best viewed as active agents in their care, which is consistent with SDT as well as the new code of biomedical ethics and medical professionalism discussed earlier. The *Patient Self-determination Act* reflects changes in our legal code that underscore changes in the importance of autonomy in health. This act was passed into law in 1990 (Omnibus Budget Reconciliation Act of, 1990), becoming the first federal law to ensure that health institutions inform patients that they have the right to accept or refuse medical treatments and to formulate advanced directives. Another active area of investigation related to autonomy is that of informed decision-making (Woolf et al., 2005). Research based on 1,400 tape recorded interviews demonstrated that patients are adequately supported to make autonomous decisions regarding their health care in only 10 % of typical medical encounters in the U.S. (Braddock et al., 1999). These results call for further research into how we can increase patient autonomy and further document its health benefits. As these studies are done, it is most important that both quality and length of life be assessed.

This increased attention to the medical interview led investigators and clinicians to create a model of the medical interview in order to map out various parts of the interview that make an encounter successful for the patient and practitioner. The three function model is an example of this work (Cole & Bird, 2000). The first function of the interview is to gather information. Accurate information collected in a timely manner is needed so that a diagnosis of patients' complaints can be made.

Without an accurate diagnosis, effective therapeutic options cannot be offered, and unneeded tests and procedures may be ordered that can do more harm than good (Institute of Medicine, 2010). This is a complex task in itself that is filled with uncertainty for practitioners and patients alike.

Recent empirical research from the communication literature demonstrates that the elements of practitioner behavior during the interview that lead to higher quality care are entirely consistent with elements of SDT's definition of autonomy support. Specifically, a team of communication researchers (Takemura, Atsumi, & Tsuda, 2007) demonstrated that practitioner facilitation (i.e., eliciting patient perspective by nodding, or encouraging patient to continue without interrupting), practitioner use of opened to closed-ended questions allowing patients to describe their symptoms in their own words, and practitioner use of summaries were correlated with more information that resulted in more information available to make the diagnosis from. These relations remained after statistically controlling for the amount of time taken in the interview. All three of these practitioner behaviors are consistent with support autonomy and relatedness by minimizing control, remaining nonjudgmental, and encouraging patients to provide their perspective in their own words and reflecting it back to them with summaries of what they said.

The second function of the medical interview is developing rapport. This function is directly relationship supportive and satisfying to patients. When rapport is good, patients are more likely to come back for treatment and be satisfied with their care. In a second study, the same team (Takemura, Atsumi, & Tsuda, 2008) demonstrated that the more practitioners reflected and legitimated what patients said, the more patients were satisfied with their care. These relations were significant even when controlling for the length of the visit. These behaviors are entirely consistent with principles of need support in SDT.

The third function is to inform patients about their problems and motivate them to engage in treatment. Both SDT (Ng et al., 2012) and informed decision-making literature (Braddock et al., 1999; Woolf, 2005) support the role that autonomy and competence behaviors result in more informed decisions are made and greater behavior change occurs when agreed to by patients. Empirical studies now support all three functions of the medical interview as being consistent with need supportive behaviors of practitioners from SDT. However, much more research is called for to link specific need supportive behaviors to the various aspects of the interview to achieve more accurate diagnoses, less test ordering, cost-effective care, and improved welfare of patients.

In summary, the health care practitioner-patient relationship is bound by the tenets of biomedical ethics and medical professionalism, which are intended to create the health contract with patients and society. Patients and practitioners have both extrinsic and intrinsic motivation for being in the practitioner and patient relationship. Further study of this relationship is needed to understand how attempts to improve care with interventions such as pay for performance affect practitioner and patient behavior, the outcomes achieved, and the quality of their lives. Enhancing patient autonomy, enhancing patient welfare, and reducing health disparities are the three highest goals of the relationship, and each are related to SDT's needs. SDT is an empirically supported theory of motivation that provides evidence which links support of human needs for autonomy, competence, and relatedness to improved mental health and healthy behavior change that can prevent chronic illness and premature death. This combination of effects is expected to result in higher levels of quality adjusted life years for patients treated in need supportive relationships. SDT provides structure on how to facilitate change in health behaviors that are difficult to alter and improve mental health. If integrated with US National Health Guidelines (e.g., Million Hearts), and principles of medical professionalism, use of an SDT approach to enhancing autonomy, competence and relatedness may enhance motivation for preventing heart disease, strokes, and other many diseases. Research and theorizing are just beginning with much more empirical study needed to assess the optimal manner in which practitioners can provide care for their patients, and which medical educators and health care systems can train and employ practitioner in a manner that is more satisfying.

References

American Academy on Communication in Healthcare. (2012). http://www.aachonline.org/. Accessed 9 Sept 2012.

American Board of Internal Medicine Foundation, American Board of Internal Medicine, ACP-ASIM Foundation, American College of Physicians, American Society of Internal Medicine, & European Federation of Internal Medicine. (2002). Medical professionalism in the new millennium: A physician charter. *Annals of Internal Medicine, 136*, 243–246.

American College of Physicians. (2005). *Medical professionalism in the changing health care environment: Revitalizing internal medicine by focusing on the patient–physician relationship*. Philadelphia: American College of Physicians: Position paper.

Beauchamp, T. L., & Childress, J. F. (2001). *Principles of biomedical ethics* (5th ed.). New York: Oxford University Press, Inc.

Beauchamp, T. L., & Childress, J. F. (2009). *Principles of biomedical ethics* (6th ed.). New York: Oxford University Press, Inc.

Braddock, C. H., Edwards, K. A., Hasenberg, N. M., Laidley, T. L., & Levinson, W. (1999). Informed decision making in outpatient practice: Time to get back to basics. *Journal of the American Medical Association, 282*(24), 2313–2320.

Centers for Disease Control. (2012). Million hearts millionhearts.hhs.gov. Accessed 10 Sept 2012.

Chiuve, S. E., McCullough, M. L., Sacks, F. M., & Rimm, E. B. (2006). Healthy lifestyle factors in the primary prevention of coronary heart disease among men: Benefits among users and nonusers of lipid lowering and anti hypertensive medications. *Circulation, 114*(2), 160–167.

Chobanian, A. V., Bakris, G. L., Black, H. R., et al. (2003). National Heart, Lung, and Blood Institute Joint National Committee on Prevention, Detection, Evaluation, and Treatment of High Blood Pressure, National High Blood Pressure Education Program Coordinating Committee. The Seventh Report of the Joint National Committee on Prevention, Detection, Evaluation, and Treatment of High Blood Pressure: the JNC 7 report. *The Journal of the American Medical Association, 289*, 2560–2572.

Cole, S. A., & Bird, J. (2000). *The medical interview: The three-function approach*. St. Louis, MO: Mosby Inc.

Deci, E. L., & Ryan, R. M. (2000). The "what" and "why" of goal pursuits: Human needs and the self-determination of behavior. *Psychological Inquiry, 11*, 227–268.

Dietary Guidelines for Americans. (2010). http://health.gov/dietaryguidelines/2010.asp. Accessed 9 Sept 2012.

DiMatteo, M. R., & DiNicola, D. D. (1982). *Achieving patient compliance*. New York: Pergamon Press.

Engel, G. L. (1961). Is grief a disease? A challenge for medical research. *Psychosomatic Medicine, 23*, 18–22.

Engel, G. L. (1977). The need for a new medical model: A challenge for biomedicine. *Science, 196*, 129–136.

Expert Panel on Detection, Evaluation, and Treatment of High Blood cholesterol in Adults (Adult Treatment Panel III). (2001). Executive summary of the third report of the National Cholesterol Education Program (NCEP). *Journal of the American Medical Association, 285*, 2486–2497.

Fiore, M. C., Jaen, C. R., Baker, T. B., et al. (2008). *Treating tobacco use and dependence: 2008 update*. Clinical Practice Guideline. Rockville, MD: U.S. Department of Health and Human Services. Public Health Service. http://www.ncbi.nlm.nih.gov/books/bv.fcgi?rid=hstat2.section.28189

Fortier, M. S., Sweet, S. N., O'Sullivan, T. L., & Williams, G. C. (2007). A self-determination process model of physical activity adoption in the context of a randomized controlled trial. *Psychology of Sport and Exercise, 8*, 741–757.

Frieden, T. R., & Berwick, D. M. (2011). The "Million Hearts" initiative—preventing heart attacks and strokes. *The New England Journal of Medicine, 365*(13), e27.

Grouzet, F. M., Kasser, T., Ahuvia, A., Dols, J. M. F., Kim, Y., Lau, S., et al. (2005). The structure of goals across 15 cultures. *Journal of Personality and Social Psychology, 89*, 800–816.

Institute of Medicine. (2010). *The healthcare imperative: Lowering costs and improving outcomes*. Washington, DC: National Academies Press.

International Society for Behavioral Nutrition and Physical Activity. (2012). *Self-determination theory and motivational interviewing in behavioral nutrition, physical activity, and health*. Series coordinator Teixeira, P. http://www.ijbnpa.org/series/Self_deter. Accessed 9 Sept 2012.

Kaplan, S. H., Greenfield, S., & Ware, J. E., Jr. (1989). Assessing the effects of physician–patient interactions on the outcomes of chronic disease. *Medical Care, 27*, S110–S127.

Kaplan, S. H., Kessler, M., & Greenfield, S. (2012). *The effectiveness of physician level interventions to improve quality of care: Pay for performance, assessment and feedback and specialty certification*. A Systematic Review (under review).

Kasser, V. M., & Ryan, R. M. (1999). The relation of psychological needs for autonomy and relatedness to health, vitality, well-being and mortality in a nursing home. *Journal of Applied Social Psychology, 29*, 935–954.

Kennedy, S., Goggin, K., & Nollen, N. (2004). Adherence to HIV medications: Utility of the theory of self-determination. *Cognitive Therapy and Research, 28*(5), 611–628.

Konold, D. E. (1962). *A history of American medical ethics 1847–1912*. Madison, WI: State Historical Society of Wisconsin.

Korsch, B. A., Gozzi, E. K., & Francis, V. (1968). Gaps in doctor-patient communication. I: Doctor- patient interaction and patient satisfaction. *Pediatrics, 42*, 855–871.

Kushi, L. H., Byers, T., Doyle, C., Bandera, E. V., McCullough, M., Gansler, T., et al. (2006). American Cancer Society Guidelines on nutrition and physical activity for cancer prevention: Reducing the risk of cancer with healthy food choices and physical activity. *CA: A Cancer Journal for Clinicians, 56*, 254–281.

Levinson, W., Kao, A., Kuby, A., & Thisted, R. A. (2005). Not all patients want to participate in decision making. *Journal of General Medicine, 20*, 531–535.

Lipkin, M., Jr., Putnam, S. M., & Lazare, A. (1995). *The medical interview*. New York: Springer.

Maciosek, M. V., Coffield, A. B., Edwards, N. M., Flottemesch, T. J., Goodman, M. J., & Solberg, reviews and analysis. *American Journal of Preventive Medicine, 31*(1), 52–61.

McGinnis, J. M., & Foege, W. H. (1993). Actual causes of death in the United States. *Journal of the American Medical Association, 270*(18), 2207–2212.

Miller, W. R., & Rollnick, S. (2002). *Motivational interviewing* (2nd ed.). New York: The Guilford Press.

Mokdad, A. H., Marks, J. S., Stroup, D. S., & Gerberding, J. L. (2004). Actual causes of death in the United States, 2000. *Journal of the American Medical Association, 291*, 1238–1245.

Moyer, V. A. (2012). Screening for prostate cancer: U.S. Preventive services task force recommendation statement. *Annals of Internal Medicine, 157*, 120–134.

Münster Halvari, A. E., & Halvari, H. (2006, August 2). *Motivational predictors of change in oral health: An experimental test of self-determination theory*. Retrieved from http://www.selfdeterminationtheory.org/SDT/documents/2006_HalvariHalvari_Oral Health_ME.pdf

Münster Halvari, A. E., Halvari, H., Bjørnebekk, G., & Deci, E. L. (2012). Self-determined motivational predictors of increases in dental behaviors, decreases in dental Plaque, and improvement in oral health: A randomized clinical trial. *Health Psychology*. Advance online publication. 10.1037/a0027062

Ng, J., Ntoumanis, N., Thøgersen-Ntoumanis, C., Deci, E. L., Ryan, R. M., Duda, J. L., et al. (2012). Self-determination theory applied to health contexts: A meta-analysis. *Perspectives on Psychological Science, 7*(4), 325–340.

Niemiec, C. P., Ryan, R. M., Deci, E. L., & Williams, G. C. (2009). Aspiring to physical health: The role of aspirations for physical health in facilitating long-term tobacco abstinence. *Patient Education and Counseling, 74*, 250–257.

Omnibus Budget Reconciliation Act of 1990. Public Law 101-508 (1990, November 5), && 4206, 4751. See 42 USC, scattered sections.

Osterberg, L., & Blaschke, T. (2005). Adherence to medication. *The New England Journal of Medicine, 353*, 487–497.

Percival, T. (1803). *Medical ethics; or a code of institutes and precepts, adapted to the professional conduct of physicians and surgeons*. Manchester, England: S. Russell.

Pesis-Katz, I., Williams, G. C., Niemiec, C. P., & Fiscella, K. (2011). Cost-effectiveness of intensive tobacco dependence intervention based on self-determination theory. *The American Journal of Managed Care, 17*, e393–e398.

Resnicow, K., & McMaster, F. (2012). Motivational interviewing: Moving from why to how with autonomy support. *International Journal of Behavioral Nutrition and Physical Activity, 9*, 19.

Rogers, C. (1951). *Client-centered psychotherapy*. Boston: Houghton- Mifflin.

Rollnick, S., Miller, W. R., & Butler, C. C. (2008). *Motivational interviewing in health care: Helping patients change behavior*. New York: The Guilford Press.

Ryan, R. M., & Deci, E. L. (2000). Self-determination theory and the facilitation of intrinsic motivation, social development, and well-being. *The American Psychologist, 55*, 68–78.

Ryan, R. M., Patrick, H., Deci, E. L., & Williams, G. C. (2008). Facilitating health behaviour change and its maintenance: Interventions based on self-determination theory. *The European Health Psychologist, 10*, 2–5.

Schroeder, S. A. (2007). We can do better – Improving the health of the American people. *The New England Journal of Medicine, 357*, 1221–1228.

Self-determination theory: An approach to human motivation & personality. (2012, October 2). Retrieved from http://www.selfdeterminationtheory.org/

Senecal, C., Nouwen, A., & White, D. (2000). Motivation and dietary self-care in adults with diabetes: Are self-efficacy and autonomous self-regulation complementary or competing constructs? *Health Psychology, 19*, 452–457.

Silva, M. N., Markland, D. A., Carraca, E. V., Vieira, P. N., Coutinho, S. R., Minderico, C. S., et al. (2011). Exercise autonomous motivation predicts 3-yr weight loss in women. *Medicine and Science in Sports and Exercise, 43*, 728–737.

Stewart, M., Brown, J. B., Weson, W. W., McWhinney, I. R., McWilliam, C. L., & Freeman, T. R. (1995). *Patient-centered medicine*. London: Sage Publications.

Street, R. L., Makoul, G., Arora, N. K., & Epstein, R. M. (2009). How does communication heal? Pathways linking clinician–patient communication to health outcomes. *Patient Education and Counseling, 74*, 295–301.

Takemura, Y. C., Atsumi, R., & Tsuda, T. (2007). Identifying medical interview behaviors that best elicit information from patients in clinical practice. *Journal of Experimental Medicine, 213*, 121–127.

Takemura, Y. C., Atsumi, R., & Tsuda, T. (2008). Which medical behaviors are associated with patient satisfaction. *Family Medicine, 40*(4), 253–258.

Temel, J. S., Greer, J. A., Muzikansky, A., Gallagher, E. R., Admane, S., Jackson, V. A., et al. (2010). Early palliative care for patients with metastatic non-small-cell lung cancer. *The New England Journal of Medicine, 363*, 733–742.

The Hippocratic Oath. Text, translation and interpretation by Ludwig Edelstein, p. 56 ISBN 978-0-8018-0184-6 (1943).

U.S. Department of Health and Human Services. (2004). *The health consequences of smoking: A report of the surgeon general.* Atlanta, GA: U.S. Department of Health and Human Services. Centers for Disease Control and Prevention, National Center for Chronic Disease Prevention and Health Promotion. Office on Smoking and Health.

U.S. Department of Health and Human Services. (2008). *2008 physical activity guidelines for Americans.* Available at www.health.gov/pageguidelines. Accessed 9 Aug 2012.

U.S. Preventive Services Task Force. (2009). Aspirin for the prevention of cardiovascular disease: U.S. preventive services task force recommendation statement. *Annals of Internal Medicine, 150*(6), 396–405. Retrieved from http://annals.org/journal.aspx

West, D. S., Gorin, A. A., Subak, L. L., Foster, G., Bragg, C., Hecht, J., et al. (2011). A motivation-focused weight loss maintenance program is an effective alternative to a skill-based approach. *International Journal of Obesity, 35*(2), 259–269.

Whitlock, E. P., Orleans, T., Pender, N., & Allan, J. (2002). Evaluating primary care behavioral counseling interventions: An evidenced-based approach. *American Journal of Preventive Medicine, 22*(4), 267–284.

Williams, G. C. (2002). Improving patients' health through supporting the autonomy of patients and providers. In E. L. Deci & R. M. Ryan (Eds.), *Handbook of self-determination research* (pp. 233–254). Rochester, NY: University of Rochester Press.

Williams, G. C., & Deci, E. L. (1996). Internalization of biopsychosocial values by medical students: A test of self-determination theory. *Journal of Personality and Social Psychology, 70*, 767–779.

Williams, G. C., & Deci, E. L. (2012). *Medical professionalism, self determination, and health.* Unpublished manuscript University of Rochester.

Williams, G. C., Freedman, Z. R., & Deci, E. L. (1998). Supporting autonomy to motivate glucose control in patients with diabetes. *Diabetes Care, 21*, 1644–1651.

Williams, G. C., Lynch, M., & Glasgow, R. E. (2007). Computer-assisted intervention improves patient-centered diabetes care by increasing autonomy support. *Health Psychology, 26*, 728–734.

Williams, G. C., McGregor, H. A., Sharp, D., Levesque, C., Kouides, R. W., Ryan, R. M., et al. (2006a). Testing a self-determination theory intervention for motivating tobacco cessation: Supporting autonomy and competence in a clinical trial. *Health Psychology, 25*, 91–101.

Williams, G. C., McGregor, H. A., Sharp, D., Kouides, R. W., Lévesque, C., Ryan, R. M., et al. (2006b). A self-determination multiple risk intervention trial to improve smokers' health. *Journal of General Internal Medicine, 21*(12), 1288–1294. PMCID 1924739.

Williams, G. C., McGregor, H. A., Zeldman, A., Freedman, Z. R., & Deci, E. L. (2004). Testing a self-determination theory process model for promoting glycemic control through diabetes self-management. *Health Psychology, 23*, 58–66.

Williams, G. C., Minicucci, D. S., Kouides, R. W., Levesque, C. S., Chirkov, V. I., Ryan, R. M., et al. (2002). Self-determination, smoking, diet and health. *Health Education Research, 17*, 512–521.

Williams, G. C., Patrick, H., Niemiec, C. P., Williams, L. K., Devine, G., Lafata, J. E., et al. (2009). Reducing the health risks of diabetes: How self-determination theory may help improve medication adherence and quality of life. *The Diabetes Educator, 35*, 484–492.

Williams, G. C., Rodin, G. C., Ryan, R. M., Grolnick, W. S., & Deci, E. L. (1998). Autonomous regulation and adherence to long-term medical regimens in adult outpatients. *Health Psychology, 17*, 269–276.

Woolf, S. H. (2008). The power of prevention and what it requires. *Journal of the American Medical Association, 299*, 2437–2439.

Woolf, S. H., Chan, E. C. Y., Harris, R., Sheridan, S. L., Braddock, C. H., Kaplan, R. M., et al. (2005). Promoting informed choice: transforming health care to dispense knowledge for decision making. *Annals of Internal Medicine, 143*(4), 293–300.

Yusuf, S., Hawken, S., Ounpuu, S., & On behalf of the INTERHEART Study Investigators. (2004). Effect of potentially modifiable risk factors associated with myocardial infarction in 52 countries (the INTERHEART study): case-control study. *Lancet, 364*, 937–952.

MIX
Papier aus verantwortungsvollen Quellen
Paper from responsible sources
FSC® C105338

If you have any concerns about our products,
you can contact us on
ProductSafety@springernature.com

In case Publisher is established outside the EU,
the EU authorized representative is:
Springer Nature Customer Service Center GmbH
Europaplatz 3, 69115 Heidelberg, Germany

Printed by Libri Plureos GmbH
in Hamburg, Germany